Science in the Art of Osteopathy

Science in the Art of Osteopathy

Osteopathic principles and practice

Caroline Stone

Stanley Thornes (Publishers) Ltd

First published in 1999 by:
Stanley Thornes (Publishers) Ltd
Ellenborough House
Wellington Street
Cheltenham
GL50 1YW
United Kingdon

99 00 01 02 03 / 10 9 8 7 6 5 4 3 2 1

A catalogue record for this book is available from the British Library

ISBN 0 7487 3328 0

Original illustrations by Oxford Designers and Illustrators.

Typeset by Columns Design Ltd, Reading, Berkshire
Printed and bound in Great Britain by Redwood Books, Trowbridge, Wiltshire

CONTENTS

PREFACE

Then Prometheus
Gathered that fiery dust and slaked it
With the pure spring water,
And rolled it under his hands,
Pounded it, thumbed it, moulded it
Into a body shaped like that of a god.

Though all the beasts
Hang their heads from horizontal backbones
And study the earth
beneath their feet, Prometheus
Upended man into the vertical –
So to comprehend balance.
Then tipped up his chin
So to widen his outlook on heaven.

Ted Hughes: Tales from Ovid
(Reproduced with permission from Faber and Faber.)

The Art of Osteopathy is the appreciation of motion; the Science is the acknowledgement of the effects of any aberration of movement within body structures and soft tissues.

Osteopathy offers a unique contribution to healthcare – not only has it encompassed and encapsulated so many of the threads of hands-on healing and manipulative practices that have been on earth as long as man, but it has additionally introduced a fuller understanding of the biomechanical aspects of the human form and its physiology. It has brought all these elements together and proffered them as a system of manual medicine that can both complement but also challenge many of the concepts of modern Western medicine.

While osteopathy has brought relief and an end to suffering to many thousands of people for a whole variety of musculoskeletal complaints, it remains more than just the treatment of such pains. Many people's experience of osteopathy has sadly not revealed to them the broadness of the potential within osteopathic practice; even many osteopaths are uncertain as to the true scope of osteopathic healthcare.

The paradigms of Western medicine are shifting – not away from but towards those already rooted in osteopathy: that all parts are interdependent and that the whole is greater than the sum of the parts. What osteopathy offers is the hypothesis that there is a somatic component to disease; that manual techniques applied to the human form affect body physiology; and thus that manipulation can intervene in homeostasis and effect the inherent healing mechanisms of the human form. It is not a panacea, and will never be capable of being 'all things to all conditions' but, that said, it is capable of a lot more than it is currently credited with, and this book aims to set the stage for a broader scope of practice.

There are many and varied types of manipulations used under the umbrella of osteopathy, and it is a truism that there are as many 'osteopathies' as there are osteopaths. However, these different styles all encompass the same underlying principles and have common threads that link them, making a very rich profession. Its diversity is in fact one of the profession's enduring strengths: **it takes an individual to treat another person individually**. Osteopathy is not about 'prescription medicine': there is no set recipe for a certain manipulation to be applied in a certain case. This is something that many onlookers find hard to accept – and something that has led to a degree of confusion as to what osteopathy is supposed to be.

I hope that this book will play a small part in helping the osteopathic profession demonstrate that it has something unique and special to offer in the evaluation and management of people suffering with a wide variety of symptoms and conditions. I hope that it will also demonstrate how the differing strands of osteopathic practice are united and how a practitioner may decide what type of intervention s/he is going to use for his/her patients.

The founder of osteopathy, Andrew Taylor Still, said:

To find health should be the object of the practitioner. Anyone can find disease.

This book is an exploration of the way osteopaths aim to move their patients from suffering and ill-health/disease towards health.

Many readers will note that there is much within this book that is also 'claimed' (as their own) by other manipulative professions. Such is the nature of using similar tools for patient care. The reader will judge for themselves whether what is outlined here in any way constitutes a 'special' or 'individual' view of man, biomechanics, health and disease – and, if so, whether it makes osteopathy a 'separate' profession or part of an umbrella of manipulative practices, with professional margins being blurred and indistinct. With increasing referral between professions, a blending and mixing of techniques, ideas and concepts is predicted, natural and healthy. What is to be hoped is that by sharing knowledge and approaches patients will benefit.

Osteopathy is at this moment an empirical science. The case discussions in Chapter 11 are not meant to be cast-iron claims of proof of treatment efficacy. Illustrating the way that osteopaths work with patients may help to give an insight into the way that healthcare workers both within and external to osteopathy might research outcomes of treatment and possible mechanisms underlying these events.

The list of patients discussed in Chapter 11 illustrates that osteopathic practice is not confined to the management of musculoskeletal symptoms, nor does it exclude treatment of children, the elderly, pregnant women nor patients suffering with a variety of medically diagnosed conditions.

Throughout their professional lives osteopaths come across a wide variety of people, with a wide variety of complaints, some of whom it is within their scope to deal with, others where it is not. It is natural that some osteopaths will gravitate towards having an enthusiasm and interest for certain areas of practice, and many osteopaths concentrate on sports injuries, some on working with children, some on obstetrics and others on such things as asthma, irritable bowel syndrome and pelvic organ problems. All osteopaths have a good grounding in the consideration and management of many 'musculoskeletal conditions' and deal with patients suffering from low back to neck pain, 'frozen shoulder' (adhesive capsulitis) to carpal tunnel syndrome, headaches to sprained ankles.

All osteopathic patients receive individualised treatment and, although there are often common factors within similar cases, there are no exact recipes for treatment. However, the application of osteopathic principles should enable the practitioner to analyse and manage a case, even if the case is complex and 'new' to his/her own experience to date; or to decide if another avenue of management/investigation is more appropriate.

What principles could link the cases discussed in Chapter 11, such that manipulation of the various parts and tissues of the body could alleviate symptoms in such a variety of people and problems?

In an attempt to answer this, the book begins by discussing some concepts of health and disease that osteopaths make use of when analysing their patients. It then goes on to discuss homeostasis and the role of the biomechanics of the body tissues (joints, muscles, fascia, organs and so on) within health and disease, and will look at the way various pathological processes can disrupt these body tissues (and the effects that this can have). It will then discuss the inter-relatedness of parts within movement patterns and a variety of effects that movement restrictions can have throughout the body.

Using these concepts, the book then discusses how osteopaths come to various decisions within their evaluation and management of a patient, and discuss a variety of treatment options, and the expected prognoses of various conditions/cases.

As an osteopathic colleague (Steve Sandler) once said: 'Osteopathy is Still looking for an answer'.

This is my contribution.

Acknowledgements

I would like to thank many people for the help and encouragement they have given me, not only to write this book, but throughout my career. Some of the following people may be unaware of their help – but I would like to thank them anyway!

I am indebted to Christopher Dyer, Colin Dove, Lady Audrey Percival, Peter Mangan, Caroline Penn, Stuart Korth, Robert Lever and the technique department at the BSO when I was a student. I would also like to say thanks to all my patients, and students, in all the schools I have worked in, and my many friends and supporters within the profession. Stephen Tyreman and Leslie Smith have been especially formative: I could not have written Chapters 1 and 2 without knowledge of Stephen's work; and without Leslie's work (and marvellous vision of fibro-blasts in particular!) the physiological interpretation would have been much more difficult. I would like to say a special thanks to Jean-Pierre Barral, for opening my eyes, to Andre Racio for his support and, in particular, to Renzo Molinari for his knowledge and help, particularly through my time at the European School of Osteopathy. I am grateful to the British School of Osteopathy and the British College of Naturopathy and Osteopathy for their support of my research, and to Frank Willard (New England College of Osteopathic Medicine) for his invaluable introduction to dissection and the art of anatomical photography, and for access to his database of references. I also thank Jane Langer and many other colleagues for their support of my work in the field of visceral osteopathy.

I would like to say thanks also to my family, for their understanding throughout everything, and lastly I would like to dedicate this book to my dearest friend and partner, who has given more than he can ever know.

Caroline Stone
Wokingham, Berkshire, May 1999

1 PLACING OSTEOPATHY IN RELATION TO HEALTHCARE PHILOSOPHIES AND SYSTEMS

IN THIS CHAPTER:

- A brief description of osteopathy
- How osteopathy relates to various concepts of health and disease
- An introduction to an osteopathic perspective on health management and a review of how osteopathy could be part of a general healthcare system.

WHAT IS OSTEOPATHY?

There have been many attempts at producing a definition of osteopathy that encompasses all elements within one rounded, easily understood statement. This has provided many variations on a theme, none of which are completely satisfactory to all concerned parties (and many not fully understandable, without further explanation).

Osteopathy seems somewhat elusive to short, snappy phrases. A strict definition is not therefore the most useful starting point when introducing osteopathy to potential students, or anyone interested in the work of osteopaths. A description or illustration may give the reader some insight into an osteopath's work, which can then serve as a guide though the more detailed analysis of osteopathic theory later in the book.

Loose description: Osteopathy has perspectives on medicine, biomechanics and traumatology.

Clinically, osteopaths have an interest in these three main areas:

- **Medicine**: people with a whole variety of identifiable pathologies/medical diseases and disorders can be helped with osteopathy.

- **Biomechanics**: osteopaths have a great interest in the subject of biomechanics; they relate form/structure with function and have a variety of opinions on what constitutes normal movement and good posture and how activity and movement in various parts of the body affect the function of other parts.
- **Traumatology**: in addition to helping people with medical conditions, osteopaths are very interested in the field of traumatology and the rehabilitation of damage ranging from minor soft tissue injuries to major soft tissue and bony trauma.

SCOPE OF PRACTICE

Osteopaths are best known for their work in this third category (traumatology), particularly in relation to minor soft tissue injury.

Some osteopaths are happy with this as the profession's general scope of practice; while some feel that a wider scope (inclusive of the first category) is the best application of osteopathy.

All osteopaths have an interest in biomechanics and treat through the medium of touch.

OSTEOPATHIC MANIPULATIONS, OR MANIPULATIONS USED BY OSTEOPATHS

Osteopathic manipulations are many and varied and consist of physical manipulation of various tissues and parts of the body. They include soft tissue massage and stretch techniques, muscle energy techniques, strain–counter-strain techniques, articulation, high-velocity thrust techniques, gentle low-amplitude mobilizations (including balanced ligamentous tension manipulations and functional techniques) and neuromuscular techniques. (These terms will be expanded upon later.)

It is true that several other manipulative professions such as chiropractic and physiotherapy also use similar types of procedures; so what makes the whole thing 'osteopathic'?

Manipulation in medicine

It does have to be said that there is already a system of physical manipulation that is used by the orthodox medical profession: that being physiotherapy. Physiotherapy is practised within concepts of disease employed by the orthodox profession. It is a therapeutic procedure and does not challenge concepts of disease development within the orthodox system. Some physiotherapists may wish to challenge the view of some consultants, for example, as to how effective and useful physiotherapy intervention can be as a therapeutic tool (although the hierarchical arrangement of the orthodox healthcare system makes this difficult in many instances).

Osteopathy, being a profession outside the orthodox system, does not have this constraint, and this makes it easier for it to proffer alternative systems, approaches and ideas.

Alternatives

In physiotherapy there has not been the same development of ideas concerning the aetiology of disease, and the interplay between mind, emotion, the physical state and condition of the body and physiological/homeostatic function, as there has been within osteopathy. Also, the fact that not all physiotherapists have been fully trained in general body manipulation means that they end up treating many conditions without necessarily using a manipulative approach or by using it only as a small part of their routine. Thus their reliance upon physical manipulations is not the most fundamental aspect of all their regimens of care. This approach is foreign to osteopaths, who use some type of manipulation in every case (and not just where the symptoms relate to the function of the musculoskeletal system – as we shall see).

This difference in modes of practice must surely illustrate that there is a difference in perception of what physical manipulation can achieve for a patient. Such differences highlight a degree of divergence regarding underlying concepts of bodily function and of health and disease, although this does not mean that there can be no similarities of opinion.

Furthermore, the patient population that the two professions deal with is not always the same: and this certainly accounts for some of the 'differences' between the two professions. The needs of the acutely ill patient are not the same as those of the chronically ill, for example. Also, osteopaths are not currently routinely used in community health and rehabilitation in the same context as physiotherapists. Thus physiotherapy is often used in differing settings from osteopathy.

The 'osteopathic' approach

The application of technique according to principles held by osteopaths is what differentiates osteopathic practice from other forms of manipulative practice. This is not to say that there are no similarities of principle between the manipulative professions, to repeat the point made above. But these professions are currently perceived to be different by their members, by their patients and other lay-people, and by healthcare providers external to those professions; views that must have some foundation. Seemingly, what an osteopath does with their patient is not exactly the same as a chiropractor or a physiotherapist, or indeed someone who practises, for example, therapeutic massage, Rolfing, Hellerwork or another type of 'bodywork', or uses some other sort of physical manipulation within their work.

Even within osteopathy there are many ways of manipulating a structure, tissue or body area, and several patients even with very similar conditions may be treated differently by different osteopaths. What is interesting is that the majority of these patients will each benefit from their differing treatments.

How is it that all these styles can be of benefit? What is it that makes people get better? Is it placebo – is simply being treated physically of benefit – with the exact procedure not being of vital importance; or are seemingly similar problems actually unique in the way they affect the person's body; or, even, does the person's body determine how a problem develops or needs managing? How can one know what osteopathy is if each application of it is different, and which one is best?

The answer to this is that the practice of osteopathy needs careful illustration. Not only to demonstrate its individuality within the general pool of manipulative practices but also to highlight how the practice of osteopathy is underpinned by a universal set of principles and concepts, which are individually applied to individual cases. The aim is to demonstrate how all the potentially different approaches within osteopathy are part of a unified system of care, and how this can coexist with other healthcare systems.

To begin the illustration of osteopathy, further 'notes' and 'commentary' are given.

OSTEOPATHY – A LOOSE DESCRIPTION (CONTINUED)

Osteopathy is a system of manual medicine: one that employs movement of the human body to help restore and maintain normal (or more normal) bodily function, so that the body is more able to 'help heal itself' from any stress/trauma/disease it may be exposed to, or develop.

This manual approach can be applied in any number of illnesses, injuries and situations (with a variation in anticipated outcomes). Whatever the cause or aetiology of the condition there is a variable role for osteopathy. In these situations there are a variety of expected prognoses and outcomes. These range from complete resolution and healing, through supporting someone through their problem, to helping them gain and maintain as much ability to live their lives well as is possible, given their condition.

These opinions have arisen because osteopaths believe that

- altered movement/restriction within the moving parts of the body, and
- altered tone, contracture, elasticity/compliance of the soft tissues of the body

can be related to physiological and mental/emotional processes within the body.

In many cases these findings (of altered movement and tension/tone in the tissues and mobile parts of the body) precede changes in emotional and physiological processes, and can be considered to be aetiological to dysfunction in these areas. The opposite is also felt to be true. Mental/emotional problems, physiological dysfunction and disease/pathology can bring about changes in soft tissue texture, tone and consistency. These changes affect the biomechanical properties of the tissues and the parts of the body they comprise. Subsequently they affect the ongoing function of the affected area/part (compounding the original problem), and also of other areas/ parts/fields of function (creating new problems and symptoms as the body tries to compensate).

Thus cause and effect can be seen to be intertwined.

These points will all be returned to later, and expanded upon.

Osteopaths feel that the presence of movement restrictions and soft tissue tension may interfere with the way the body adapts to, accommodates, heals itself from and resolves a variety of illnesses, pathologies and traumas (both physical and emotional). Clinically, improving body movement is thought to help mental/emotional health and physiological efficiency, and therefore overall bodily health.

This perspective allows osteopaths to consider that they can influence health and disease rather than just help manage the effects of ill-health, disease or dysfunction.

Describing osteopathy

Some useful 'landmark' comments, by way of summary:

- Osteopathy appreciates the interplay

between mind, emotion, the physical state of the body and physiological function and homeostatic balance.

- It considers that the biomechanical arrangement of the body could aid homeostasis and health (if the biomechanical movement is efficient).
- It also considers that the biomechanical arrangement of the body could be detrimental to homeostasis and health (if the movement is 'inappropriate' – a term that will be interpreted later).
- Osteopaths treat people who have various biomechanical constraints within their tissues (aetiological to, or consequent to, or somehow related to, any symptoms that they may have).
- Osteopaths rationalize their treatment intervention through relating biomechanical restrictions in the tissues and articulations of the body to symptoms and problems that the patient presents with, or has experienced previously.
- Osteopaths provide healthcare through touch and manipulation of the body and its tissues, with the aim that, if the biomechanics of the body and its tissues can be returned towards efficiency, then some or all aspects of the patient's symptoms/problem will be resolved.
- Touching people can be beneficial on many levels (physiologically and psychologically); a concept that osteopaths incorporate within their work.
- It is not known precisely how osteopathy achieves its results, and there are several theories that attempt to rationalize this intervention (some of which will be reviewed later).
- Osteopathy is related in a number of ways to other healthcare systems: as complementary care, supplementary care and also alternative care.

Many of these points require clarification and expansion (which will be a theme throughout the book) but one way to gain further insight into the osteopathic perspective at this stage is to pose a few questions.

What is the aim of osteopathy for its patients? For example:

- Is it to remove the disease process?
- Is it to remove symptoms?
- Is it to get them back to work?
- Is it to improve their ability to do various things?
- Is it to make them feel more comfortable (mentally and physically)?
- Is it to maintain a status quo?
- Is it to supplement other care they may be receiving?
- Is it to replace other types of care?

These are all important questions, and perhaps the answers lie in what one's views of health, disease and healthcare provision are and where one places osteopathic care within this overall picture.

OSTEOPATHIC CONCEPTS OF HEALTH AND DISEASE

In the Preface the following statement was quoted:

To find health should be the object of the practitioner. Anyone can find disease.
A. T. Still, founder of osteopathy

'Health' thus seems to be one of the aims of osteopathic intervention. So, what is it?

Health

In a philosophical debate concerning the nature of health René Dubois said: 'Health and disease cannot be defined merely in terms of anatomical, physiological, or mental attributes. The real measure [of health] is the ability of the individual to function in a manner acceptable to himself and to the group of which he is part.'

In this comment, the disease process itself does not seem to be the most important thing – or, if

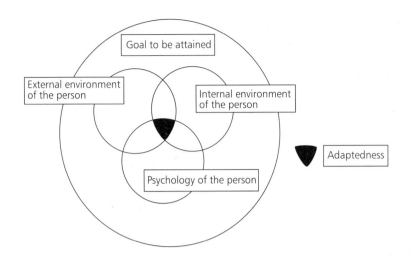

Figure 1.1

Adaptedness is the measure of the ability of the internal and external environments of a person, and their psychology, to interact to attain the desired goal.

it is important, other concepts, such as the quality of life and potential for action of the patient, seem to be equally important in defining health. In this context, the health of the patient can be improved by means other than by simply treating the disease itself (although this does not imply that the disease should be excluded from treatment).

In essence, what Dubois is saying is: the more able a person, the more healthy.

What governs one's ability to be healthy?
Nordenfelt said:

> *Success of an action is dependent on three types of things: the agent with his or her biology and psychology, the nature of the goal to be attained or maintained, and the nature of the circumstances surrounding the action. A person may be prevented from success by the manipulation of all three kinds of factors, and he or she may be helped to success by the manipulation of all [or any] of these factors.*
>
> Nordenfelt, 1995

He also used the term 'adaptedness', which was first coined by Porn, in his article 'Health and adaptedness' (Porn, 1993). The adaptedness of a person is seen as the overarching construction/measure for health in a person who has a number of abilities to meet goals in a number of different environments and situations. This is illustrated in Figure 1.1.

The term 'adaptedness' is perhaps an awkward one, and its usage here needs to be understood. 'Adaptedness' means how well adapted one is to the task in hand (emotionally, physically or physiologically). Adaptedness is a measure of the number of tasks one is potentially adapted to do: the greater the number of tasks possible given the make-up of the individual, the greater the adaptedness of that person. The more individual abilities a person has (to perform tasks) the greater the adaptedness of that person. If one has a degree of adaptedness, then it means that one can accommodate several differing demands and needs, and one can perform them all easily and without distress to one's emotional, physical or physiological health. If one is 'unadapted', then one cannot cope as well as might be desired with whatever stress or strain or demand is placed upon one, and the body may suffer distress as a result.

There seems to be a growing concept of health being defined as 'adaptedness to be able to perform a desired action', where help to achieve adaptedness may need to be on a physical, biological or mental/emotional level.

Figure 1.1 shows that there is a triad of circumstances in which a person has to demonstrate adaptedness. This concept of relationship triads

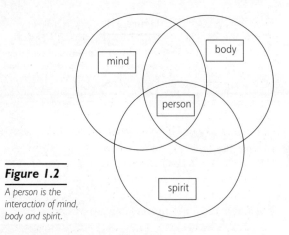

Figure 1.2

A person is the interaction of mind, body and spirit.

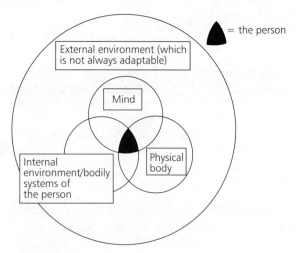

Figure 1.3

The health of the person is a balance of the mind, the physical body and the internal environment of the person, all interacting with the environment external to that person.

is used with different permutations by many different groups of people, who consider the person to be a melding/interlocking relationship of mind, body and spirit. A general example of this is shown in Figure 1.2.

This view is holistic in perspective and has been called a 'triad of health'. This inter-relationship is one that osteopaths respect, along with those described above.

On the basis of these pictures or analogies, health (and adaptedness) requires that all three parts should function appropriately. A problem or dysfunction in any one will compromise health. Additionally, a problem in one part may be expressed through dysfunction in another – hence the mind can affect the body, the body can affect the spirit and so on.

A system of healthcare that subscribes to such ideas places strong emphasis on providing care for all aspects of the person. Looking at orthodox healthcare systems perhaps reveals that their prime interest is not in the interplay of all these factors but in a more confined model of pathology and its management. Orthodox medicine is perhaps more concerned with the inter-relation between the internal and external environment, as shown in Figure 1.3, although this view may now be broadening.

Management plans within orthodox medicine are aimed at correcting differences from normal within the internal environment, which is done through a limited number of intervention options.

This approach may not address all the relevant factors, and indeed, if resolution is not achieved through these measures, then what? Within orthodox systems, for example, if something cannot be 'removed' or 'treated with medication', what then? What other strategies are there for helping the patient?

However, osteopathy, which as stated subscribes to the 'triad of health' concept, while not disagreeing with much of orthodox medicine's opinions on pathology has additional and differing perspectives on how pathology arises, and how its management can be most effective. Osteopathy considers that 'treatment' needs to be broad, in order to encompass the overall nature of a person's distress, illness or dysfunction and to address all components of their 'unadaptedness' to function (and thus improve their health).

Therefore, although it may be necessary to identify a pathological process, it may not be sufficient to pursue its eradication only through surgery or medication (for example); these procedures may not be sufficient to resolve the patient's difficulties completely.

By reflecting on a broader number of parameters for health, practitioners should appreciate more possible aetiologies for the ill-health of a patient, thus allowing more courses of treatment and management to emerge for that patient.

Because 'circumstances' are by their nature very variable, the healthcare planners and providers must organize an adaptable system. Man does not live in an isolated bubble, and Dubois illustrated the problems this causes when he went on to say:

> A perfect policy of public health could be conceived for colonies of social ants or bees whose habits have become stabilized by instincts. Likewise it would be possible to devise for a herd of cows an ideal system of husbandry with the proper combination of stables and pastures. But, unless man became robots, no formula can ever give them permanently the health and happiness symbolized by the contented cow, nor can their societies achieve a structure that will last for millennia. As long as mankind is made up of independent individuals with free will, there cannot be any social status quo. Men will develop new urges, and these will give rise to new problems, which will require ever new solutions. Human life implies adventure, and there is no adventure without struggles and dangers.
>
> Dubois, 1979

In this sense, it is likely that, in order to achieve freedom to pursue their goals, most people may require help on several different levels, and also be required to help themselves. It may also mean that what helped them at one stage is not necessarily going to help them at another time or in another situation. A broad, flexible and interchangeable healthcare model is required to constantly adapt to this idea of shifting healthcare needs.

Within this framework, it is unlikely that the same treatment will be as successful for all people suffering the same disease process; and individual assessment and management is called for. Osteopaths certainly subscribe to the opinion that treatment must be individually tailored to each person who presents for care. (Even in similar cases, the treatments are not the same, which makes it a difficult method of practice to investigate using double-blind randomly controlled clinical studies, for example.)

At this point, it can be appreciated that one cannot simply give the same treatment to each person and expect the same outcomes. This is why each application of osteopathy is so different, and explains why some observers of osteopathy, who do not come from the same perspectives of health and function, are often confused by this individualistic approach within osteopathy.

Dubois's comments highlight the philosophical aspect of the debate concerning what is health and disease. Philosophical considerations can reflect on the well-being of a person, their autonomy and self determination, and can place these within the context of the human (and individual) experience of disease, or 'non-health'. These considerations have led to a change in the nature of the provision of general healthcare, as those within orthodox systems (with perhaps more confined perspectives on health) gradually realize that some 'parts of their jigsaw' are missing. Many complementary/paramedical professions have been partially 'incorporated' into the mainstream healthcare system in an attempt to bridge these 'gaps'.

Osteopathy as a complementary system

A lot of osteopathic work involves making people more comfortable with themselves and their limitations, and working with them to achieve as much as their constraints will permit and, in a manner of speaking, to 'push back the barriers created by these limitations'. Managing chronic arthritic conditions, helping people adapt to physical deformity or trauma, or helping people overcome a poor body image associated with a painful, restricted and uncomfortable part of themselves can all be a part of manual medicine; and, although not addressing a specific disease, all lead to better life experiences for the person concerned. Thus, osteopathy, like many other systems of healthcare, can provide ways to help the person manage their life within the context of their disease/problem, this being considered beneficial to their level of health.

In this sense, osteopathy is a complementary system and may offer one of the few avenues of help to patients in conditions where currently orthodox medicine has little further to offer.

The relation of health and disease

'Health' has been the topic of consideration so far, and the term 'healthcare' has been much used. But, what exactly are the aims of a health-care system? Is it to promote health, or to elimi-nate disease? The use of the term 'healthcare' seems to imply that health is of prime considera-tion, leaving disease to be a small area of con-cern. Indeed, all of the above discussions on 'concepts of health' can highlight many interest-ing and meaningful things without being required to define the nature of disease at all.

The exact nature of the relation between health and disease has been the subject of much debate over centuries and is not fully rationalized even today. For example, are health and disease separate and independent of each other or are they somehow related? Are health and disease different points along the same continuum? Does a healthy body become diseased because of some factor external to the person or is there some-thing within the person that turns them from being healthy into being not-healthy and thus diseased?

Although the relationship is not fully defined, if one accepts the premise that, at some point, health and disease **do** have a relation, then such a perspective on disease is relevant to the debate concerning health.

Additionally, one's perspective on disease must subsequently be reflected in what one considers to be the purpose of a healthcare system or how a healthcare system must be set up. Thus an osteopathic healthcare system, with its own perspective on health and disease, is bound to be different from an orthodox one.

Defining disease

This is problematic, as disease is described differ-ently by different people.

Traditionally, western healthcare systems have been established to resolve disease that is thought to arise in accordance with external theories of disease.

Being diseased means having an infection or a tumour or some factor that interferes with the tissues of the body, causing disruption to the structure of those tissues and disturbing the way those tissues maintain the internal environment of the body through homeostatic mechanisms.

Western orthodox medicine has developed a science that is devoted to the recognition of such disease states. That science is called 'pathology', which in fact grew out of histopathology – a study of the microscopic changes found in sick people that was largely pioneered by Virchow. Disease is categorized by changes in tissue histol-ogy and by any changes in normal physiological processes and mechanisms of homeostasis. Diagnostic criteria in this context include such things as microscopy, clinical and laboratory test-ing of homeostasis, and various imaging tech-niques looking for signs of tissue change and disruption (Cawson *et al.*, 1982).

Medical care aims to resolve the disease processes and minimize tissue disruption so that normal physiological function can be rein-stated and homeostatic balance re-established. The corresponding system of healthcare is pri-marily interested in the effects of the disease and how these can be managed. Any pre-existing inefficiencies in the body's own homeostatic mechanisms or immune function seem not to be recognized as being of major importance in disease aetiology, only as factors to be managed.

The management concept seems to be that once 'diseased' the body cannot bring itself back to health and requires 'external help', for example in the form of surgery or drugs, to resolve the consequences of disease. In other words, once a tissue is diseased, i.e. histologically altered, this means that the body's own self-help mechanisms have failed and need external help. They cannot themselves be made to work in a such a way that they resolve the abnormal tissue state. Tissue pathology is deemed irreversible, requiring that the adverse effects this has on homeostatic balance be 'externally managed'.

> Western concepts consider how disease can interfere with homeostasis but perhaps do not recognize that failure of homeostatic mechanisms constitutes a disease in its own right, nor the idea that homeostatic mechanisms can function in such a way that they induce/contribute to histologically recognizable disease states, or that histological change is potentially reversible.

Orthodox analysis of the origin of the disease relates mostly to epidemiological factors, and recognizing genetic and autoimmune components of the disease. The host of the disease – the person – is almost a passive individual in such an analysis, awaiting the outcome of diagnosis into what is afflicting them.

Thus the role of the person in the disease process is not fully recognized in the above view of disease and its associated system of diagnosis and management. Thus the orthodox approach to disease and management can leave many people feeling isolated from their disease process, and also from the care that they are receiving. (It is perhaps this point that has led to the incorporation of 'complementary' therapies such as acupuncture into orthodox care, as mentioned earlier.)

To expand this point, if there is no histologically demonstrable disease then it is difficult for western medical practitioners to prescribe treatment (which should normally follow on from a diagnosis of disease). This may mean that many people in distress may be offered no explanation for their condition, and no methods of help or management. If these people are to be helped, then what constitutes 'disease' and lack of health must be revised and expanded.

Other views of disease
Certainly, some examples of disease can be imposed from the outside, as in infection and exposure to environmental irritants; and others can be internal, as in the lack of an essential enzyme, or an autoimmune disorder. However, as science has progressed and our understanding of the minutiae of physiological processes has expanded, it is clear that things are rarely that black-and-white, and there may be several factors that summate to create a disease state in any given person (the implication being that different factors may summate to give similar effects in different people).

Claude Bernard, the father of experimental biology, coined the term *milieu internal*, which was expanded into the term 'homeostasis' by Walter Cannon. They both recognized the essential nature of dynamic, regulated equilibrium of the body's internal environment and its key role in normal, healthy body function.

Taking up this point, Dr Jonathan Miller states in his book *The Body in Question*:

> *By the time anyone feels ill enough to call in a doctor, he has already been receiving free treatment from a private physician whose personal services have been available to him from the moment of his conception. By inheriting the premises in which we are condemned to spend the rest of our lives, we are born into a hospital whose 24 hour services are, paradoxically, designed to overcome and counteract the risks of living in such a dangerous tenement. It is a hospital staffed by its only patient, and although we take no conscious part in our own therapeutic activities, the fact that we have ourselves on call around the clock means that we can overcome most common emergencies without having to summon outside help.*
> Miller, 1978

The effectiveness of this internal self-help environment may play a role in determining at what stage external help is required, or in influencing the extent to which such help is needed. Osteopathy is inherently interested in the efficiency of this self-help environment.

Alteration of the internal environment may affect the stability of the person's health and contribute to ill-health or disease. For example, if the internal environment of the body is efficient and well regulated, then the body is more likely to be able to resist infection and heal from trauma quickly and effectively, whereas if homeostasis is poorly regulated then infection is more likely and recovery from trauma is poorer.

Such ideas recognize that the state of the person prior to the demonstration of frank disease is important and, moreover, is influential to the disease process and its progression.

In this context, analysis of the disease must include analysis of the person and, consequently, management of the disease process must incorporate resolution (when possible) of whatever state within that person predisposed them to the disease process.

Such an analysis considers that any alteration in the internal environment comprises a 'change in the host' and predisposes to disease. This gives an internal perspective to the issue of disease and ensures that the person becomes centrally placed in any healthcare system based on this premise.

Osteopathy is such a healthcare system.

There is now greater appreciation of the possible merit in considering the internal environment of the person's body a little more closely, as maintaining a good level of 'internal' health may well offset the need for much 'external' care. Certainly, where healthcare based on the external theory of disease has not met the patient's needs or expectations, the orthodox professions have been encouraged to consider the value of other theories and approaches.

Osteopathy and the 'internal' theory of disease

Osteopathy is a system of healthcare that bases many of its concepts and modes of practice in the context of an internal theory of health and disease and, as such, offers opinions on a part of the equation between health and disease that have previously been lacking within the orthodox system. (The internal theory of disease will be reviewed in the next chapter.)

Osteopathy offers these other opinions without necessarily refuting the orthodox description and analysis of disease. Osteopaths will still use aspects of the orthodox system of diagnosis and use the same types of disease classification within osteopathy's own modes and methods of practice to identify and describe what state the body has developed into. This makes pathology a very important subject for osteopaths, although they do consider other things as well.

> Recognizing a disease state is a good way of analysing how dysfunctional the body's homeostatic and immune mechanisms have become. Also, recognizing the extent of tissue change and disruption is important as these factors in themselves interfere with homeostatic and immune function, further compromising the ability of the body to heal itself and resolve the disease process.

Therefore 'pathology' is a very important subject for osteopaths but does not constitute the extent of the osteopathic evaluation of a person.

Osteopaths try to analyse how the homeostatic mechanisms of the body could have 'allowed' the body to become diseased in the first place. This includes exploring the state of the soft tissues of the body – from the muscles, ligaments and articular capsules to the state of connective tissues and fascial sheaths and the state of the tissues of the internal organs of the body – and how these interfere with homeostasis. (Later chapters will discuss the details of how it is that physical restrictions in the body might relate to physiology, homeostasis, health and immunity, and also dysfunction, disease and pathology.)

Osteopaths make unique evaluations and interpretations of how such soft tissue factors relate to the state of the internal environment of the body, based on palpatory awareness and observations of how the person can express movement and activity. This, combined with a consideration of the pathological status of the tissues, forms a special perspective on the person and their problems and helps the osteopath to formulate an individual management plan for that person's care.

Differing perspectives therefore have effects on the healthcare delivery system.

Any healthcare system that incorporates this broader view of disease would therefore need to have additional criteria and modes of management to those that relate to the classic perspective on disease.

COMPOSITE THEORIES AND MANAGEMENT SYSTEMS

If one component of a composite theory of disease is external, it will require a different healthcare arrangement from any components that are not (i.e. are internal). An external component of the disease might require the taking of medication and the internal component might require the person taking more exercise or more sleep, or some other course of action designed to help the functioning of their internal environment, such as manipulating their soft tissues. The autonomy of the person, their perspective on what their problem is, and what they would judge as improvement and help, need also to be considered; and such things as how they can be helped to help themselves may be an important element of the overall management of their problem.

In this overall situation, treatment may need to be on several levels (i.e. in accordance with all components of the disease theory) for the person's problem to be effectively managed.

Collaborative care systems

Not all healthcare providers may be able to deliver all types of care, and so it is useful when different providers can collaborate with one another, and with the patient, concerning the most appropriate combination of care for the patient at that time. This approach can be described as 'patient-centred care'.

In reality, the concept of patient-centred care is one that is gaining increasing importance and relevance, even within orthodox systems – where it now seems to govern many aspects of quality control and assessment. Fulford (Fulford *et al.*, 1996) discusses the nature of patient-centred care, and states that a model that '[incorporates] values and facts, the lived experience of illness and scientific knowledge of disease ... is required for genuinely patient-centred health care'.

Osteopathy, like other healthcare systems, endeavours to achieve this.

Thus osteopathic care could be complementary to orthodox systems, as it works on (sometimes) different components of health and disease, or on similar components in a different way. Osteopathy, then, might be best placed in a cooperative system of healthcare where teamwork and interprofessional dialogue is efficient, so that the best compilation and balance of treatment approaches can be rationalized, generating care that is more centred on all levels of the patient's problem.

THE OSTEOPATHIC CONTRIBUTION

The contribution of osteopathy is patient-centred in that it looks at how that individual is relating to their environment and disease (or dysfunction/trauma) and in what way and on how many levels they need help. The osteopath assesses them as individuals and how their physical body is relating to their actions and environments, giving a unique (non-orthodox) assessment of that person's dysfunction (even if within that some reference is still made to, for example, a particular disease process).

The osteopathic contribution to the management of the patient is to offer treatment of their physical body, to help the person improve their levels of adaptedness.

The way that osteopaths put this into practice (as briefly introduced at the beginning of the chapter) is to manipulate various body tissues and parts and to use the therapeutic medium of touch, in the belief that this will influence the internal environment of the body and help offset/resolve any disease process that is in any way related to some sort of problem within the internal environment.

In other words, manual medicine (physical manipulation of the body) aims at helping the body to perform the 'self-help' process as depicted in the excerpt from *The Body in Question*, by Jonathan Miller, given earlier.

The osteopathic delivery of healthcare

Disease processes, injuries and various problems and dysfunctions of the body, and a person's 'non-adaptedness' to function, are treated by the osteopath not by applying medication but by manipulating the body and then standing back and observing how the disease process progresses or recedes. (Note that 'standing back' does not imply lack of monitoring for important clinical signs that could indicate the need for rapid orthodox medical intervention.)

This means that osteopaths consider that inefficiency and compromise in homeostatic mechanisms constitutes a category of disease, and that poor body movement may interfere with homeostasis and produce a situation where the person is unadapted for good function. Such unadapted homeostasis may lead to disease and pathology. It also means, though, that this situation is considered somewhat reversible. Manipulation is applied to improve adaptedness to function, i.e. to improve the function of the internal environment and allow the 'disease' to 'recede'.

Further manipulations can be applied as required or, if this is unsuccessful, other avenues may be resorted to, such as orthodox systems where help given is 'from the outside' (e.g. medication or surgery).

This means that osteopathic treatment may not be undertaken as a first choice but perhaps later used as a supplementary form of care, or subsequent to other forms of treatment, or even not at all. But it does suggest that there may be a situation where osteopathic approaches are felt to be valid alternatives to standard orthodox care procedures. The ethical and practical decision concerning whether osteopathic care is the most appropriate for the patient at any given time is one that is taken by the osteopath, incorporating within his/her decision-making process a reflection of the disease state/situation that is concurrent with orthodox differential diagnostic thinking and methods of management.

Both osteopaths and the orthodox healthcare system have to consider the appropriateness of osteopathic care in certain situations/disease processes, and this can create a dilemma for either party. As explained already, the two systems incorporate different concepts within their practice, and it is only natural that each should practise within its own theoretical boundaries. However, it is hoped that each can do so while trying to appreciate the potential benefits and scope of practice of the other.

This debate on which approach may be the most immediately beneficial to the patient can be quite clear and uncontroversial to both osteopaths and orthodox medical practitioners for a variety of scenarios and circumstances, such as in severe trauma and the acute care thereof or in surgical procedures for ruptured or infarcted organs, or space-occupying lesions. However, the dividing line indicating which system to apply when is more controversial in other areas.

What is the best way to manage someone with gastrointestinal dysfunction? How is respiratory disease best resolved? What is the most efficient method of fracture management? Is dentistry the mainstay of resolving temporomandibular joint pain and dysfunction? Is the best way to prevent infection to give long-term antibiotic medication?

Certainly, it is not always easy for the orthodox profession to see the validity of the claims of some osteopathic practitioners (e.g. when the patient is suffering from neuropathy consequent to degenerative change within the cervical spine, from gastro-oesophageal reflux, from meniscal injury within the knee or from urinary incontinence due to detrusor instability). For osteopaths, it can be difficult to put across a different perspective, and the idea that their approach may be more beneficial to the patient than the orthodox treatment – or at least a viable alternative to such care.

In addition to this sort of dilemma, though, remembering that many aspects of health relate to emotional well being, autonomy and the ability to perform as many normal and natural tasks as possible, osteopathy is uniquely placed to help people manage many aspects of their lives more comfortably and effectively.

The belief in the interaction of mind, body and spirit that underpins osteopathic care means that osteopaths have a 'handle' upon many subtle and not easily defined components of health, which, through the medium of touch and manipulation, can bring enormous relief to people in many differing situations.

Thus osteopathy is not concerned solely with eradicating disease but also with managing other aspects of health and well-being.

Ultimately, though, in whatever way the osteopath is trying to help the person and whatever the circumstance of their condition, the needs of the patient have to be safeguarded in a given situation, both ethically and legally. Whatever care the person receives, it must be appropriate to their needs.

Anyone who introduces new ideas or proposes alternative methods of management, care or treatment must be able to illustrate their benefit and effects; and these must be considered carefully with regard to potential benefits or harm to the patient. It is incumbent on the introducers to rationalize their concepts and to provide some sort of evidence for their opinions.

This is the current position of osteopathy – in need of rationalization, clarification, evidence, supportive literature; all in a package that can be communicated to others outside the profession. Osteopathic care, therefore, can only 'hover at the edges of orthodox care systems' until such things are provided; and only then can osteopaths partake in a healthcare system that accommodates and respects its concepts and autonomy.

The role of today's osteopaths is to illustrate how their care in any given situation would be different; what advantages they could bring to the patient and to the healthcare system; and to clarify the situations in which they could have a positive influence.

The next chapter will illustrate the concepts of health and disease that osteopaths use within their work and philosophies. It will introduce the osteopathic perspective on health and disease and the abstract aims of osteopathic interventions. It will also explain the basis for the development of management plans.

REFERENCES

Cawson, R. A., McCracken, A. W. and Marcus, P. B. (1982) *Pathologic Mechanisms and Human Disease*, C. V. Mosby, St Louis, MO.

Dubois, R. (1979) *Mirage of Health*, Harper Colophon, New York.

Fulford, K. W. M., Ersser, S. and Hope, T. (1996) *Essential Practice in Patient-Centred Care*, Blackwell Science, Oxford.

Miller, J. (1978) *The Body in Question*, Jonathan Cape, London.

Nordenfelt, L. (1995) *On the Nature of Health. An Action-Theoretic Approach*, 2nd edn, Kluwer Academic, Dordrecht.

Porn, I. (1993) Health and adaptedness. *Theoretical Medicine*, **14**(4), 295–303.

FURTHER READING

Barrington, B. (1944) *Greek Science – Its Meaning for Us (Thanes to Aristotle)*, Pelican Books, London.

Bradford, S. G. (1958) The principles of osteopathy: a credo. In: *Academy of Applied Osteopathy Year Book 1958*, American Academy of Osteopathy, Newark, NJ.

British Medical Association (1993) *Complementary Medicine. New Approaches to Good Practice*, Oxford University Press, Oxford.

Education Department, General Council and Register of Osteopaths (1993) *Competences Required for Osteopathic Practice*. General Council and Register of Osteopaths, Reading, Berkshire.

Feather Stone, C. and Forsyth, L. (1997) *Medical Marriage*, Findhorn Press, Forres, Morayshire.

Fulford, K. W. M. (1990) *Moral Theory and Medical Practice*. Cambridge University Press, Cambridge.

General Council and Register of Osteopaths (1958) *The Osteopathic Blue Book (The Origin and Development of Osteopathy in Great Britain)*, General Council and Register of Osteopaths, London.

King Edward's Hospital Fund for London (1991) *Report of a Working Party on Osteopathy Chaired by Sir Thomas Bingham*, King Edward's Hospital Fund for London, London.

Proby, J. (1956) The theory of osteopathy. In: *Osteopathic Institute of Applied Technique Year Book 1956*, Osteopathic Institute of Applied Technique, Maidstone, pp. 7–20.

Shaw, R. (1995) Mind body dualism: a historical perspective, and its prevalence within contemporary medical discourse. *British Osteopathic Journal*, 17, 35–38.

Stiles, E. G. (1976) Osteopathic manipulation in a hospital environment. *Journal of the American Osteopathic Association*, 76, 67–82.

Wilson, P. T. (1979) Internal medicine: an osteopathic approach. *Osteopathic Annals*, 7, 11–28.

2 PERSPECTIVES ON HEALTH, DISEASE AND INTERVENTION

INTRODUCTION

From the last chapter, we have the following perspective:

Health → adaptedness → integration between mind, body and spirit → dysfunction/disease as 'unadaptedness' → ineffective integration between parts.

As we have discussed, the role and state of the body is central to osteopathic healthcare practice, and we should consider the person more from this level in order to appreciate the details of the osteopathic approach (without forgetting the over-all balance of inter-relation of mind–body–spirit).

We have heard that to remain healthy is a challenge as humans are constantly having to adapt to their environment. Human beings do not live in a vacuum and need to constantly balance different factors in order to remain as adapted/adaptable as possible to whatever function is desired.

There are three main environments that the body is exposed to, which have an effect upon its state and arrangement. These are:

- the mental/emotional environment (EE);
- the chemical environment (nutrition and external environmental factors; CE);
- the physical environment (PE).

The relations between these three factors and the body are shown in Figure 2.1.

This inter-relation implies that any one of these environmental factors could compromise adaptedness by interfering with the body in some way.

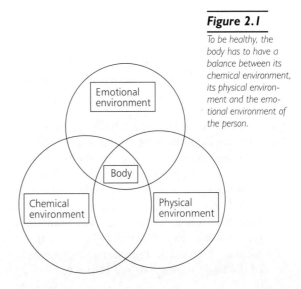

Figure 2.1

To be healthy, the body has to have a balance between its chemical environment, its physical environment and the emotional environment of the person.

Figure 2.2

*The balance between the chemical, physical and
mental/emotional environments of the body is also
related to the intersection and balance between
the physical, chemical and environmental factors
external to the body.*

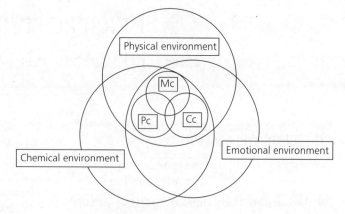

To appreciate the effect that these environments can have, one needs to see that the body itself is made up of three components:

- a mental component (MC);
- a physical component (PC);
- a chemical component (CC).

This additional set of relations is shown in Figure 2.2.

Two points now emerge:

- **Any aspect of bodily function/any of its component parts can be challenged by any of these three environments**, e.g.
  - a mental problem might cause a chemical problem, as when stress releases various hormones and chemical messengers that lead to altered bodily reaction/function;
  - a chemical problem might cause physical damage, as when pollution contributes to poor lung function and asthma, or poor diet contributes to rickets, leading to poorer bodily function;
  - a physical problem might cause emotional distress, such as the mental anguish of chronic pain following tissue damage, or as a result of disfigurement following trauma or surgery;
- **Health/adaptedness to these environments requires that the integration between the mental, chemical and physical components of the body is effective and balanced.**

Homeostasis is the measure of the effective integration of these three systems.

Health → adaptedness → effective homeostasis → effective integration of these three components.

One thing should be remembered, though: homeostasis is not a steady state. The constantly changing environment means that the state of the body at any one time is different from the next. Homeostatic mechanisms must allow changes in balance but must be able to bring these changes back towards an optimum level, to provide an optimum baseline of function.

Human beings are in a constant state of flux.

As we shall see later, disease is considered by osteopaths to be a failure of communication between the component parts of the body, such that homeostasis is disturbed, leaving the body unable to adequately adapt to changes in the environments to which it is exposed.

To further appreciate the concepts of health, ill-health and disease/dysfunction that osteopaths adhere to, two abstract theories of integration should be considered. These are **holism** and the **general systems theory** (which discusses entropy). These theories help to illustrate ways of thinking about inter-relatedness, and cause-and-effect relationships, that can be extrapolated into a clinical situation. These two theories will be briefly discussed but their clinical significance will be drawn out more fully in the following chapters.

HOLISM

Holism is an observation of the way things are. Holism is interested in the subdivisions of the units that make up things. Not all the units have to be the same ones but, when the units/parts are collected together, the whole is greater than the sum of the parts. As soon as you put the bits together, they take on an identity and symbolism of their own. The holistic maxim is that an organization as a whole is not resolvable into interdependent parts (systems, organs, tissues) because, in one way or another, the whole is more than the sum of its parts, and if one part of the whole changes, then this has an influence on the whole, and therefore the whole changes.

This vision can be applied directly to the human body and the person within it. A truly holistic view of a person's state would incorporate an acknowledgement of any factor that may affect the organism, and how dysfunction in each part would affect the others. Osteopathy is holistic in the sense that, more than most other systems of manual medicine, it looks at all parts of the human form/structure before deciding how to treat a certain problem, rather than confining attention to the symptomatic area. This is a departure from medical practice in that if an osteopath specializes in something, he/she does not confine his/her attention to one body system. Osteopaths would say that any one body system does not work in isolation and that symptoms (failure) within a body system are likely to have come in some part from dysfunction in another system, requiring that the other system is treated in order to resolve the presenting symptoms in the first system. Orthodox medical 'specialities' do not seem to rely on such a perspective.

Osteopathy is also holistic in that it recognizes that emotional factors can have a profound effect on physiology and homeostasis. It recognizes that many disease processes are profoundly associated with emotional or psychological problems. Orthodox medical science is now demonstrating how this might in fact occur, and this knowledge has enabled the orthodox medical profession to acknowledge the influence of emotion, even if their system does not always have adequate management strategies to resolve such problems. In this way orthodox medical practice is moving towards what osteopaths and other 'holistic' practitioners have been recognizing for a long time.

It is also increasingly recognized these days that environmental factors can have an influence on disease processes, which osteopathy also acknowledges; clearly, it doesn't matter how much manipulation you give someone if their problem is due to environmental poisoning – the osteopathic treatment won't fully resolve their problem unless something is also done about the external factor! Osteopathy is not practised as a complete holistic system, as it does not deal as a matter of course with all these environmental and dietary factors. However, a recognition of the role of these other types of factor is vital for any healthcare practitioner. (Unfortunately, a discussion of the environmental/nutritional aspects of health and disease is outside the scope of this book.) If some problem does arise through environmental or dietary factors, though, osteopathy may still have a role to play in the management of the effects of that exposure (and in limiting their impact).

Naturopathy and osteopathy

It is pertinent to note in this context that many osteopaths have managed to incorporate a broader perspective (inclusive of some of the above) by combining their work with naturopathic principles, giving quite an effective combination of treatment approaches for many situations. These, because of confines of space, will not be discussed in this book.

> **Summary of holism**
> - The whole is made up of parts or units that influence it
> - The whole has a function or identity of its own
> - The parts/units are influenced/affected by the whole

- Alteration of one part/unit will alter the whole
- A change in the whole will affect each part/unit to a greater or lesser extent

Summary of the general discussion so far

Adaptedness to function can be viewed as a constant juggling of needs and demands to maintain the body in as efficient a state as possible, given all circumstances. Maintaining equilibrium that has a wide operating range is a key feature of osteopathic practice, which attempts to be as holistic as possible in the way that it looks at the person and their body, as a whole. (How this is achieved will be expanded upon later.)

SUMMATION OF EFFECT

Maintaining equilibrium is an active process and may require considerable energy, depending upon what challenges the person is exposed to.

Why should equilibrium be such a struggle, though?

It seems that as the body adapts to challenges it is subtly changed by them, so that the next challenge is met by a body that is slightly different from the previous one. If the body can bring itself fully back into equilibrium before the next challenge arrives, then this situation will not arise. However, given the pace of modern life and the huge number of potential challenges that humans face, the body is often meeting new challenges before it has fully resolved the effects of previous ones.

In this way small perturbations in function gradually (or even quickly) summate to have large effects, which end up being greater than each of the small problems viewed in isolation. The body thus becomes progressively compromised.

Summation of effect is an important consideration within osteopathic practice.

To appreciate this, there is a missing component in the debate so far – a discussion of where this particular 'acorn to oak tree' imaging stems from.

This discussion centres on the general systems theory, which leads into an internal theory of disease. Reviewing these theories should help indicate why osteopaths don't solely concentrate on the symptomatic area of the body during assessment and treatment. (This section includes a recap of some points made in the previous chapter.)

From the background of the discussion so far, a certain concept of pathophysiology emerges (pathophysiology = when a tissue is not functioning physiologically). This concept of pathophysiology is allied to the general systems theory. This theory explains the nature of the incredible organization found in life, with regard to thermodynamics and the equilibrium (dynamic) that is maintained in all living things and that is required for the organism to remain whole, functional and alive.

THE GENERAL SYSTEMS THEORY

This revolves around the concept of **entropy**.

The entropic (random) state is the most probable state to be found in a system. A closed system leads to a true equilibrium, where there is no entropy/randomness. Note that the human body is not a closed system but an open one: there is constant exchange with the environment, which is controlled and should be of benefit to the organism. Opening a system immediately creates randomness and thus increases the entropy. In practice, the open system tends towards a dynamic equilibrium, or **steady state**, but requires energy to halt the ever-increasing tendency to randomness. Entropy takes less energy the more entropic (random) it becomes.

For humans this open state involves food and air being taken in from the environment, and heat and metabolic products being produced. Somewhere along the line the heat and the metabolic by-products are given back to the environment. It also involves the body being exposed to a variety of environmental factors that must be prevented from invading the body, or dealt with if they do. All these exchanges must be controlled to some degree, to prevent the human body dissolving into complete randomness.

Hence although humans have a level of entropy, it should always remain at approximately the same level, or be able to be brought back to similar levels if it has temporarily deviated from them. This is **homeostasis**.

With ageing and various types of distress and trauma to the body, it is thought that entropy increases – randomness within the body increases, problems/'symptoms' start to occur and disease/pathological processes can become established.

However, even in a situation of maintained dynamic equilibrium, where there is little external stress or trauma, the steady state achieved may not be completely stable. This is because there is an inherent instability within the equilibrium, and the body must 'strive' continuously towards stable function. This opinion has its foundation in the second law of thermodynamics: small eddies randomly appear (without there being a particular trigger) that then shift overall function of the body in new directions, to which it must adapt, or which it must resolve, in order that overall function is maintained in an optimum state. So, even if all things do remain equal, so to speak, function does not remain stable without effort.

Entropy can be considered as somewhat of a balancing act, requiring energy, adaptation and change to maintain its equilibrium.

In this type of analysis, one might be able to see that, if there are several small areas of dysfunction, each of these might set up small 'eddies' and ripples of randomness/altered function within the person, leading to an increasingly unstable internal environment, unless something changes to reduce these eddies.

Clinically, this type of cause and effect might be capable of being traced via a standard analysis of physiological function. Often, the exact route of summation is not straightforward and may need to be taken 'on trust' (perhaps through a current lack of complete physiological understanding), the over-riding element being that whatever is present is reducing efficient function somewhere and therefore (by default or logic)

will not help the person resolve any new or ongoing situation. These small findings reduce the adaptedness and adaptability of the body and so adversely affect health and promote disease.

The extensive history taking carried out by osteopaths endeavours to identify these 'eddies' (which will be illustrated later in the book).

This suggests a particular question: If one decreases entropy, does a healthy state return naturally, or not?

Osteopaths would believe so, at least within certain limits. Questions arising from this opinion that are currently being explored within the profession are: What are these limits, and when are other methods of care/treatment necessary to bring the body back to its appropriate level of entropy and therefore health?

These points are explored in the next section (where the concept of 'inherent health' is introduced) after a discussion on the 'internal theory of disease'. The idea of an inherent 'instability' of the body, which has emerged from the general systems theory, has contributed to appreciation of a long-standing/historical concept of an internal theory of disease.

THE INTERNAL THEORY OF DISEASE

This theory considers that disease is a disturbance of man's mind, body or soul. In it the body is credited with having a natural healing power. In other words, there is a power within the body, always trying to keep the body healthy; to balance out/cancel threatening things. Health is the natural state: the power keeps everything normal – in a status quo. Followers of this school of thought tried to understand the factors that governed the natural healing processes within the body and posed the question: Why is this person healthy when that one is diseased? The answer seemed to lie in some sort of difference within the person, rather than in an external factor that made them unhealthy/more susceptible to disease. The self-image of the person with the disease is also quite different: the patient acknowledges that if they are diseased, then there is something wrong within themselves. They do not particularly blame anything but seek advice from an experienced person, i.e. a doctor/physician. The patient asks 'How can I be made healthier?' and ends up gaining an insight into their body/way of life/attitudes/methods of caring for themselves and so on.

These insights enable the person to address whatever factors can be changed. This enables them to improve the function of their own internal environment and so help themselves to combat the disease process/dysfunction. The idea is that the patient can therefore get well on their own, with help and advice from the doctor.

Within the internal theory of disease, the concepts of health and disease should be viewed as a continuum, in that health is the optimum state for a person to be in and disease is a movement away from health. If a person moves away from optimum functioning, they progress along a type of human function curve, towards increasing inefficiency in their homeostatic mechanisms. In such cases these mechanisms cannot maintain health, and symptoms emerge as a result. Good function turns to dysfunction, and the person moves towards pathology. This then implies that pathology is not an externally applied process but one that comes from within – as a consequence of increasing inefficiency or compromise within the body's homeostatic mechanisms. As stated above, in this situation environmental or infective agents may then be able to have a more devastating effect upon the person (in said dysfunctional state) than they might otherwise have done.

Such things as emotional factors, dietary factors, poor circulation, poor mobility (and others) are all thought to have an influence on homeostatic balance (through a variety of mechanisms). Action invites reaction, and the presence of these factors requires that the body has to continually adjust to their effects and attempt to resolve any physiological consequences of their presence. These types of factor can be thought of as some sort of stress/strain/extra demand upon the body's self-healing and regulating mechanisms. They can be thought of as reducing the overall capacity for further adaptation within the system (body). They can be thought of as providing 'barriers' to effective function, influencing homeostasis and thus affecting function in some way.

This brings us to the following consideration: in the internal theory, disease is better understood as the failure of the adaptive mechanisms of an organism to counteract adequately the stimuli/stresses to which it is subjected, resulting in a disturbance in function or structure of any part, organ or system of the body.

This disturbance of function can be thought of as a disease process or pathology in its own right or as contributing to recognized pathologies/dysfunction, where the changes can make the body less resistant to infection (viral or bacterial), for example. Depending on where the function begins to break down, the symptoms that arise from this could be many and varied: they could be within an organ system, the muscles or articular structures; or within the person's emotions or mental state; or some combination of all of these.

To appreciate the level of distress within a person, it is therefore necessary to find out as much information about their lifestyle, situation, current and past history as possible. In this way the summation of various factors potentially leading to the presenting state of the person can be reviewed and reflected upon.

CLINICAL OBSERVATION OF 'SUMMATION OF EFFECT' MADE BY OSTEOPATHS

In a clinical setting, in order to come up with this type of analysis, the history taking and examinations performed by osteopaths are often much more extensive than patients and observers might expect. All history is relevant. (And, as shall be discussed in a later chapter on clinical decision making, management plans are formulated with respect to case-history and examination findings.)

A typical patient presenting with low back pain would be questioned routinely about their general health and how their other body systems are performing at the time of presentation and in the immediate past. This is not only to act as a differential diagnostic screening along orthodox lines but to investigate what types of insult the body has previously suffered and where dysfunction has previously manifested itself. The full past history of a patient is also important in this respect, and the osteopath tries to identify as many factors that could have compromised function in any area at any given time. This may even include questions about the patient's own birth (a concept that will be reviewed in a later chapter).

Osteopaths take the trouble to do all this because they perceive that everything takes its toll and most things leave behind some sort of legacy.

For example, previous injury may have left scarring and poorer function of the affected part and may have led to altered function in distant parts as the body adapted to the resolved trauma. This requires that the adapting parts work slightly differently, which, over time, might lead to fatigue and dysfunction in this second part (presenting with some sort of symptom pattern/picture).

In many cases, the osteopath would not only acknowledge the state of the person as they present (and the nature of this presenting condition in terms of standard pathology) but also the chain of events that led up to it or contributed to its aetiology. This gives a potential avenue for correction without simply having to manage the 'end state of affairs'.

Additionally, the osteopath might be able to predict where dysfunction might manifest at a later date, due to the presenting state of the patient, and the implications this has for ongoing physiological, homeostatic and biomechanical function. This makes it an important screening tool and education vehicle.

Osteopaths frequently say such things as: 'Well, you have trouble in your neck because of an old ankle injury,' or 'The fractured ribs you sustained during your rugby years are now compounding function in your respiratory system,' or 'The whiplash you had combined with the bruising and trauma to your breast bone (sternum) is related to your indigestion.' They do so to try to explain to the patient why they might be suffer-ing, and also to indicate reasons why they might propose treating areas of the body that are not currently symptomatic.

Many patients require at least a bit of an explanation of these cause-and-effect relationships, but most are grateful for an attempt to rationalize their problem, rather than having someone dismiss their symptoms as incidental or having no apparent cause!

(These themes will be returned to later, and the rationale behind such cause-and-effect statements will be more obvious after further information in later chapters is reviewed.)

Most of all, though, these considerations are made in an attempt to understand the underlying health/potential for change within a person, as this is thought to have relevance for their ability to recover and become more healthy.

All of the above sets the stage for the concept of inherent health.

INHERENT HEALTH

Inherent health is thought to be something that one has if all one's body systems are working efficiently, harmoniously and according to one's needs.

It is something that can become compromised through increasing randomness, disease, trauma, ageing and many other barriers to effective function, as already briefly discussed. It is also something that can be re-established – to varying degrees, depending on what those barriers are – by removing or resolving them. In many cases, this means that the body may require no external help in its recovery, or that if it has been receiving care based upon the end effects of any in-situ barriers, then removing these barriers should to some extent remove the need for external aids such as drugs.

In cases where external help is being provided, one can consider that the person is in a state of maintained health rather than inherent health. Maintained health, by its nature, may diminish again once that external help/treatment is withdrawn.

This leads us on to a consideration of what level one is aiming to work at, in any given clinical situation.

Levels of intervention: prevention or cure? management or maintenance?

Recognizing the aim of the intervention and identifying possible prognoses and outcomes is a vital part of any clinical practice, and one that has already been alluded to in the preceding chapter.

Two areas will be considered: where there is already disease, and where disease has not yet manifested clinically.

If disease is already established

Is the aim of treatment to control the symptoms of the disease, or is it to reverse the disease process so that the symptoms go away?

Returning to the concepts of the general systems theory for a moment: if, during treatment, one simply supports the system rather than trying to alter its entropy level, then one is in reality just managing the symptoms rather than addressing the cause. If one just treats the symptoms and not the cause, how is one to prevent a return of symptoms once the 'treatment' is withdrawn? What has been altered that will reduce the chances of the patient sooner or later being in the same situation as before the original treatment started?

Commonly, in a lot of cases, once a treatment regimen is withdrawn, the symptoms flare up again, until they are once more damped down. This is the syndrome of maintained health mentioned earlier. Irritable bowel syndrome, certain types of asthma, gastric ulceration or oesophageal reflux, migraine, repetitive strain injury to the musculoskeletal system, and so on, are all examples of this. Long-term/permanent (i.e. ongoing) treatment of these cases is expensive and demoralizing as the patient is ultimately not 'getting anywhere', and has to 'learn to live with it' and to manage their lives around their 'condition'. These outcomes are not fully satisfactory to all concerned. If the cycle of their condition could be broken, even slightly, then the situation would not be so chronic and without hope of long-term resolution.

If one could find other ways of reducing the disease process itself, surely these would be valuable things to consider? (There are not many people, whatever their profession, who would disagree with such a desire.) The point is that osteopaths feel that, in many such cases, the disease process can be 'reversed'/addressed and thus the need for medication should only be temporary/should be able to be reduced over time. Osteopaths can state this as they feel that currently many people do not have sufficient factors or barriers to their recovery addressed within their orthodox management routines.

Thus, applying osteopathic principles means the disease itself can be managed alongside its effects, such that gradually the disease comes to resolution – with no further (or reduced) requirement for any management of symptoms that arose from it.

In this way, osteopaths would consider that the orthodox view is not the only valid approach to a variety of diseases and disorders.

Of course, not all elements of a disorder/ aspects of pathology return once drug therapy is discontinued. This would depend upon the disorder being managed and what the aim of intervention was. For example, drugs are often used to damp down symptoms until the body does indeed heal itself, as in the use of analgesic and non-steroidal anti-inflammatory drugs prescribed for soft-tissue injury. However, are drugs the only way to damp down symptoms in these cases and, in fact, is it always wise to limit symptoms in all cases? These are interesting questions for ongoing reflection and study, and will be returned to when osteopathic management plans are discussed later in the book.

Point for reflection: If the views held by osteopaths prove to be relevant with respect to the aetiology of disease and dysfunction, it may be that osteopathic methods of management and care of patients may come to play a very vital role in healthcare in the future. Thus it may be that it is the medical profession that is negligent in not recognizing these factors, rather than osteopaths for not carrying out various orthodox treatment prescriptions. Also, the increasing recognition of the different levels upon which patients can gain relief/be helped with their lives and their problem means that recognition of therapeutic systems that work with these other factors should also be clinically important.

If there is no demonstrable disease

Here one needs to consider prevention: preserving inherent health. If this could be done by maintaining an efficient function of the movement of the body parts and, as much as is possible, a normal physical state of the tissues of the body (by using manipulation and other adjuncts, such as exercise and diet, for example) the inherent health of the person could be maintained. In such a situation, osteopathy could (and indeed does in the eyes of many osteopaths and their patients) play a role in the maintenance of health and the prevention of dysfunction, disease and ill-health.

Barriers to inherent health: the 'physical component'

Whatever level one is working on, barriers to health need to be identified so that they can be understood and addressed. 'Barriers' can be appreciated in a number of ways: as **'predisposing and maintaining factors'** to poor health/function, for example.

As mentioned earlier, osteopaths primarily work through the medium of touch and treat people by manipulating their physical body, and as such are particularly interested in those barriers to function that can be found within the physical field/state of that person.

Barriers within the physical field (the soft tissues, moveable parts and articulations of the body) causing alterations in texture, tone, tension and motion (as previously introduced) can therefore be thought of as either predisposing factors for disease or ill-health/dysfunction or maintaining factors for the same, as they are thought to be able to influence physiological processes and homeostatic balance.

Much osteopathic analysis is concerned with categorizing identified physical barriers as either predisposing or maintaining factors for inherent health and the patient's capacity for recovery, and rationalizing the potential effects of their removal – in other words, appreciating the physiological effects of these tissue states and reflecting on their relevance to the presenting situation of the patient and what their removal might mean for that person's recovery. (The ways in which physical states/restrictions/tensions in the body might interfere with such processes are dealt with in the following chapters.)

Implications for clinical management by osteopaths

As already indicated, this means that treatment will be directed at areas of the body that are not necessarily symptomatic at the time of presentation. It may also mean that the osteopath suggests ongoing treatment even when the presenting symptoms have passed. The aim of this would be to reduce the likelihood of any recurrence of symptoms by reducing the number of factors that led to the problem developing in the first place. This is thought to reduce the long-term treatment needs of the patient. Many practitioners suggest that one way of trying to ensure the preservation of a symptom-free state is to have fairly regular treatment on a 'preventative', or 'maintenance' basis.

Even when trying to alleviate immediate presenting symptoms of the patient, most osteopaths believe that this is most effectively done by working on some or all of any general restrictions/problems found within the patient at the same time as those that are giving rise to the immediate symptoms.

UTILIZING OSTEOPATHIC CONCEPTS ON A PRACTICAL BASIS

One of the original questions posed in this book was: What do osteopaths do?

Summary: osteopathic practice based upon all the above concepts

- The osteopathic approach to treating the person is to improve the function of their internal environment; restoring their inherent health and so helping the person to resolve the disease process for themselves.

- This involves exploring various factors, including changes in tissue texture, tone and tension, and assessing the biomechanics of the articulations and moveable parts of the body, looking for changes in normal function.

- Any factors found are described as 'barriers' to function, with some supposed to have more profound effects than others with respect to the patient's presenting state. (In other words: any tissue change or movement alteration/aberration is thought to interfere with normal body function at some level, and can be described as a barrier.) Osteopaths consider that physical restrictions within the tissues and moving parts of the body lead to increasing randomness within the person's internal environment, thus reducing the efficiency of the internal environment and the ability of the body to help itself.

- The treatment revolves around physically manipulating the body parts and tissues of the person and attempting to remove or reduce the barriers to motion. As will be discussed later, these barriers to motion are thought to affect circulation, movement of body fluids, neural function and the production of various hormones, for example. Physical manipulation of them (in an attempt to resolve the barriers and improve motion) is thought to reduce such influence, and so bring about a greater efficiency in the homeostatic regulation of the internal environment and therefore the function of the body's own healing mechanisms.

- Physical restrictions can be seen as 'barriers to physiological health' and as 'barriers to emotional health'. Physical restrictions can also place barriers to a person's health in the sense that they can limit the ability of the person to (literally) move; to express

themselves, their thoughts and ideas; and to converse and participate in social contexts and situations. Inability to do any of the above in a way or to an extent that the person would commonly expect can affect their emotional well being and so contribute to emotional distress and dysfunction. Therefore, by removing physical barriers within that person's body and tissues, the osteopath hopes to improve the mental, emotional and physiological well being of the person, helping them towards greater health and function as a human being. There is no doubt that this can also be spiritually rewarding for both patient and practitioner.

What do osteopaths do?

In order to put these ideas into practice, osteopaths would go through the following types of routine with their patients.

They would first take a thorough case history from the patient, and then begin to examine them using observation, palpation and physical examination.

Diagnostic criteria used by osteopaths include standard orthodox concepts of pathological change and descriptions of disease processes. Thus much differential diagnostic thinking is similar to orthodox practice. Osteopaths can thus have a role to play as a screening/sieving layer for the healthcare system, as they are aware of the potential confusion between the presentation of various medical conditions and of various biomechanical problems. This is particularly important, as the osteopath is often the first person to examine a patient and their symptoms: many people present to osteopaths without having seen an orthodox medical practitioner in advance.

The above is reflected within the differential thinking processes employed by osteopaths (which will be explored later in the book) and may also prompt the osteopath to investigate the patient's symptoms by using a stethoscope, sphygmomanometer or otolaryngoscope, for example.

Clinical presentation

Patients presenting for treatment fall broadly into three camps: those with symptoms in their physical field (the musculoskeletal system), those with symptoms in their emotional field and those with symptoms in their chemical field (their internal environment; comprising their organs and internal body systems); although many present with symptoms in several fields at once.

Clinical decision making

In any clinical situation one of the most important things to work out is: 'How can this person be helped?'

Deciding this involves investigating the following:

- the pathological state of the tissues;
- the origin(s) of this condition;
- maintaining factors that will limit or hinder recovery from the pathological state of the tissues;
- predisposing factors to the condition, which if left unresolved might lead to a recurrence of the pathological state of the tissues – this presumes that the person can survive the presenting condition, giving time to work on prevention of future episodes;
- rationalizing management strategies.

Management

This falls into three main areas:

- **Acute care**: the most effective way to immediately relieve the patient's symptoms or limit the progression of the problem;
- **Medium- to long-term care**: ensuring that there are as few maintaining factors for the problem remaining as possible – thus optimizing chances for recovery;
- **Preventative care**: attempting to eliminate the combination of factors that led to the development of the original problem, thus aiming to reduce the possibility of a recurrence of that condition in future. This can

involve treatment and education, and self-help regimes for the patient.

Influencing clinical situations

Within the above progression of analysis, there are two things that are important determinants of the direction in which the decision making goes. These are:

- the considered nature of the pathological condition, and how it emerged;
- how reversible one considers are the factors uncovered, either in the short or long term, that contributed to the pathological condition.

This is where the preceding discussion of the inter-relatedness of parts and the importance of a regulated internal environment is relevant, as these concepts relate to the consideration of pathology. One can't perform any of the above analyses without a perspective on pathology.

Diagnostic criteria used by osteopaths that differ from/expand upon those used by other professions

Diagnosis is carried out through physical exploration of the body. Osteopaths look for any departure from normal or expected movement ranges, and explore soft tissue textures and responses to active and passive mobility testing and consider if these are normal/as expected or not.

Having found any movement aberrations/restrictions/changes in soft tissue state and tension, they reflect on how these might be relevant to the physiology and homeostatic balance of the body and the efficient control of such things as circulation and fluid drainage and communication/function within the neuroendocrine–immune systems. From this consideration they can analyse how the soft tissue and articular changes may be related to the symptomatology of the patient, and thus rationalize how their physical manipulations might influence this process. They conclude whether they can offer the patient anything of therapeutic value and, in putting this to the patient, explain whether what is proposed is the primary line of care or whether there is a need for other intervention instead of, supplementary to or complementary with whatever the osteopath is offering.

Thus they enter into a contract of care with the patient and, in implementing it, continuously reflect upon their continued involvement with that patient, changing/adapting the care as required.

The actual delivery of the physical manipulation is tailored to the overt needs and tolerance of the patient, and there are many different styles and methods of manipulation that osteopaths can draw upon to achieve their aim of restoring good mechanical function of the tissues and articulations of the body. There are no absolute hard and fast rules for deciding when to apply what manipulation in which situation. However, there are some relative and some absolute contraindications that apply to some manipulations in some conditions. These mainly concern the use of high-velocity thrust techniques in cases of, for example, spinal fracture, osteoporosis, severe degenerative change and other pathological conditions of the bone such as carcinoma; or the use of highly vigorous manipulations of tissues in the presence of aggressive infective processes or where there is damage to the vascular system. However, there are many other manipulative techniques that can be applied in many of these situations with safety and that are considered to have a therapeutic value. In this sense, all contraindications are relative.

Exactly where and to which bits of the body the manipulation is applied can also vary depending on the condition, the nature and extent of the various changes found and the particular experience and belief system of the osteopath involved – the agreement of the patient also being a consideration. Thus one osteopath's proposed care of a particular patient may differ from another osteopath's assessment of the same patient; but both osteopaths will have something to offer and both may be working on different aspects of the patient's overall problem.

CONCLUSION

This chapter and the previous one have been about placing osteopathy in context in relation to a number of philosophies of health and disease and various systems of healthcare delivery.

It is interesting to highlight the fact that, for many osteopaths, their philosophy of care becomes a vehicle for their own views, actions and ideals, or a mirror for aspects of themselves that they feel warrant recognition and exploration.

Osteopathy thus becomes for some a way of appreciating many facets of their own actions and experience. To illustrate this, the following is offered, which was written by a student of osteopathy part-way through their undergraduate training. It may be a long way from where some people imagined osteopathy to be.

Osteopathy should be looked at as broadening your mental state. Why? Because everything around is in motion, not stasis. The world is not static. Since I have started my course I have begun to understand what osteopathy is really about ... or what I think it is about!

I definitely look more within myself and if I reflect on how I was at the outset I can recognize differences that are emerging in the way that I am now, and probably will be at the end of the course. Life is in perpetual motion: motion is life. Which one leads the other? People must work in balance to be able to exist/function properly. This is what I am beginning to understand: to be able to adapt yourself to any possible eventuality is a worthy goal, and one that often takes a lifetime to achieve.

Knowing this has allowed me to become more grounded in certain fields, and is increasing my understanding and tolerance of individuals. Trying to understand how both they and myself function allows me to appraise them more openly. Even if their system/body is not perfect or my system to help them is not complete, at least the quest 'to help' should continue; and it may be that this is only possible within a supportive philosophical framework .

There must be a diversity of people involved within osteopathy; as it is only with such diversity within the profession, and the diversity within ourselves that this encourages, that we will be able to do what is most appropriate for our patients (and ourselves). The practice of osteopathy is therefore something of an art.

There is increasing science within osteopathy, but let this not be at the expense of the art within it: the Art of Motion.

FURTHER READING

American Osteopathic Association (1997) *Foundations for Osteopathic Medicine*, Williams & Wilkins, Baltimore, MD.

Bynum, W. F. and Porter, R. (1993) *Companion Encyclopaedia of the History of Medicine*, Routledge, London.

Craige, B. J. (1992) *Laying the Ladder Down*, University of Massachusetts Press, Amherst, MA.

Hanson, B. G. (1995) *General Systems Theory – Beginning with Wholes*, Taylor & Francis, Washington, DC.

Money, M. (1993) *Health and Community*, Resurgence Books, Totnes, Devon.

Prigogine, I. and Stengers, I. (1984) *Order Out of Chaos*, Bantam Books, London.

Skytther, L. (1996) *General Systems Theory*, Macmillan, Basingstoke.

3 COMMUNICATION IN THE HUMAN FORM

IN THIS CHAPTER:

- Communicating networks
- Disease as a breakdown in communication
- Definition of osteopathy and the concept of barriers to function
- Cellular signalling mechanisms and their variability and flexibility
- Neural signalling mechanisms and their adaptability – 'use it, but don't abuse it'
- Axonal transport
- Cellular health and fluid dynamics
- The extracellular matrix – its role in fluid movement and immunity
- The general osteopathic treatment (GOT)
- Body movement and its role within extracellular matrix mechanics
- Mechanical signalling mechanisms acting in and around cells, affecting cell function
- The regulatory role of the extracellular matrix.

INTRODUCTION

The preceding two chapters have so far dealt with abstract principles. Giving detail to such abstract concepts should provide an introduction to why osteopaths feel that they can influence the recovery of people in a number of different clinical situations.

The whole basis of the previous discussions was inter-relatedness and how one part of the body can affect another. This inter-relatedness depends on each and every part and system of the body being in communication with every other part, and often with the external environment as well. **Communication is the key to health and effective function.**

This chapter provides an introduction to current understanding of some of the mechanisms that might underpin osteopathic philosophy and practice. It uses communication as the key premise, and focuses on cell signalling. It begins to demonstrate the inherent flexibility within signalling mechanisms, and sets the stage for later chapters, which attempt to illustrate how 'confusion' can arise within tissue signalling mechanisms and so provide a potential pathway for homeostatic imbalance and physiological dysfunction.

The efficiency of the internal environment of the body – the homeostatic mechanisms within us all – helps to determine the state of the body and its ability to be healthy and to fend off and cope with disease. This chapter aims to expand on the ideas in Chapter 2, showing that the homeostatic mechanisms within us are adaptable but that this may not always be to the benefit of the person as a whole.

As knowledge and understanding grow, so do interpretations and validations. It is only right that concepts should be allowed to develop. Consequently, much of what osteopaths used to say about these mechanisms is no longer correct, and no doubt much of what is here will be superseded as understanding continues. However, it is incumbent on any profession to make strenuous efforts to rationalize what might underpin its practice – it is a part of professional maturation and allows much more effective interprofessional communication as a consequence, through trying to describe philosophies in terms that are recognizable to others.

COMMUNICATING NETWORKS

Disease as a breakdown in communication

The term 'adaptedness' was introduced in the preceding chapter. It relies on communication between parts, and 'unadaptedness' in such a context implies a breakdown in communication such that function cannot be adapted to demands. Communication between parts is a very important theme within osteopathic principles (Keuls, 1988).

The concept of communication needs further discussion. Previously a triad of influences upon the body was introduced, and it is shown again in Figure 3.1.

This illustrated that the health of the body depends on a balanced integration between these three areas.

Communication ensures adaptability, and this adaptability should be on several levels:

- emotional stability and flexibility;
- physical (structural/biomechanical) stability and flexibility;
- chemical (visceral/endocrine/immune) stability and flexibility;
- neural stability and flexibility.

(As we have stated, these 'divisions' are artificial and do not operate *in vivo*.)

Considering the inter-relatedness of parts in the above illustration, dysfunction in any one part could manifest within its own part or in any other part.

In order for this inter-relatedness to operate, there must be various methods of communication between these areas, to permit influence to be transferred from one system to another.

Figure 3.2 indicates that there are three main pathways for communication: neural, chemical and mechanical.

These three terms require clarification:

- chemical relates to the endocrine-immune and the visceral systems (and to external/environmental agents);

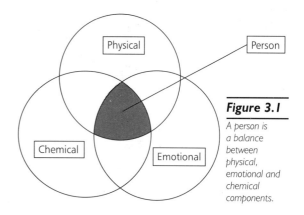

Figure 3.1

A person is a balance between physical, emotional and chemical components.

- neural relates to the nervous system;
- mechanical relates to the musculoskeletal system, and also to all other soft tissues within the body (as will be discussed later).

The emotions can have an influence at all levels, hence their place as the outer, encompassing field. (This point will be returned to later in the book.)

The areas where the circles overlap indicate the sphere of influence that one of these systems can have over another (the 'neuroendocrine—immune system'; 'neuromusculoskeletal system'; 'neurovisceral system'). Brief examples of this would be:

- effect of neurotransmitters on muscle cell action;
- environmental toxins acting on neural tissue;
- central nervous system function mediating the action of the enteric nervous system and hence visceral function;
- proprioceptors within the musculoskeletal system influencing neural control of motion;
- metabolic demands of muscle action influencing the visceral system;
- the endocrine system influencing calcium metabolism in bone.

Note: Within the context of a book introducing the application of osteopathic principles to

Figure 3.2

Communicating networks – the 'discrete' communicating networks between the neural, chemical and mechanical components of the body, within the encompassing influence of emotional factors.

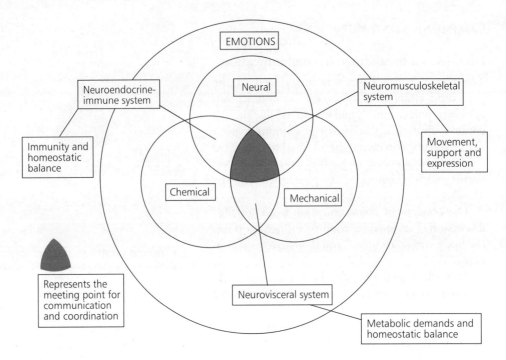

the workings of the internal environment of the human body, there is not the space to discuss the effect of such external factors as environmental chemicals and compounds, and so the term 'chemical' as introduced above will not include these terms.

The musculoskeletal system as a communicating network

The decision to include the musculoskeletal system as a communicating network may seem unusual, as this is not how it is traditionally viewed. However, within osteopathic principles the musculoskeletal system is uniquely placed as it is considered both as an aid to effective communication and also a potential origin for interference in this same communication, while constituting the means by which man can participate in life.

In fact one must consider all soft tissues of the body in this way. Fascial structures, smooth muscle structures (including the organs of the body), indeed all tissues that are either innervated or connected to the circulatory system in

some way, can interfere with communication.

Because of their prime interest in the physical structure of the body, osteopaths assess problems within all three fields – emotional, physical and chemical – through the state of the body tissues and movement therein.

These points will be returned to later.

Changes in communicating networks

It is very important to note that signalling mechanisms are designed to be very adaptable and flexible. These pathways are not 'hard-wired' and are constantly being adapted so that their function shifts within the parameters of 'normal function'. But how far can these signalling mechanisms shift before they become inefficient at information processing and deliverance? How will the whole body be affected if either a small part or a large part of the communicating network(s) coordinating homeostasis, immunity and locomotion (for example) becomes overloaded or inefficient? At what point does a breakdown in communication become manifest as dysfunction or disease; can such a thing occur? Finally, how significant is a breakdown in communication networks in the recovery from pathological or biomechanical distress?

These are all things that we now need to consider if we are to understand the hypothesis of disease being related to a breakdown in communication within and between body systems.

EFFECTIVENESS IN COMMUNICATION

Key point: Signals must reach their destination.

Communication is a result of the summation of chemical, electrical and mechanical factors acting upon and around a cell, which sits in a fluid environment. Regulation of this fluid environment, by controlling circulation and fluid dynamics, ensures the effective deliverance of signalling mechanisms that are fluid-borne.

Altering communication

Anything that interferes with electrical activity, mechanical activity or fluid dynamics will have an effect on cellular health, signalling efficiency and therefore effective communication. Ineffective communication brings the body closer to disequilibrium, and closer to disease and dysfunction.

Altering levels of electrical activity within the nervous system have the potential for altering the control of homeostatic mechanisms, immunity and circulation. Altering circulation has the potential effect of interfering with hormone and other fluid-borne signalling mechanisms, and so interfering with cellular health and function, and immunity. Emotions affect levels of neural activity, and hence function, in the muscular, homeostatic and immune mechanisms of the body.

Osteopaths consider that changes in the mechanical activity of tissues (i.e. within the musculoskeletal framework of the body, coupled with changes in mechanical activity in all other soft tissues) are capable of altering levels of electrical activity, and also fluid dynamics. Altering the mechanical activity within tissues creates a barrier to communication and thus interferes with homeostasis.

This is osteopathy in a nutshell.

A key tenet within osteopathy is: **Structure governs function**. This is better written as: **Motion relates to physiology**.

To appreciate this you need a knowledge of dynamic anatomy, and systemic and cellular level physiology. Then one can understand that:

- soft tissue biomechanics can affect homeostasis;
- altered movement reflects pathophysiology.

In terms of evaluation:

- soft tissue quality reflects physiological efficiency.

In the rest of this chapter, and many of the rest, there will be a lot of detail given about tissue function, be it neural, fascial, muscular or whatever. The key aim in this coming dialogue is to point out how changes in soft tissue activity can affect neural communication, or fluid movement and communication. They create barriers to communication.

Barriers

Soft tissue changes of any sort – and many types will be discussed over the next few chapters – should be thought of as **mechanical barriers**.

Mechanical barriers alter neural reflex loops and levels of activity. When neural activity is altered, communication becomes adapted, which can be described as a **neural barrier**.

Neural barriers can alter levels of activity within the soft tissues (e.g. smooth or skeletal muscles) and compound or create **mechanical barriers**.

Neural barriers can alter glandular, visceral or arterial wall activity (vasoconstriction) and so create 'chemical' or fluidic barriers.

Mechanical barriers can affect circulation of all body fluids, either locally or more generally, creating stasis within nerves, organs, glands, muscles ligaments or fascial structures, thereby creating 'chemical' or fluidic barriers.

'Chemical' or fluidic barriers affect neural function and soft tissue function and so compound or create neural or mechanical barriers.

Osteopathy is about removing tissue barriers and allowing better communication between parts to re-establish itself.

The anatomical relations discussed through the rest of the book are to highlight links between parts and relations to physiology, so that, when movement is affected, a pathophysiological interpretation can be made.

In order to appreciate this potential, it is necessary to first remind ourselves of the flexibility and normal function within cell-signalling mechanisms, and to appreciate how fluid dynamics are controlled at a cellular level. This will serve the purpose of illustrating that the human form is constantly changing and that the recycling of our function, our homeostasis and our health is dependent on these mechanisms not being overloaded by stressors (be they chemical, electrical, mechanical or emotional).

As stated, an overview of cellular signalling mechanisms will be explored to begin with, followed by a discussion of fluid mechanics and subsequent delivery of fluid-borne signalling messengers. The role of the extracellular matrix in fluid transport will be discussed, as will its role as a mechanical signalling system between cells and tissues.

This latter discussion should introduce the concept of movement as a form of communication, which is fundamental within osteopathic theory.

COMMUNICATION NETWORKS: CELL-SIGNALLING MECHANISMS

The communicating networks within the body need to pass immense amounts of information and would comprise an enormous system if one nerve or one chemical messenger could carry only one signal or lead to only one response. In many life forms, signalling mechanisms have evolved to be capable of performing several different tasks, to convey differing types of information at different intensities, and at different times. This means that the overall signalling network can be 'smaller' but that each part must be more flexible. Also, signalling mechanisms have evolved over time so that primitive systems have been overlain by more and more sophisticated systems, and a hierarchy of controlling influences now operates in complex biological organisms.

Each cell is programmed during development to respond to a specific set of signals that act in various combinations to regulate the behaviour of the cell and to determine whether the cell lives or dies and whether it proliferates or stays quiescent. Cell signalling requires both extracellular signalling molecules and a complementary set of receptor proteins in each cell that enable it to bind and respond to them in a programmed and characteristic way.

However, plasticity within the signalling pathways means that the cell response can change and adapt through life, so that ongoing function is ensured. If cells could not adapt, or vary their responses, then homeostatic balance would not be maintained, learning could not be initiated and human beings could not perform a wide variety of tasks in a wide variety of environmental and internal physiological situations.

Through summation of signalling mechanisms acting upon the cell and its environment, each cell can react in a variety of ways, which may or may not be wholly predictable. However, to induce different action by the cell, the signalling mechanisms must act on or through the cell membrane, in order to reach the internal structures of the cell, and in particular the nucleus of the cell, so that the ongoing activity of that cell can be adapted.

Cells are 'self-contained'.

Because of the structure of the cell membrane, it acts as a barrier to the passage of many molecules. This barrier function is crucially important as it allows the cell to maintain concentrations of solutes in its cytosol that are different from those in the extracellular compartment and in each of the individual cells (membrane-bound compartments). In response to this barrier, there have developed many different ways that the information/molecules can be transported both into and

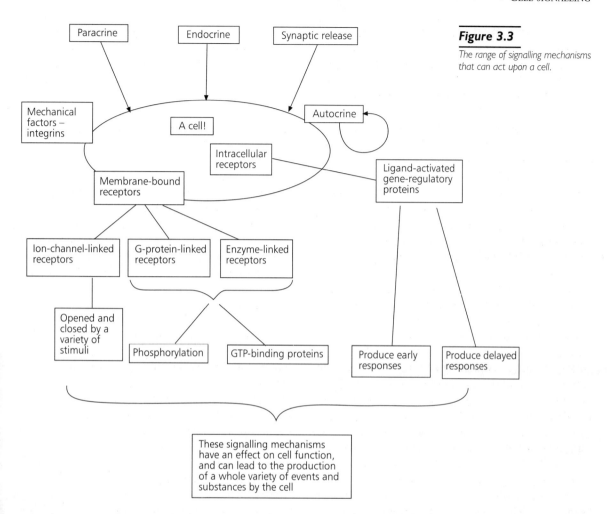

Figure 3.3

The range of signalling mechanisms that can act upon a cell.

out of the cell. Cells must have their action regulated by signals. These initiate a variety of processes, and other molecules and substances are produced (whether they be waste products, secreted signals to other cells or some other product), which must then be transported out of the cell and away from it, so that overall function can be maintained.

SIGNALLING MECHANISMS: THEIR FLEXIBILITY, 'RANDOMNESS' AND ADAPTABILITY

Cell signalling and membrane transport mechanisms take many forms but there are various 'families' or 'groups' into which they can be broadly categorized. Looking at these mechanisms helps to illustrate the enormous potential for variation in response that is needed to maintain function, equilibrium and homeostasis through all events and challenges in life.

Note: The following is only to illustrate certain points, and is not meant as a definitive discussion of the mechanisms introduced.

CELL SIGNALLING

Figure 3.3 indicates the range of signalling mechanisms that can act upon a cell.

Bearing in mind that in Figure 3.3 each of the cells producing the paracrine, endocrine or synaptic releases of substances has already had its function induced by a similar process of multi-stage signalling mechanisms to those shown in the illustration, one can see that the whole cycle of information processing depends upon, and can possibly be affected at, a large number of stages between the initiation of a signal and the eventual response to that signal.

So, cell activity depends on signalling messengers arriving at the cell.

Leaving aside synaptic transmission for a moment, the other modes of signalling mechanisms indicated in Figure 3.3 are transported to the cells in two ways: either by entering the circulation (a general fluid medium), then entering the interstitium (a local fluid medium) and so coming into contact with the cell (which might be quite distant from where the signal was produced); or by being produced straight into the interstitium, travelling through the interstitium and acting on the cells in that vicinity.

Paracrine and endocrine signalling requires effective circulation at a general and an interstitial level. The effectiveness of capillary circulation and the dynamics of the extracellular matrix are essential for these types of signalling.

However, whether by paracrine, endocrine or synaptic release, once secreted, the extracellular signalling molecules act upon the cell membrane through two types of receptor:

- membrane-bound receptors;
- intracellular receptors.

Signalling by membrane-bound receptors

There are three classes of cell-surface receptor: ion-channel-linked receptors, G-protein-linked receptors and enzyme-linked receptors.

Ion-channel-linked receptors are often involved in rapid synaptic signalling between electrically excitable cells. These let various ions cross the cell membrane. They can be opened or closed by a variety of mechanisms. They are thus 'gated' in a variety of ways:

- by mechanical stress: mechanically gated channels;
- by the binding of a ligand: ligand-gated channels (note: the ligand can be a neurotransmitter, an ion or a nucleotide);
- by changes in voltage across the membrane: voltage-gated channels;
- by phosphorylation.

Note: The neurocrine signalling within synapses mentioned earlier uses (neuro)transmitter-gated-ion channels. (The neurotransmitter acts as a ligand to affect/gate the ion channel.)

The other two types of membrane-bound receptor, the **G-protein-linked receptors** and **enzyme-linked receptors**, themselves generally act within the cell through two main types of action:

- signalling by phosphorylation;
- signalling by GTP-binding protein.

The variability within these pathways and stages

Communicating networks do not operate a binary system of one input–one output. One input, under a variety of circumstances, may lead to a variety of outputs.

Multiplicity of outcome is possible through several things, such as: the combination of signalling messengers that arrive at the cell at any one time, triggering a variety of receptor activity; the length of time that channels are open (and thus the amount of signalling molecules allowed into the cell); the possible variability in the first and second messenger cascades of phosphorylation; and the nature of the mechanisms that replicate genes (one of the main reasons the signalling molecule was permitted into the cell in the first place) – gene transcription.

It may be helpful to briefly discuss some of these factors.

Gene transcription

Of all of these, it is at the level of gene transcription that there is the greatest potential for variability. Remember we said earlier that communication is a summation of signalling messages acting upon a cell? Depending on the combination and nature of signalling mechanisms that act upon a cell, the nature of gene transcription may be affected, thus adapting cell function. Unfortunately, it is not fully understood how or why a cell transcribes a certain section of gene compared to another, and what the differences in activity may be from each of a number of subtly different cell products. However, as understanding grows, it may be possible to see how variability in gene transcription might be initiated, and what the clinical relevance might be.

Within the cell, in order for the cell to react to stimuli, coded information is required that is held within the gene. Sections of gene need to move out of the nucleus so that cell activity can be triggered. The 'original' gene cannot be used, as clearly the cell would have a very short life span, and so 'copies' of the gene are made, and it is these copies that are transported out of the nucleus to initiate cell activity.

A certain section of the DNA is copied and is called messenger RNA (mRNA). To produce the right signal, various different bits of the DNA code are copied and then spliced together in a particular sequence.

In lots of different cells, the genes are obviously all the same and so would produce identical mRNA were it not for the action of certain enzymes that each cell contains. The enzymes in the cell determine which parts are spliced and which are not. These differently spliced mRNAs lead to the production of different proteins (although they all came from the same gene originally). The summation of a variety of different signalling messengers acting upon and within the cell are thought to influence the splicing patterns of the mRNA, and so influence the nature of the cellular products, and hence action.

Hypothetical example
Imagine that there are six genes that give actin (which we could call actin 1–6). Each of these can be spliced differently to give different variants: 1a, b, c, d; 2e, f, g, h and so on.

Many different organs contain and utilize actin variants: in the liver, for example, the type that is required could be actin 1b, whereas in the ovary it could be actin 4x. This differentiation is strongly predetermined. Under certain circumstances, though, depending on the demands placed on the cell, the actin that is 'called for' can change. Under these changed circumstances the liver might require another type of actin than previously; a need that will have been communicated to the gene-transcription mechanisms by some means. Hence the 'liver' can adapt to external influences and its ongoing function may be slightly changed.

The clinical ramifications of this are unknown. The point being made is that cellular activity is not the product of a simple one input–one output system.

Note: One of the factors that may influence transcription is neurally mediated signalling mechanisms, which under altered levels of neural activity may lead to slightly adapted gene transcription. Altered levels of neural activity are discussed below and also in Chapter 4

Length of time channels are open
Different channels, when opened by different signalling molecules, remain open for different lengths of time. This allows a greater proportion of the channelled substance into the cell, which would have an effect on subsequent cell action. This occurs with certain calcium channels, among others.

Example
In the central nervous system, some cells, if their calcium channels are open for a long time, gain a certain high concentration of intracellular calcium. This leads to the activation of genes to give protein synthesis, to promote cell growth. This enables dendrites to grow out of the cell and make connections with other cells, and so promotes mechanisms for learning and memory, through the establishment of these developed connections.

Phosphorylation
The exact nature of the cascades within the processes of phosphorylation will not be

discussed, but their complexity is such that some of the signalling proteins (often referred to as 'intracellular mediators' or 'second messengers') within the cascades act as integrating devices, equivalent to microprocessors in a computer. In response to multiple signal inputs, they produce an output that is calibrated to cause the desired biological effect, giving unique responses to individual situations.

Signalling by intracellular receptors

Intracellular receptors are another group of signalling mechanisms introduced in the overview diagram of cell-signalling mechanisms and yet to be discussed.

Intracellular signalling is carried out through the 'intracellular superfamily', which is composed of the steroid hormones, thyroid hormones, retinoids and vitamin D. They bind to intracellular receptors that are ligand-activated gene regulatory proteins, and can produce two types of change, early and delayed.

Gene transcription

The gene transcription triggered by this process gives a quick response or one that is more slow acting. In this way, a simple hormonal trigger can cause a very complex change in the pattern of gene expression.

Longevity

Neurotransmitters and non-steroid hormones have only short periods of time in which they can be active. For example, the non-steroid hormones are water-soluble and so very quickly removed and/or broken down on entering the blood stream, and the neurotransmitters are removed from the extracellular space even faster – within seconds or milliseconds. The steroid hormones, being water-insoluble signalling molecules, persist in the blood stream for many hours or even days (in the case of thyroid hormones).

Again, many factors can influence levels of neural activity that lead to the release of various hormones, such as emotions and stress. Such things can lead to shifts in homeostatic function, with consequent influence on health and immunity.

SYNAPSE ACTIVITY

Levels of activity in the nervous system can produce general effects throughout the body (e.g. through the hypothalamic–pituitary–adrenal axis or the neuroendocrine–immune system), or direct effects on local tissues (such as blood vessels and specific skeletal muscle cells). Neural signalling mechanisms are capable of undergoing considerable plastic change, which can be both very useful (for learning mechanisms) and very damaging (as in centrally maintained pain phenomena). Details of the way osteopaths reflect on neural activity in general will be discussed in Chapter 4 but the basic mechanisms of neural signalling are outlined below by way of an introduction.

NEURAL SIGNALLING MECHANISMS

Normal neural structure and function

There are three main types of neural cell:

- **the 'classic neurone'**, which has neurotransmitter receptors and releases neurotransmitters;
- **the neurosecretory cell**, which has neurotransmitter receptors and releases hormones (hormones released into a synapse are called neuropeptides and those released into the circulation are called neurohormones);
- **the steroid-hormone-sensitive neurone**, which has neurotransmitter receptors, membrane steroid hormone receptors and a nuclear steroid hormone receptor, and can have adaptable neurotransmitter or hormone release.

These categories are based upon the nature of the receptors that trigger nerve cell activity, and of the types of product/signalling mechanism that the nerve cell produces.

The interesting outcome of having these various structures is that the function and level of activity of individual nerve cells can be adapted by a number of factors, which leads to a great diversity in possible outcomes following a stimulus. For example, variability in circulating hormones or in the level or nature of initial stimulus to a nerve cell can lead to a different signal outcome from the same nerve cell.

Additionally, where a neurone releases signalling molecules into the circulation, then their delivery is dependent on the circulatory efficiency of the person and on the perfusion of the target tissues. Any compromise in tissue/cellular level circulation around those release sites or within the target tissues might affect the effectiveness of the signalling process, and so the subsequent activity of the target tissue and of any feedback loops that monitor responses to the original signal.

Synapse activity

Synapses are electrical junctions. By contrast with the propagation of an action potential (which can occur in either direction along a nerve or muscle fibre), junctional transport is unidirectional. And although even the fastest chemical synaptic responses are slower than the electrical synaptic responses, chemical synaptic transmission has the advantage that a single action potential releases thousands of neurotransmitter molecules, allowing amplification of the synaptic response. Perhaps because it is a multistage process, chemical transmission is more easily modified than electrical transmission. Another point of contrast is that junctional transmission is much more liable to fatigue. Because of this, and the fact that much junctional transmission is chemically mediated, transmission can be blocked or enhanced by means of chemicals similar in structure to the transmitter chemical: the junctions between excitable cells provide the sites at which many therapeutic agents (drugs) act.

Activity-dependent synapse function

Each time a signal passes along the nerve, this releases a neurotransmitter from the presynaptic membrane. Normally, there are a number of receptors waiting for this transmitter on the postsynaptic membrane. Up to a certain level, as more transmitter passes into the synaptic cleft, the postsynaptic membrane is triggered to produce more and more receptor sites so that the signals (contained within the transmitter molecules) can be passed on more readily. This should make signalling more efficient. If the signal dies down, less transmitter is released, and the receptors are no longer maintained and are allowed to degrade. So, synaptic activity keeps receptor population high and decreased synapse activity allows receptors to degrade.

Normal adaptive processes

Synapse activity can adapt in other ways than by increasing or decreasing the number of receptor sites. The level of reactivity/responsiveness can also be adapted such that the same level of incoming stimulus can create either a greater response (sensitization) or a lesser response (habituation) than before. These changes are normal adaptive responses.

Sensitization: In response to increasing stimulus, the nerve cell activity is increased, so that each time the stimulus is given there is a bigger response. If the signal stops, then, after a while, when it restarts, the response is 'back to normal'.

Habituation: If the stimulus does not stop, then the synapse tires and each time the stimulus is given there is less and less response to it. Left alone for a while, the synapse recovers and, when it reappears, the signal triggers a normal response.

Such factors mean that ongoing neural processing is either heightened or damped down according to need. These processes are involved in short-term learning processes within the nervous system.

'Use it, but don't abuse it'

Both the above phenomena are short-lived events. However, in the presence of repeated bombardment of signals, the nerve structures and synapses can undergo more long-standing changes.

The phrase 'use it, but don't abuse it' seems quite apt to neural function, as under some conditions function can be altered in the longer term by incorporating structural changes to the synapses themselves.

Long-term adaptation

Long-term potentiation (LTP) and long-term depression (LTD) are long-lived events, where the changed response of the synapse to increased activity does not return to normal after a short period of respite from the signal.

In **long-term potentiation**, even after some time of resting, when the original signal comes along the synapse still creates a much bigger response than it should do under normal circumstances.

In **long-term depression**, when the signal comes along the synapse does not react as fully as it should and, in effect, stops the signal from being passed on adequately.

Such factors mean that ongoing neural processing is altered, not in accordance to need, but because of structural changes in the synapses.

Both these events may be important strategies for neural function but have important clinical relevance (Malinow, 1994) and are important for osteopathic hypotheses and practice. These points will be reviewed later.

Experimental exploration of these processes has often concentrated on pain mechanisms, as pain is one of the most common presenting symptoms for many patients. Pain mechanisms seem to be affected by afferent synapse activity governed by nociceptive activity in the periphery. The spinal cord (for example) can undergo, as a result, distinct and long-lasting modulation of synaptic activity, which appears physiologically relevant for the transmission and integration of sensory information, including pain (Randic *et al.*, 1993). People who have suffered nociceptive insults in the periphery may be transmitting higher levels of activity throughout their nervous system as a result and may thus be experiencing greater levels of pain than would be expected from the level of injury/insult alone. This can create a cascade of effects throughout the whole of the nervous system, as all the synapses within the spinal cord and brain (which number millions and millions) are maintained under similar circumstances.

Note: There is still debate as to whether these (long-term) changes occur at the presynaptic membrane, the postsynaptic membrane or both (Malgaroli, 1994). However, it does seem evident that these processes are involved in longer term learning processes within the nervous system (Kandel *et al.*, 1991). In this way the body can learn to function at quite different levels from before, and the long-term changes imply that function may not naturally revert to previous levels without some further impetus to re-adaptation.

Other mechanisms involved in learning and memory

Dendritic spines: the number of interconnections a nerve cell can make

In learning and memory studies, increasing stimuli resulting from constantly using a certain part of the body, continually thinking the same thought or some such repetitive action will, through cellular events within the nerve, lead to a change in the structure of that nerve. It will literally grow more dendrites, and these branch out, create connections with other nearby neurones and interneurones, and so strengthen the association between parts. Now, when the original stimulus comes along, many more neurones are informed and stimulated than before. This reinforces learning and memory.

Thus synaptic plasticity and dendritic growth are both mechanisms that can influence the patterning and reflex responses of the nervous system and, once initiated, a chain of events may spread throughout the whole nervous system if the stimulus is either sufficient or prolonged, or induces structural change in the neurones involved. Patterning is a major subject in later chapters.

OTHER MECHANISMS OF NEURAL COMMUNICATION

Axonal transport

We have discussed (in very simple terms) the potential for change within synaptic structures and the effects that this may have for neural processing; it is now time to discuss another form of neural transmission – axonal transport – to complete our discussion of variability within neural signalling mechanisms.

Many neurotransmitters are synthesized in the cell body yet are released from nerve terminals that may be a long way from the cell body. The neurotransmitters are transported to nerve terminals by the active processes of axonal transport. Not only are neurotransmitters transported this way, but so are various other subcellular components necessary for the process of neurotransmission (such as the specialized cell membrane at the nerve terminal, the vesicular membrane and various enzymes used by the Golgi apparatus and the endoplasmic reticulum). Furthermore, the systems necessary for the recycling of transmitter at the nerve terminals and re-uptake of synaptic vesicular membrane are also transported from the cell body to the terminals. Finally there is also retrograde transport of substances from the terminals back to the cell body.

Neurotrophic function
The neurotrophic function of nerves concerns axonal transport mechanisms. As mentioned, various substances are passed along the length of the nerve, both in an anterograde direction (away from the cell body) and in a retrograde direction (towards the cell body).

Anterograde transport
Activity in the nerve that triggers anterograde activity will pass molecules into the target tissue that help maintain the integrity of that tissue.

Retrograde transport
This is very important. The tissue that the nerve innervates produces a variety of substances, one of the best known of which is nerve growth factor. These molecules must be picked up by the nerve cell on a regular basis in order for the nerve to remain in intimate contact with that tissue. If the nerve receives no nerve growth factor from the tissue, then the nerve will degrade (so that the body can no longer fire a signal into that tissue

from that nerve). The tissue must remain healthy and in use for its nerve supply to remain intact.

Note: Certain concepts of neural function will be discussed in Chapter 4, such as spinal facilitation (which is related to the sensitization and habituation, LTP and LTD mechanisms listed above). Osteopaths feel that this type of altered neural activity could lead to changes in neurotrophic function that may be deleterious for target/end tissue function.

Peripheral compression of nerves
Peripheral nerve injury can occur through many different mechanisms, including fascial entrapment and intervertebral compression resulting from space-occupying lesions such as disc protrusions and osteophytic spurs. This can also have dramatic effects on axonal transport mechanisms. Peripheral neuropathy will be discussed in Chapter 9.

RECAP

The sections above have briefly described a number of neural communication mechanisms and introduced the idea that each of the mechanisms/pathways can become adapted/altered under a variety of circumstances. The very wide range of possibilities of adaptation within the neural system make it capable of some very complex and particular interactions. These may or may not be to our advantage, as will hopefully be illustrated in Chapter 4.

CELLULAR HEALTH AND FLUID DYNAMICS

To complete our review of signalling pathways and cellular activity, we need finally to review fluid dynamics and the extracellular matrix (ECM). This allows us to appreciate factors that can influence the delivery of fluid-borne signalling molecules and the role of the ECM as a mechanical signalling device in its own right.

Cell activity depends upon sufficient nutritional factors and signalling messengers arriving at the cell, and on the transport away from it of waste products and signalling messengers produced in that cell. In other words, the composition and regulation of the extracellular fluid is vital for cell function.

'Extracellular fluid' is all fluid that is outside the body cells, and is found in various places:

- between the microscopic spaces between the cells of tissues, where it is called **interstitial fluid**;
- within the blood vessels and lymphatic channels of the body, where it is called **plasma** and **lymph**, respectively;
- within the peritoneal, pleural, pericardial and cerebrospinal spaces.

All the fluid compartments of the body (which includes cells) do not exist as fixed spaces with identical fluid compositions but rather are in constant interchange with each other, and the fluids within each of them often have strikingly different compositions (Wiggins, 1990). For the body's cells to survive, the pressure and composition of the fluid within and surrounding the cells must be maintained precisely at all times (Hill, 1990).

All cells need a balance between nutrition and elimination to survive, and the circulation of extracellular fluid (through the extracellular matrix) helps to provide this. If cells are required to work harder, then the extracellular fluid/ matrix system comes under greater pressure to maintain adequate nutrition and elimination, and any failure within it will compromise homeostasis and therefore tissue health (Plante *et al.*, 1995). If such homeostasis is disturbed sufficiently the person may find their body expressing signs and symptoms of this dysfunction. If the body fluids are not eventually brought back into balance, death may occur. Also, if cell function is compromised through poor regulation of the extracellular fluid compartment, then signalling messengers may not achieve the desired responses from the 'unhealthy' cell. This has ramifications for ongoing homeostatic regulation and physiological function.

There is increasing orthodox interest in the study of the microcirculation and interstitial compartment physiology and its role in body fluid balance (Shields, 1992). Some of these researchers are beginning to appreciate the critical role of microcirculation dysfunction, which they can present as the basis of disease. For example, these researchers discuss the circumstances in which various factors can lead to oedema (interstitial or cellular), which impairs the traffic of nutrients and waste products to and from the cellular mass, leading to organ damage (Portincasa *et al.*, 1994).

This is what osteopaths have been saying for a long time, without the science to base it on!

Littlejohn's equation of nutrition and elimination

Littlejohn was the founder of the first osteopathic college in Britain (London 1917), and he discussed (among many things) the need for an appropriate balance between nutrition and elimination at a cellular level for healthy function. He took the broad components of the approach of A. T. Still, the founder of osteopathy in America in the late 19th century, and interpreted them using his background as a physiologist and as a naturopath.

Littlejohn felt that, whatever the physiological problem within the body, in order that the body's own self-regulating and self-healing mechanisms could operate at an optimum, one needed to ensure an effective tissue circulation and an effective eliminative function. He expressed this as an equation between nutrition and elimination. He felt that, on the whole, one should always improve the eliminative side of the equation first before trying to address the nutritional side of things (for example, by working on the autonomic nervous system or improving diet/reducing exposure to environmental factors).

Littlejohn's equation is illustrated in Figure 3.4.

Note: This type of cellular dynamic is also discussed by Katherine Keuls (1988).

Tissue 'toxicity'

One of the outcomes of such a disturbance in local cellular balance might be that the local

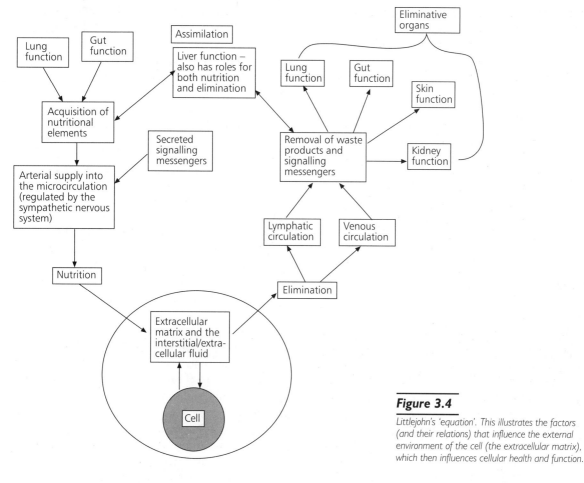

Figure 3.4

Littlejohn's 'equation'. This illustrates the factors (and their relations) that influence the external environment of the cell (the extracellular matrix), which then influences cellular health and function.

tissues would become unhealthy in some way. This has often been referred to in osteopathic texts as 'toxicity'. One effect of altering the local environment of the cell could be to affect the pH of its environment. If the intracellular pH was to become altered, this could have an effect on cell function, leading to a number of aberrant cellular reactions and resistances to various hormones and medications: a classic behaviour of diseased cells (Carlin and Carlin, 1994). Poor fluid dynamics and poor function of the eliminative organs, and hence poor regulation of the local cellular environment, is thought by many osteopaths to cause 'toxicity' within the body (literally, a 'poisoning' of the body), which then affects health and homeostasis (Miller, 1950).

Managing the equation

Continual shifting and circulating of fluids brings a much greater exposure of regulatory/eliminative organs to body fluids. Effective circulation leads to a greater potential for the body's own self-regulating mechanisms to naturally bring the body fluid composition to normal levels and maintain homeostatic balance without external intervention. Osteopathic management of this 'equation' of body fluid composition centres on manipulations designed to move fluids between the compartments of the body and the different sections of the circulatory system, and on improving the function of the eliminative organs, through local manipulation or by influencing the activity within the autonomic nervous system, for example. Promoting fluid movement through compartments requires an effective and efficient function of the connective tissues of the body – through which the body fluids must move. To understand this we will shortly be looking at the composition of connective tissues and the extra-cellular matrix.

The orthodox management of body fluid composition is somewhat different.

If body fluids have too much or too little of a particular substrate, then this can often be remedied pharmacologically, with the result that a lot of orthodox medical practice revolves around maintaining the internal environment by external means. This can be remarkably success-ful and useful. It can also be extremely expensive, and may prove complicated in the long run, in that drug supplementation to sustain one body system might lead to dysfunction in another body system, requiring further and different pharma-cological intervention to redress this new im-balance. Iatrogenic dysfunction can be a major problem in long-term care situations. Most of these 'risk–benefit' equations are resolved by rationalizing that the original intervention was necessary and vital, and that any side-effects are offset by the fact that life has been sustained.

The osteopathic approach is somewhat differ-ent in that, although the aim of having an effi-cient internal environment is not contested and the benefits of homeostasis being regulated are not in question, the method by which this may sometimes be achieved is.

One of A. T. Still's tenets was: '**The rule of the artery is supreme**'. The discussion above gives some indication of what he meant by that statement.

Summary at this point

The osteopathic perspective is that, for effec-tive regulation of the internal environ-ment to occur, one of the most basic requirements is that the fluids within the body must be transported through all tissues, and therefore to those organs whose specific action is to regulate the composition of those fluids. Without this fluid movement, regulation of the internal environment will be compromised and signalling mechanisms that can affect cellular activity and compartment physi-ology will not be effectively transported from the organs/structures where they are produced to the tissues in need.

THE EXTRACELLULAR MATRIX (ECM)

The ECM is a three-dimensional, web-like struc-ture that contains the interstitial fluid of the body. As movement passes through the ECM, the web twists, and this is one factor that helps to promote fluid movement through the intersti-tium. In fact, fluid dynamics are aided by several factors, but these include two mechanical mecha-nisms: the squeezing of individual water mole-cules and other substances, which are gradually moved into the venous system or the lymphatics; followed by entry into the initial lymphatics being aided by the tension of the extracellular matrix pulling apart the collecting ducts, allow-ing fluid to enter.

Because they are transported through a fluid medium, anything that disturbs circulation, either general or interstitial, could have an effect on the deliverance of signalling/immune mole-cules. The structure of the ECM may be capable of affecting fluid movement favourably or unfavourably.

It is important to note at the outset of any discussion of the ECM that it has viscoelastic properties. This gives it a very dynamic structure, which acts sometimes like a fluid and sometimes like a solid (Janmey *et al.*, 1991). This inherent internal adaptability has implications for ECM regulation of fluid dynamics and cell function, which we will discuss below. Other factors to bear in mind are that biological fluid dynamics invariably involve the interaction of elastic flexible tissue with viscous incompressible fluid, and the fact that in many cases the tissue is not only elastic but is also active (i.e. capable of doing work on the fluid; Peskin and McQueen, 1995). And finally,

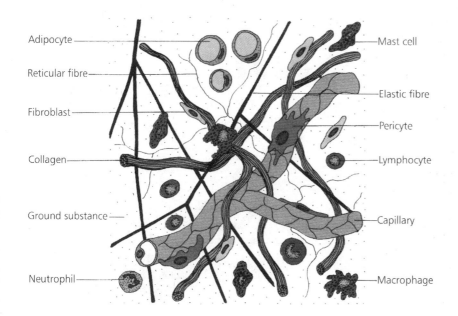

Adipocyte

Reticular fibre

Fibroblast

Collagen

Ground substance

Neutrophil

Mast cell

Elastic fibre

Pericyte

Lymphocyte

Capillary

Macrophage

Figure 3.5

Loose areolar connective tissue, a three-dimensional matrix containing collagen, elastic and reticular fibres and a variety of cells. (Reproduced from Hubbard and Mechan, 1997.)

if the extracellular fluid viscosity changes, this will also have implications for cell membrane function and secretion, and for the regulation of cellular and biochemical processes in general (Yedgar and Reisfeld, 1990).

The 'problem' as far as signalling mechanisms within the interstitium are concerned is that, because of the properties listed above, sometimes the ECM is 'stiff' and sometimes it is not. This does in fact help fluid movement in most cases, but osteopathic theory holds that the ECM can sometimes end up being too stiff/inert, or too twisted/distorted, and so become a 'trap' for fluids rather than a pump.

Figure 3.5 shows the arrangement of loose areolar connective tissue.

This contains all the characteristic components of connective tissues, and gives some indication of the arrangement of the extracellular matrix, to which it is often linked. Fluid passes from the capillaries within the loose connective tissue, and enters the interstitial circulation, which is contained within the ECM. Fluid molecules, immune cells and other molecules must all pass through the network of fibres that make up the ECM.

Figure 3.6 shows the ECM itself.

It is made up of a network of fibres that each have different physical properties. For example, collagen fibres give tensile strength to the matrix, hyaluronan (with the water molecules that it attracts) gives compressive resistance and elastin fibres provide stretch and recoil properties. The ECM links the loose areolar tissue we saw in Figure 3.5 to the cellular membrane through special connections called integrins, and from there to the cytoskeleton (the internal scaffolding of the cell).

ECM movement and blood circulation

The web-like arrangement of the ECM is very useful to the function of the capillary beds that it supports. The ECM, coupled with special stress fibres within the microvascular endothelium, serves as an external tensile scaffold and an internal cytoskeletal scaffold, respectively, which stabilizes the tubular, three-dimensional geometry of microvessels and supports their function (Guilford and Gore, 1995). The natural motion of the ECM (caused by body movement, respiration and so on) can help to promote flow within these vessels, as well as within the interstitium. Additionally, vasomotion (the neurally induced

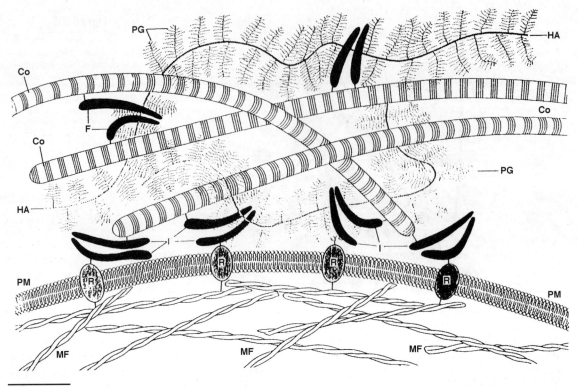

Figure 3.6

Possible extent of cross-linking between collagen fibres (Co), proteoglycans (PG), hyaluronic acid (HA) and fibronectin (F) in the extracellular matrix of animal cells. Fibronectin also ties the network to surface receptors (R) in the plasma membrane (PM); the surface receptors are transmembrane glycoproteins that bind at their cytoplasmic ends to microfilaments (MF) of the cytoskeleton. Reproduced with permission from Wolf (1995).

activity of blood vessels) produces a vibratory, wave-like motion that passes through the ECM. This is thought to set up a periodic oscillation that helps to determine the distribution of flow in blood vessels where they branch (Ursino *et al.*, 1996) – which helps general tissue perfusion.

Incidentally, blood flow can create pressure against the vessel walls, and the stability provided by the ECM to the capillary beds can help the endothelium resist the shear forces created by blood flow and by collision with red and white blood cells (Nehls and Drenckhahn, 1991). These shear forces do seem important for vessel integrity, and some vessels seem more prone to damage in this way simply on account of the amount of turbulence present because of where they are sited (Glagov *et al.*, 1992). To add to this there also seems to be a large body of evidence that implicates fluid dynamic forces in

the genesis and progression of atherosclerosis (Friedman, 1993). The vascular endothelial cells may help to combat these shear forces (Ando and Kamiya, 1993), and may indeed act as some form of mechanoreceptor (Rubanyi *et al.*, 1990). It should be noted, though, that it is not only small calibre vessels such as capillaries that might be affected by shear stresses: the carotid arteries (Perktold and Rappitsch, 1995) and the aorta itself are also vulnerable and, if flow is disturbed here, that will have an effect on renal and mesenteric flow, as well as iliac flow (Chandran, 1993).

Although there are many factors that influence blood flow at this level, it seems that the orientation of the tubes and vessels themselves may have some effect upon red blood cell movement. As red cells must deform to pass through these vessels, any deformation of the vessel may impede this. Any transient or longer-lasting deformations contribute to increased flow resistance in the microcirculation and may lead to small areas of relative tissue ischaemia (Secomb, 1995). This will have implications for cellular health and function. Also, the level of viscosity of blood is important for microcirculatory efficiency (Intaglietta, 1997).

ECM movement, fluid dynamics and immune function

There are many diverse components to the immune system and, although there are clearly many factors that influence immune activity, it is worthwhile reflecting on the influence of fluid dynamics on immunity (and of body movement on fluid flow), to bring certain components of the immune system into contact with potential antigens.

Fluid movement aids the activity of B-cells (one of the many components of the immune system). Movement of the interstitial fluid into the initial lymphatics, and from there to the lymph nodes, is important as this is where much immune processing can occur.

B-cells

Expressed very simply, once a B-cell is mature, it leaves the bone marrow, with its bit of IgD sticking out of itself, and goes out on patrol. If it doesn't meet its antigen in a few days, it dies. It is really interested in 'soluble' antigens – i.e. ones that are in plasma, lymph or extracellular matrix fluid. It won't 'go after bacteria' as it is not equipped for that.

B-cells like to sit in lymph nodes, as most things eventually waft past/through a lymph node, so it is a good place to sit and wait. For this reason, to get the lymph circulating through to where the B-cells are waiting, one requires good fluid mechanics at a general and at a cellular level.

If the B-cell does meet the antigen it is specific for, then the antigen sticks on to the protruding IgD molecules on the B-cell. This coupling (IgD/antigen) sinks into the cell, where it is broken down by a lysosome that fuses to it, and bits of it get taken back to the surface of the cell 'under escort' of another molecule – a class II MHC (major histocompatibility complex). In this state, the B-cell can present itself to a T-cell and ask if it can divide, so that it can produce many molecules capable of combating the immune challenge.

The ECM may also influence other aspects of immune function, by interfering both with cell activity (and responses) and with the necessary mobility of certain immune cells.

Cell responses

Mechanical forces seem to have an effect on immune function, in that, if any of the complex controlling mechanisms of cellular interaction (the adhesion molecules, integrins, tissue matrix and so on) become disturbed, this perhaps affects the development of the inflammatory response (Carreno et al., 1995; mechanical forces are discussed later).

Immune cell movement

Immune cells (such as T-cells, macrophages and neutrophils) have to 'walk' through the network of fibres that make up the ECM to get to their target area in the tissue. Immune cells are naturally deformable, which helps them to pass through the ECM (Hochmuth et al., 1993). But where the ECM is stiff or tense, the network is more like a jungle and the immune cell is fighting through rather than walking through. The ECM may impede immune function in this way. Also, the ECM network may impede the flow of fluid molecules through the area – which may affect inflammatory oedema clearance.

Exposure through fluid movement is thus a key feature of immune success.

Ensuring mobility in tissues and using articulation to promote fluid movement is thought to help the efficiency of the immune system, by helping ECM manipulation of these immune cells. The extent of the clinical relevance is, however, currently unevaluated.

Nevertheless, osteopaths have always had a very strong interest in fluid dynamics, including the efficiency of the lymphatic system, and continue to reflect on how body mechanics may disturb lymph flow.

So, before looking at other aspects of cellular signalling, it is worthwhile appreciating some of the dynamics of fluid movement through the body as a whole. This enables us to gain a broader picture of the osteopathic perspective on fluid movement, in advance of returning to a cellular level and fine detail once more.

BODY MOVEMENT INFLUENCES FLUID CIRCULATION

Fluid movement in all tissues

The fluid movements we are discussing not only relate to skeletal muscle cells and their lymphatic drainage but are relevant for all tissues. In particular, by having an influence on the movement of such things as peritoneal, pleural and cerebrospinal movement and the drainage of lymph from the abdominal, pelvic and thoracic cavities, the musculoskeletal system aids physiological and immune function within the organ systems.

The way in which particular parts of the musculoskeletal system are involved in promoting fluid movements in different body areas/tissues will be discussed in detail in a separate chapter. What follows is by way of an introduction.

Fluid movement is strongly associated with movement in fascial structures (from compartments to the extracellular matrix).

A. T. Still, the founder of osteopathy, was constantly emphasizing the importance of the functions of fascia and its clinical significance. One of his reported musings on the subject of fascia is as follows:

> *As soon as we pass through the skin we enter the fascia. In it we find cells, glands, blood and other vessels, with nerves running to and from every part. Here we could spend an eternity with our present mental capacity, before we could comprehend even a superficial knowledge of the powers and uses of the fascia in the laboratory of animal life.*
>
> Magoun, 1960

In this and many other quotes, Still was in essence discussing the role that fascia has in determining fluid flow at a cellular level, and hence the regulation of the internal environment.

Relation to models of osteopathic practice

Osteopaths consider that microbiomechanics affects fluid movement at a cellular level (with normal body movement, e.g. during locomotion, gradually passing down to this cellular level). Therapeutically, osteopaths consider that gentle movement applied to an affected tissue can increase the health of that tissue, by improving the function and physiology of fascia (Northop, 1952) and speeding up recovery from pathology or injury by helping to maintain appropriate fluid movement and hence tissue physiology.

The clinical relevance of this approach has yet to be adequately researched (and is perhaps not as recognized by the orthodox profession as it is by osteopaths and other manual practitioners), but has many fascinating and potentially very useful outcomes if validated.

It is a concept that osteopaths have always held very dear to their hearts. So much so that many osteopathic manipulations have been developed with the aim of influencing fluid movement. The general articulatory techniques within a system of treatment called the 'general osteopathic treatment' (GOT) can be performed in a way that is thought to promote fluid movement. The articulation within the GOT should be performed rhythmically, in an oscillatory fashion, at a certain rate and amplitude, to affect movement in tissues deep to the surface of the body. This point has also been discussed in detail in a book by Eyal Lederman (1997).

Note: As will be amply illustrated in Chapter 6, osteopathic techniques have changed over the years and it is probable that not all current members of the profession are as well versed in the style of GOT that will induce better fluid movement as they might be, which is very sad.

Over the years, the full application of this procedure, which takes time and skill to perform properly and effectively, was gradually put aside by some parts of the profession in some sort of drive for greater efficiency, and because some felt it was an 'unexciting' technique to perform (compared to high-velocity thrust techniques, for example) or because (for some reason) they could not see its relevance for the types of condition with which their patients were presenting. What is left of this part of the GOT procedure for these sections of the profession is a more locally applied technique that has more limited effects on whole-body fluid movement than the original technique (according to the osteopaths who still practise it in its entirety).

General techniques

However, general articulatory techniques, rhythmic movements and general mobilization techniques will all have some effect on fluid movement, and have a major role in the clinical management of many disorders.

Fluid movement throughout the body is needed whether one's patient has a sprained ankle, a compression neuropathy of a peripheral nerve in the intervertebral foramen, a cold/the flu, muscle strain and spasm, chronic fatigue syndrome, cardiovascular problems such as high blood pressure, varicose leg ulcers or chronic prostatic congestion, for example. Any tissue in distress needs to receive effective signalling, receive nutrition, have its waste products removed and receive any required immune components; and this can only be achieved through fluid movement (with appropriate care for the pathological nature of the tissue state or condition being managed – one example for a case of extreme caution is when there is bacterial infection involved; another is carcinoma).

Restoring an interest in fluid dynamics within standard treatment procedures to those parts of the profession that have 'lost touch' with the broad detail of this concept would be a very positive outcome of this book. Other authors are also making a similar plea – such as Eyal Lederman in his lectures and books (1996, 1997); he has 'come separately' to many of the original osteopathic perspectives on body movement, manipulative techniques and fluid movement.

HOW THEN MIGHT BODY MOVEMENT INFLUENCE FLUID DYNAMICS?

Body movement and its influence on fascial compartments and the extracellular matrix (ECM)

To appreciate the role of the musculoskeletal system and body movement upon fascial structures and hence fluid movement, we need to 'borrow' an image from a discussion of tensegrity in a later chapter. In this discussion an analogy is introduced to illustrate the architectural arrangement of man: we will use a picture of a man with many membranes inside him, stiffened out by multijointed rods, forming many compartments and spaces, which are either filled up with organs or with fluid. The movement patterns of the multijointed rods caused by muscle contraction would continuously change the shape, tension and orientation of these membranes. (Man functions as a tensegrity structure: movement in one part is automatically and instantaneously transferred to all other parts.)

As these membranous compartments are elastic, any body movement subtly distorts their shape on a moment-to-moment basis, which creates a pumping effect on the fluids within the compartments. This helps to move the fluid from one compartment to another, as these are not 'sealed' but somewhat permeable to fluid and its constituents. This creates a movement-orientated circulation of body fluids throughout the whole structure of the human form.

If our posture and biomechanics are efficient, and all parts of the body move well, then fluid circulation throughout all tissues should actually be helped and not hindered. (Various studies show evidence of a redistribution of body fluids following activities such as change of position, and due to the influence of gravity upon the body (Maw *et al.*, 1995; Lillywhite, 1996).) (As an interesting aside, high altitude also seems to affect fluid flow in body compartments – Anand *et al.*, 1993.)

On a cellular level the fluid compartments are controlled by the connective tissue extracellular matrix – which will be reviewed in a moment – and some lymphatic pumps are formed through deformation of the tissue that the initial lymphatics are embedded in. So the general body movement, by engaging all the connective tissue membranes, will eventually induce movement at a cellular level.

Fluid dynamics in the interstitium: the influence of body movement on the extracellular matrix

Where does motion stop and start? If you move one part, where else is the effect of that motion felt? If one part of the body is generally less mobile, will this filter down to a cellular level and affect tissue drainage in any way? Questions such as this are the subject of endless debate among osteopaths, and the following picture may help the reader appreciate the conundrums these pose for osteopaths.

Refer back for a moment to the properties of tensegrity structures – movement passes through all tissues. The connective tissue structures of the ECM and the cytoskeleton act as component parts of the tensegrity structure of the whole body, passing gross movement through all parts of the body down to a cellular level.

Figures 3.5 and 3.6 illustrated the way internal structures of the cell are in intimate connection with surrounding connective tissue structures; in the first instance the extracellular matrix and thereafter, through the perfusion of connective tissue throughout and between all component parts of the body, all cells can be thought of as being physically connected with each other.

As stated earlier, the ECM forms a sort of three-dimensional web, which, as the tissue is twisted and torsioned, will create a propulsive force on the fluid molecules within it. The movement induced will open up some parts of the web and close down or constrain other parts. So the physical arrangement of the ECM affects cellular level fluid transport (which of course also relates to the transport of information). (Note: Physical forces acting upon the cell membrane via the ECM can also be influential to cell membrane function. This point will be taken up later in the chapter.) The ECM movement also helps to regulate the viscosity of the extracellular fluid, as the level of viscosity is an important determinant of cell function (Dintenfass, 1990).

This arrangement of the ECM (in addition to the chemical and other forces promoting molecular movement) helps to ensure not only that fluid movement through the ECM is effective but also that the entry of interstitial fluid into the lymphatic vessels is promoted (Schmid-Schonbein, 1990). Movement passing through the ECM acts upon the initial lymphatics, which are embedded within it. If there is poor movement through the extracellular matrix, then drainage of tissue fluid into the initial lymphatics may be compromised (Aarli and Aukland, 1991). It is interesting to note that the output of lymphatic pumps seems to depend on the rate of flow into the pump, which is similar to the mechanics of blood circulation: cardiac output depends on the rate of blood flow through the veins into the heart and on the pumping characteristics of the heart itself (Gallagher *et al.*, 1993). This means that one needs to consider all components of the lymphatic system together and not just concentrate on the initial lymphatic mechanisms discussed below. (Note: Further similar commentary on the lymphatic system is included in Chapter 9.)

Initial lymphatics

As a general rule, initial lymphatics are located in wide connective tissue regions with collagen bundles and 'anchoring filaments', which serve to provide dilatation rather than compression of these structures in oedema (Aukland and Reed, 1993; Aarli *et al.*, 1991). General movement and external pressures can facilitate fluid movement through the interstitium (Aukland and Reed, 1993). The anchoring filaments act as springs and exert a pulling force on the outer surface of the capillary wall of the lymphatic vessels (Reddy and Patel, 1995). Good compliance of the interstitium will aid fluid movement and entry into the initial lymphatics (Aarli and Aukland, 1991). Figure 3.7 shows the initial lymphatics.

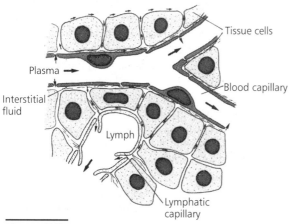

Figure 3.7

The circulation of fluids in the tissues. Fluid is filtering into the interstitial spaces on the left-hand side of the diagram (representing the arterial end of the capillary bed) and returning to the blood on the right (representing the venous end). About 10% of the fluid flows into the lymphatic capillaries. (Reproduced from Hubbard and Mechan, 1997.)

Effects of poor movement/interference with compartment action on fluid dynamics

Clinically, damage to the fluid compartments or the membranes that form them can be devastating for fluid movement; for example, the scarring in the axillary and upper chest region caused by irradiation in the treatment of breast cancer can cause upper-limb lymphoedema.

On a 'less pathological' level, 'puffy ankles' at the end of the day can be due to fluid stasis caused by too little moving about, and hence inefficient pumping of the fluids from the periphery to the centre of the body. Gravity is a difficult force to overcome – and active promotion of fluids by passive pumping techniques is a necessary aid to fluid circulation.

Other types of circulatory problems within the limbs can occur through different mechanisms. If the fascial sheaths of the limbs are too tight, then fluid dynamics can still be compromised, as in 'compartment syndrome' or 'shin splints'. In these conditions tight fascia constricts the muscle blood flow during activity, leading to ischaemia and hence pain.

Torsion of the body, scarring, and tightness in fascial sheaths and planes can all disrupt the 'fluid compartments' throughout the rest of the body. Osteopaths are very interested in such consequences, and the chain of events that perpetuate them.

Connective tissue structure and function is therefore very important for fluid dynamics.

Note: The effects of scarring, inflammation and poor mobility on connective tissue structures will be reviewed later.

MECHANICAL SIGNALLING MECHANISMS ACTING ON AND WITHIN CELLS

To conclude our chapter on cell signalling, one final component of communication related to the extracellular matrix has yet to be discussed. That is the concept of mechanical signalling through the structural parts of the matrix, through the cell membrane and into the internal scaffolding of the cell and its constituent parts.

The extracellular matrix, the cytoskeleton and cell function

The important interaction between cell function, cell health and fluid dynamics is not the only way that the ECM can affect cell signalling. Movement itself acts upon components within the ECM, and may prove to have a very important role in cell communication.

The concept of tensegrity was briefly alluded to earlier, and we return to it now as it helps to illustrate the concept of inter- and intracellular communication through movement and physical force applied to a cell.

The concept of tensegrity suggests that motion in one part or tissue will be transmitted throughout the rest of the structure of which that tissue is a part.

There is an inter-relatedness of parts with respect to movement.

The arrangement of tensional and compressional elements within a tensegrity structure (which is how the human body can be described) will ensure that all parts move together (Robbie,

1977). It is impossible to move one part without it affecting the mechanics of even quite distant parts of that tissue/the body. Thus, consequent to a few general movements of the body (e.g. locomotion), or such things as peristalsis or respiration, there is always a continuous micromotion being applied to all tissues of the body that is somewhat self-perpetuating – the body never really stops moving at all.

There is always some shifting of tension in some tissue somewhere. The body makes use of this movement in a number of ways.

The fact that physical force seems to act at a cellular level may be very significant to cell function.

Key concept

The structural arrangement of the cell and of the extracellular matrix is well suited for the transmission of physical force through to the cell nucleus. It seems that physical forces acting upon the cell are a necessary and important component of cell function.

Osteopathy is concerned with movement, and with consequences of altered movement patterns and altered physical forces acting through and within tissues.

The following discussion is a review of the potential effects of physical forces upon the extracellular matrix, the cell membrane and the internal architecture of the cell – the cytoskeleton – with a view to appreciating how tissue mobility may affect cell function and how, ultimately, movement disorders within the body may affect cell function, and ... **how physically manipulating the tissues may affect cellular level activity.**

The extracellular matrix and the cytoskeleton and the effects of external forces

What will hopefully emerge from this part of the discussion is a picture of cells bound together in special ways and contained in a tissue system that connects right through from the inside of the cell out into the area surrounding adjacent cells and on into other adjacent parts of the body. If the tissues are pulled, the ECM acts to resist this, 'huddles the cells together' against the stress and

helps them remain intact. The ECM may have to remodel the shape of the cells to withstand prolonged stress, and it may have to shore itself up by making itself more rigid. The 'scaffolding' properties of the ECM come from particular cells – fibroblasts. As we shall see later, fibroblasts may be very useful to cell function but they can also be the source of dysfunction in the 'right' conditions. However, they are also the route by which many osteopathic manipulations of tissues may have a positive effect (in restoring normal function).

Even with the vast amount of biological and biochemical data that exists, little is known at a molecular level about physical mechanisms involved in attachments between cells or about consequences of adhesion on the material structure. The functions of the extracellular matrix, though, are beginning to be understood, and it is known that the extracellular matrix can affect a number of important cell functions such as cell motility (certain cells need to 'walk around the body', for example immune cells) and angiogenesis (the formation of new blood vessels, for example in tissue healing). The ECM is also thought to have a role in the physiological efficiency of tissues, as the structure of the extracellular matrix, of adhesions between cells and the structure of the cytoskeleton are intimately involved in biological cell function (Evans *et al.*, 1995), which we shall discuss in a moment.

We will consider these different functions separately, starting with support.

The supporting role of the ECM

The physical support of cells in tissues is an important function of the ECM. It helps the tissue group/organ/structure to remain intact.

Tensile forces acting on the cell

One distinguishing feature of 'life' is that the physical forces between biological molecules and membrane surfaces are highly specific, in contrast to other non-specific interactions (such as van der Waals, hydrophobic and electrostatic (coulombic) forces) that act in/within tissues (Helm *et al.*, 1991). This specificity means that they can exert very particular effects on the cells.

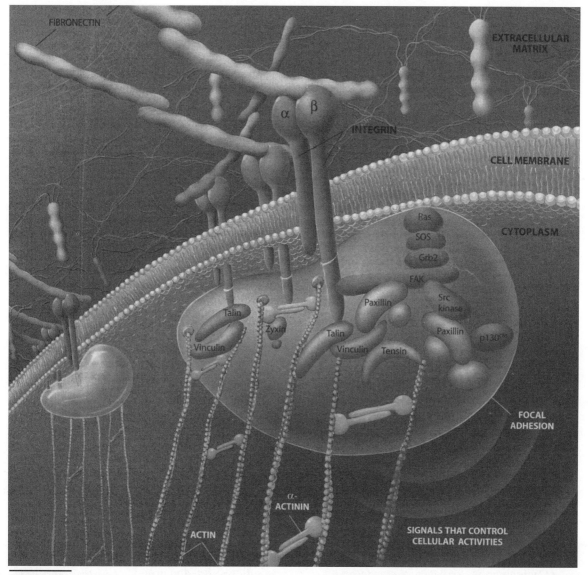

Figure 3.8

Integrins span cell membranes. They hold a cell in place by attaching at one end to molecules of the extracellular matrix (or to the molecule of other cells) and at the other end to the cell's own scaffolding, the cytoskeleton. They connect to this scaffolding through a highly organized aggregate of molecules – a focal adhesion – that includes such cytoskeletal components as actin, talin, vinculin and alpha-actinin. (Reproduced from Horwitz, 1997.)

Where physical/tensile forces act upon the cell, there is increasing evidence that the cytoskeleton and the structure of the extracellular matrix are mutable – in other words that they change according to the tensile forces applied to them (Dufort and Lumsden, 1993).

The mechanisms behind this may relate to the properties of collagen gels (within the extracellular matrix), which can adapt to changes in physical forces acting upon them, altering their viscoelastic properties and hence the cell function (Ozerdem and Tozeren, 1995). Figure 3.8 shows some of the special links between the ECM and the cytoskeleton, which are called **integrins**.

In effect, the integrins act as mechano-receptors, transmitting mechanical forces to the cytoskeleton, and as interdependent struts and strings that reorient globally in response to localized stresses applied (Wang *et al.*, 1993).

In this way, the physical support both of the tissue and within and around individual cells is a gently varying thing that shifts and adapts and reorients according to the needs of the body. This connecting web does more than provide support, though: it provides a unique communication network.

ECM communication

What will hopefully emerge from this part of the discussion is the way that movement is a type of conversation between cells, and the fact that, without movement, the cell is left 'in the dark' and cannot work in a way that is coordinated with the rest of the body.

Cells are known to use integrins for communication among themselves in the extracellular matrix and also for communication with the 'outside world' (in other words, adjacent tissues and structures, and ultimately the rest of the body; Nietfeld *et al.*, 1994). Integrins seem to be very important for regulating health and influencing disease processes (Horwitz, 1997).

How far this communication goes and what potential there is for physical forces to affect cell activity is perhaps summed up by the following:

> *Cells and intracellular elements are capable of vibrating in a dynamic manner with complex harmonics, the frequency of which can now be measured and analysed in a quantitative manner by Fourier analysis. Cellular events such as changes in shape, membrane ruffling, motility, and signal transduction occur within spatial and temporal harmonics that have potential regulatory importance. (These vibrations can be altered by such things as growth factors and the process of carcinogenesis.)*
>
> *It is important to understand the mecha-nism by which this vibrational information is transferred directly through the cell. From observations it is proposed that vibrational information is transferred through a tissue-tensegrity matrix which acts as a coupled harmonic oscillator operating as a signal transducing mechanism from the cell periphery to the nucleus and ultimately the DNA.*
>
> *The vibrational interactions occur through a tissue matrix system consisting of the nuclear matrix, the cytoskeleton, and the extracellular matrix that is poised to couple the biologic oscillations of the cell from the peripheral membrane to the DNA through a tensegrity-matrix structure.*
>
> *Tensegrity has been defined as a structural system composed of discontinuous compression elements connected by continuous tension cables, which interact in a dynamic fashion. A tensegrity tissue matrix system allows for specific transfer of information through the cell by direct transmission of vibrational chemo-mechanical energy through harmonic wave motion.*
>
> Pienta and Coffey, 1991

Thus DNA activity can be influenced by mechanical forces. Variability in gene transcription processes are discussed later, and it may be that movement is one of the key determinants influencing the manufacture of cell products and hence homeostatic/physiological function (Carter *et al.*, 1991).

Mechanical forces have other effects on the cell membrane, such as altering the electrical field activities within and around cells (McLeod, 1992) and altering the membrane potential (by the influence of mechanically activated ion channels; Craelius *et al.*, 1993), although the study of electrical forces in and around cells *in vitro* is difficult and, as a study, is in its infancy (McLeod, 1992).

Thus the effects of physical forces on cell membranes, excitability, protein channels and myriad other aspects of cell activity is a growing area of scientific investigation that may prove to be deeply influential to the understanding of body function and physiology. Whatever the effects of mechanical forces are ultimately understood to be, the fact of cell communication through the extracellular matrix is established.

THE REGULATORY ROLE OF THE ECM

As indicated in the preceding sections, then, the extracellular matrix plays a role in regulating the behaviour of cells by the fact that matrix proteins can engender changes in cell shape and movement, bind growth factors and facilitate cell–cell and cell–matrix interactions (Schnaper and Kleinman, 1993). The ECM may also regulate specific responses of axons and dendrites, influencing their development *in vitro* (Lafont *et al.*, 1993).

In other words, it helps the cell membrane with very many signalling mechanisms. The ECM can help to orientate various signalling molecules to the right bits of the cell membrane, which have the receptors in them that the molecules are looking for.

When mechanical forces are applied to cell surface receptors, the cytoskeletal stiffness (ratio of stress to strain) increases in direct proportion to the stress applied, and this causes intact microtubules and intermediate filaments as well as microfilaments to respond. This helps to orient the receptor to the signalling molecule and also to control the passage of the molecule as it passes into the cell, to its destination. (It is a bit like having a series of flexible fingers that grapple the molecule and drag it through the dense structure of the cell.)

To illustrate the potential effects of differing ECM stiffness and mobility, the following image may be useful:

> The cell membrane needs to be supple in order to allow the signalling molecule to pass through it. Try to picture the membrane for a moment as a sort of elastic membrane with holes in it, which is trying to act like a two-way gate/barrier. Now picture an enormous number of molecules jostling against that gate trying to get in or

out, and soon the membrane becomes a heaving sheet of tissue that is bulging and twisting all over as molecules push into it trying to find the gap that they are supposed to go through. In all the twisting and distortion of the membrane, some of the relative positions of the gaps (receptor sites) become changed in relation to each other, and some are pulled open or shut as a result, and one can imaging that actually getting a signal across the cell membrane is harder than it originally appeared!

MANIPULATION AND THE ECM

Manual therapy is considered to have effects upon connective tissue (Threlkeld, 1992) and manipulations may eventually be found to operate at a cellular level. Osteopaths are working practically with tissue tensions every day, and eagerly await further progress in this field to expand their appreciation of what it is that they are actually doing.

> Even now, though, during their practice, many osteopaths often describe how they want to 'restore integrity and communication' between parts of the body, and between different areas within a tissue. They are looking for the right mechanical response in the tissues as they feel through them, and they use their palpatory sense to interpret whether communication between parts is 'reasonable' or not. The fact that movement is a form of communication may mean that such interpretations may not be so 'fantastic' after all!

SUMMARY

This chapter started by illustrating that, in order for effective human function to be as unhindered as possible, efficient signalling mechanisms must be in place that are adaptable to various stressors/events.

The effects of fluid dynamics and connective tissue activity on cell communication have been introduced and the potential for a variety of shifts in function within the nervous system has been illustrated. Changes in body movement may influence these factors, leading to adaptation in signalling effectiveness or signal transport.

The idea of the musculoskeletal system as a communicating mechanism has been introduced, as has the idea that it can interfere with a number of other signalling/communicating networks. Although the full implications of the way in which it could interfere with neural signalling mechanisms (and the subsequent control of homeostasis and immunity) are yet to be explored, it is hoped that some appreciation of how the musculoskeletal system and its actions could relate to health and dysfunction processes has been achieved.

The osteopathic perspective on dysfunction and disease development therefore centres on fluid dynamics, their effects on cellular health and immunity, and changes in mechanical and electrical signalling mechanisms, which may become adapted (perverted) by such things as changes in general body biomechanics and the state of the musculoskeletal system.

It is sad but true that the scientific appreciation of osteopathy and the effects of manual procedures on physiological processes is in its early (or even fetal) stages, but that should not hinder the exploration of ideas.

The next chapters aim to expand on the image of movement and communication through the body and discuss further the neurological implication of altered movement patterns and activity within the musculoskeletal system.

REFERENCES

Aarli, V. and Aukland, K. (1991) Oedema-preventing mechanisms in a low-compliant tissue: studies on the rat tail. *Acta Physiologica Scandinavica*, **141**, 489–495.

Aarli, V., Reed, R. K. and Aukland, K. (1991) Effect of longstanding venous stasis and hypoproteinaemia on lymph flow in the rat tail. *Acta Physiologica Scandinavica*, **142**, 1–9.

Anand, I. S., Chandrashekhar, Y., Rao, S. K. *et al.* (1993) Body fluid compartments, renal blood flow, and hormones at 6000m in normal subjects. *Journal of Applied Physiology*, **74**, 1234–1239.

Ando, J. and Kamiya, A. (1993) Blood flow and vascular endothelial cell function. *Frontiers of Medical and Biological Engineering*, **5**, 245–264.

Aukland, K. and Reed, R. K. (1993) Interstitial–lymphatic mechanisms in the control of extracellular fluid volume. *Physiological Reviews*, **73**, 1–78.

Carlin, K. and Carlin, S. (1994) Diseased cells and pH. *Medical Hypotheses*, **42**, 299–306.

Carreno, M. P., Rousseau, Y. and Haeffner-Cavaillon, N. (1995) [Cell adhesion molecules and the immune system]. *Allergie et Immunologie*, **27**, 106–110.

Carter, D. R., Wong, M. and Orr, T. E. (1991) Musculoskeletal ontogeny, phylogeny, and functional adaptation. *Journal of Biomechanics*, **24**(Suppl. 1), 3–16.

Chandran, K. B. (1993) Flow dynamics in the human aorta. *Journal of Biomechanical Engineering*, **115**, 611–616.

Craelius, W., Ross, M. J., Harris, D. R. *et al.* (1993) Membrane currents controlled by physical forces in cultured mesangial cells. *Kidney International*, **43**, 535–543.

Dintenfass, L. (1990) A new outlook on body fluid viscosity and cell function: concluding remarks and discussion. *Biorheology*, **27**, 611–616.

Dufort, P. A. and Lumsden, C. J. (1993) Cellular automaton model of the actin cytoskeleton. *Cell Motility and the Cytoskeleton*, **25**, 87–104.

Evans, E., Ritchie, K. and Merkel, R. (1995) Sensitive force technique to probe molecular adhesion and structural linkages at biological interfaces. *Biophysical Journal*, **68**, 2580–2587

Friedman, M. H. (1993) Arteriosclerosis research using vascular flow models: from 2-D branches to compliant replicas. *Journal of Biomechanical Engineering*, **115**, 595–601.

Gallagher, H., Garewal, D., Drake, R. E. and Gabel, J. C. (1993) Estimation of lymph flow by relating lymphatic pump function to passive flow curves. *Lymphology*, **26**, 56–60.

Glagov, S., Vito, R., Giddens, D. P. and Zarins, C. K. (1992) Micro-architecture and composition of artery walls: relationship to location, diameter and the distribution of mechanical stress. *Journal of Hypertension (Supplement)*, **10**, S10I–S104.

Guilford, W. H. and Gore, R. W. (1995) The mechanics of arteriole–tissue interaction. *Microvascular Research*, **50**, 260–287.

Helm, C. A., Knoll, W. and lsraelachvili, J. N. (1991) Measurement of ligand-receptor interactions. *Proceedings of the National Academy of Sciences of the United States of America*, **88**, 8169–8173.

Hill, L. L. (1990) Body composition, normal electrocyte concentrations, and the maintenance of normal volume, tonicity, and acid-base metabolism. *Pediatric Clinics of North America*, **37**, 241–256.

Hochmuth, R. M., Ting-Beal, H. P., Beaty, B. B. *et al.* (1993) Viscosity of passive human neutrophils undergoing small deformations. *Biophysical Journal*, **64**,1596–1601.

Horwitz, A. F. (1997) Integrins and health. *Scientific American*, **May**, 46–53.

Hubbard, J. and Mechan, D. (1997) *The Physiology of Health and Illness, with Related Anatomy*. Stanley Thornes, Cheltenham.

Intaglietta, M. (1997) Whitaker lecture 1996: microcirculation, biomedical engineering, and artificial blood. *Annals of Biomedical Engineering*, **25**, 593–603.

Janmey, P. A., Euteneuer, U., Traub, P. and Schliwa, M. (1991) Viscoelastic properties of vimentin compared with other filamentous biopolymer networks. *Journal of Cell Biology*, **113**, 155–160.

Kandel, E. R., Schwartz, J. H. and Jessel, T. M. (1991) *Principles of Neural Science*, 3rd edn, Prentice Hall, Englewood Cliffs, NJ.

Keuls, K. (1988) *Osteopathic Principles*, Keuls & Associates, Brighton.

Lafont, F., Rouget, M., Rousselet, A. *et al.* (1993) Specific responses of axons and dendrites to cytoskeleton perturbations: an in vitro study. *Journal of Cell Science*, **104**, 433–443.

Lederman, E. (1996) *Harmonic Technique*, 3rd edn, E. Lederman, London.

Lederman, E. (1997) *Fundamentals of Manual Therapy: Physiology, Neurology and Psychology*, Churchill Livingstone, Edinburgh.

Lillywhite, H. B. (1996) Gravity, blood circulation, and the adaptation of form and function in lower vertebrates. *Journal of Experimental Zoology*, **275**, 217–225.

McLeod, K. J. (1992) Microelectrode measurements of low frequency electric field effects in cells and tissues. *Bioelectromagnetics (Supplement)*, **1**, 161–178.

Magoun, H. I. (1960) Fascia in the writings of A. T. Still. Privately published, pp. 159–173.

Malgaroli, A. (1994) LTP expression: hanging like a yo-yo? *Seminars in Cell Biology*, **5**, 231–241.

Malinow, R. (1994) LTP: desperately seeking resolution. *Science*, **266**, 1195–1196.

Maw, G. J., Mackenzie, I. L. and Taylor, N. A. (1995) Redistribution of body fluids during postural manipulations. *Acta Physiologica Scandinavica*, **155**, 157–163.

Miller, E. S. (1950) On the nature and treatment of toxicity. *Unknown.*

Nehls, V. and Drenckhahn, D. (1991) Demonstration of actin filament stress fibers in microvascular endothelial cells in situ. *Microvascular Research*, **42**, 103–112.

Nietfeld, J. J., Huber-Bruning, O. and Bylsma, J. W. (1994) Cytokines and proteoglycans. *EXS*, **70**, 215–242.

Northop, T. L. (1952) Role of connective tissue in acute and chronic disease. In: *Meeting of the Academy of Applied Osteopathy, Atlantic City*, Academy of Applied Osteopathy, Newark, NJ, pp. 67–69.

Ozerdem, B. and Tozeren, A. (1995) Physical response of collagen gels to tensile strain. *Journal of Biomechanical Engineering*, **117**, 397–401.

Perktold, K. and Rappitsch, G. (1995) Computer simulation of local blood flow and vessel mechanics in a compliant carotid artery bifurcation model. *Journal of Biomechanics*, **28**, 845–856.

Peskin, C. S. and McQueen, D. M. (1995) A general method for the computer simulation of biological systems interacting with fluids. *Symposium of the Society for Experimental Biology*, **49**, 265–276.

Pienta, K. J. and Coffey, D. S. (1991) Cellular harmonic information transfer through a tissue tensegrity–matrix system. *Medical Hypotheses*, **34**, 88–95.

Plante, G. E., Chakir, M., Lehoux, S. and Lortie, M. (1995) Disorders of body fluid balance: a new look into the mechanisms of disease. *Canadian Journal of Cardiology*, **11**, 788–802.

Portincasa, P., Di Ciaula, A., Baldassarre, G. *et al.* (1994) Gallbladder motor function in gallstone patients: sonographic and in vitro studies on the role of gallstones, smooth muscle function and gallbladder wall inflammation. *Journal of Hepatology*, **21**, 430–440.

Randic, M., Jiang, M. C. and Ceme, R. (1993) Long-term potentiation and long-term depression of primary afferent neurotransmission in the rat spinal cord. *Journal of Neuroscience*, **13**, 5228–5241.

Reddy, N. P. and Patel, K. (1995) A mathematical model of flow through the terminal lymphatics. *Medical Engineering and Physics*, **17**, 134–140.

Robbie, D. L. (1977) Tensional forces in the human body. *Orthopaedic Review*, **6**, 45–48.

Rubanyi, G. M., Freay, A. D., Kauser, K. *et al.* (1990) Mechanoreception by the endothelium: mediators and mechanisms of pressure- and flow-induced vascular responses. *Blood Vessels*, **27**, 246–257.

Schmid-Schonbein, G. W. (1990) Microlymphatics and lymph flow. *Physiological Reviews*, **70**, 987–1028.

Schnaper, H. W. and Kleinman, H. K. (1993) Regulation of cell function by extracellular matrix. *Pediatric Nephrology*, **7**, 96–104.

Secomb, T. W. (1995) Mechanics of blood flow in the microcirculation. *Symposia of the Society for Experimental Biology*, **49**, 305–321.

Shields, J. W. (1992) Lymph, lymph glands, and homeostasis. *Lymphology*, **25**, 147–153.

Threlkeld, A. J. (1992) The effects of manual therapy on connective tissue. *Physical Therapy*, **72**, 893–902.

Ursino, M., Cavalcanti, S., Bertuglia, S. and Colantuoni, A. (1996) Theoretical analysis of complex oscillations in multibranched microvascular networks. *Microvascular Research*, **51**, 229–249.

Wang, N., Butler, J. P. and Ingber, D. E. (1993) Mechanotransduction across the cell surface and through the cytoskeleton. *Science*, **260**, 1124–1127.

Wiggins, P. M. (1990) Role of water in some biological processes. *Microbiological Reviews*, **54**, 432–449.

Wolf (1995) *Cell and Molecular Biology*, Wadsworth.

Yedgar, S. and Reisfeld, N. (1990) Regulation of cell membrane function and secretion by extracellular fluid viscosity. *Biorheology*, **27**, 581–588.

FURTHER READING

Brown, A. G. (1991) *Nerve Cells and Nervous Systems. An Introduction to Neuroscience*, Springer-Verlag, New York.

Brown, R. E. (1994) *An Introduction to Neuroendocrinology*, Cambridge University Press, Cambridge.

Holmes, O. (1993) *Human Neurophysiology. A Student Text*, 2nd edn, Chapman & Hall, London.

Kandel, E. R., Schwartz, J. H. and Jessell, T. M. (1991) *Principles of Neuroscience*, 3rd edn, Appleton & Lange, Norwalk, CT.

4 COMMUNICATION AND TISSUE CHANGE: THE NERVOUS SYSTEM

INTRODUCTION

This chapter continues the theme of providing an overview to current understanding of some of the mechanisms that might underpin osteopathic philosophy and practice. It focuses on communication within the nervous system, and expands the concept that a breakdown in communication may have a role to play in dysfunction and disease. The chapter highlights how neural communication networks may become 'confused' and therefore less well adapted to coordinating function. As part of this dialogue it discusses the traditional osteopathic hypothesis that irritation and dysfunction within the somatic structures (and other soft tissues) of the body might be a contributory factor to neural 'confusion' and hence homeostatic imbalance and physiological dysfunction.

The chapter discusses the range of neural barriers to communication and introduces the factors that could create/aggravate such barriers. The number of factors and tissue changes that could create barriers to effective neural communication is very great, and the reader must follow through Chapters 4–9 to gain a full appreciation of this concept. There is some repetition within this and subsequent chapters, for reinforcement.

As knowledge and understanding grow, so do interpretations and validations. It is only right that concepts should be allowed to develop. Much of what osteopaths used to say about these mechanisms is no longer correct, and no doubt much of what is here will be superseded as understanding continues. The reader should note that ideas expressed here may be novel to many outside the profession. However, as mentioned before, it is incumbent on any profession to make strenuous efforts to rationalize what might underpin its practice – it is a part of professional maturation and allows much more effective interprofessional communication as a consequence, through trying to describe philosophies in terms that are recognizable to others.

This chapter cannot stand alone, and constitutes just a part of how osteopaths consider body function, health and disease. It is only when the ideas throughout this book have been put together that one can appreciate the overall nature of the osteopathic perspective on health and disease, and begin to see how manipulation of the body tissues may help the person to recover from the problems and dysfunctions within their bodies, and their lives.

THE GENERAL ARRANGEMENT OF THE NERVOUS SYSTEM

In Chapter 2 we discussed how systems may operate in dynamic equilibrium and how this may become chaotic or disordered in some circumstances. The arrangement of the nervous system seems to be ideally suited to operate in this manner. The nervous system is made up of many different components that are networked together in numerous complex and often subtle ways. There are many potential routes for integrative function and for one part to have influence on others. There are increasing numbers of studies that look at this complexity of networks (Katz, 1996; Derryberry and Tucker, 1990) and our understanding of them is increasing all the time, although not all levels of organization and inter-relation are as yet fully understood. This networking is on an anatomical level, and also on a chemical level, and works in a very flexible way, as hinted at in the preceding chapter.

The following quote from Paul Grobstein reinforces the concept that neurology is not a fixed science and that function is open to adaptation:

According to the Harvard Law of Animal Behaviour, 'under carefully controlled experimental circumstances, an animal will behave as it damned well pleases'. An informally propagated and often ironically intended summary of large numbers of observations, the Harvard Law in fact has quite concrete and deep significance for understanding the basic information processing characteristics which underlie the behaviour of all organisms, humans very much included. An appreciation of this requires drawing together threads from a variety of lines of enquiry, and is facilitated by a perspective which treats both behaviour and the nervous system as nested sets of interacting information-processing boxes each with a more or less clearly defined inputs and outputs. Briefly put, the Harvard Law provides the basis for a desirable and productive fusion of scientific and folk perspectives on the determinants of behaviour, one which acknowledges that some degree of unpredictability is not only inevitable but desirable.

Grobstein, 1994

In categorizing the nervous system as similar to a 'chaotic system' he goes on to say: 'It is now well recognized that the behaviour of even relatively simple systems involving small numbers of interacting non-linear elements (such as neurones) can be highly unpredictable. ... An additional noteworthy feature of chaotic systems is a "strong dependence upon initial conditions". Very small changes in the starting conditions can lead to very large differences in subsequent behaviour.'

This idea of one input leading to a possibly unpredictable output(s) is key to the osteopathic interpretation of neural function.

Connectionist models

While many commentators might not describe the nervous system as chaotically as Grobstein, most modellers of neural function have turned from serial systems to parallel distributed models, which they call **connectionist models**. The following quote illustrates that there is a high degree of potential variability within such systems, which could, until we understand the interconnections more completely, lead to a picture of chaos and confusion:

Connectionist models use interconnected computational elements that, like neural circuits, process information simultaneously and in parallel. The preliminary insights that have emerged from such models are consistent with physiological studies, and illustrate that individual elements in the model do not transmit large amounts of information. It is the connections between the many components, which make complex information processing possible. Individual neurones can carry out important computations because they are wired together in organized and different ways. It is the distinctiveness of the wiring and the ability to modify this wiring through learning that create a brain in which relatively stereotyped units can endow us with individuality.

Kandel *et al.*, 1991, p. 32

One osteopathic interpretation of this is that, although adaptation has been built into our nervous systems – to our advantage – depending on what structural changes occur (e.g. within the synapses) this adaptation may be capable of compromising function rather than aiding it. It is not so much that the wiring goes wrong, *per se* – it is that continued adaptability might lead to output that is not as effective at regulating homeostasis and function as it might be.

To appreciate the overall role that neural connections and their interactions can have in health and disease, the general arrangement and the interconnections between different parts of the nervous system need first to be reviewed.

DEDICATED FIBRE SYSTEMS, TOPOGRAPHY AND INTERCONNECTIONS BETWEEN PARTS

On the whole, different parts of the body use dedicated sections of the nervous system for their information processing. Also, different types of information (particularly sensory information) use dedicated fibre types. Such topography and fibre dedication holds true within the peripheral nervous system and the spinal cord. Topographical arrangements are also important in higher structures such as the cerebellum and thalamus. However, as one gets further and further into the brain, so to speak, the idea of having dedicated cells in discrete groups becomes a little less valid. In the cortex, for example, large slabs/layers of neural tissue, which contain areas of nerve cells relating to a number of particular functions, do not just use discrete one-to-one contacts but instead also rely on flooding that whole slab of brain with neurotransmitter (with each layer of the slab being activated by a different family of transmitters). This leads to a lot of general engagement of neural areas, compared to the cord (where signals activate much smaller areas of neural tissue in comparison).

The central nervous system has many interconnections between these dedicated systems. They do not 'stand alone' but are interlinked with an extensive system of interneurone pools that allow many levels of activity and function to be smoothly integrated and adapted to needs as they arise.

The fact that there are so many interconnections means that signals in one part of the system are relayed to many other areas, and one could consider that the nervous system is continuously 'aware' of activity in all parts, adjusting the whole network depending on the summation of inputs that originate in the discrete sections.

NEURAL INTERCONNECTIONS

There are a whole variety of normally operating interconnections and reflex loops, which include:

- **somato-somatic**: the neural control of motion; involving sensation, integration and activation;
- **somato-emotional**: associative correlation concerning somatic events and emotional interpretation and memory;
- **viscero-visceral**: autonomic nervous system adjustment and regulation of function of the enteric nervous system (based on sensory feedback from the gut, for example), and within other visceral systems;
- **viscero-somatic**: protective requirements, e.g. splinting; integrated functioning between visceral and somatic structures, as in respiration and the function of the pelvic floor muscles and bladder;
- **somato-visceral**: feedback from the somatic structures, e.g. muscles, to the endocrine

and visceral areas of the brain, to trigger an autonomic nervous system response to adjust visceral function in tune with somatic demands;

- **viscero-emotional**: pain and sensations of dysfunction triggering emotive responses.

These reflex loops do not act in isolation during normal function, nor in cases of dysfunction or trauma, as the following demonstrates.

CLINICAL HYPOTHESIS: CONCERNING THE INTERCONNECTIONS BETWEEN PARTS

A single event or incidence (such as pain signals arising from a damaged tissue) can have widespread influence through the rest of the nervous system and body (Wallace, 1992; Lund *et al.*, 1991)and the consequences of the reaction to that event can cascade through many levels of function, adaptation and activity.

Pain associated with movement will trigger a variety of things:

- **changes in relative muscle action**, with some muscles now being inhibited or excited more than before, or coordinated into a different pattern of action and reaction;
- **emotional associations**: the person develops fear if that part is moved;
- **autonomic associations**: the visceral system responds to give a fear-fight-or-flight type of response (the general adaptive syndrome), which affects heart rate, sweating and other bodily functions).

Consequence of altered muscle patterning

Changes in locomotor control leads to altered biomechanical arrangements and altered responses to movement commands from the brain.

Descending control from the cortex to the ventral horn of the cord is altered, and this affects the level of activity in the interneurone pool at a segmental level. This leads to altered activation of cord patterns (see also Consequences of autonomic association, below).

Now, other areas of the body move differently, and this might induce stress, strain or fatigue in those areas if the pattern is not re-adapted (see also Neurotrophic consequences, below).

Consequences of emotional association

Whereas, before the change, the person was not afraid of having that body part touched or moved, now they are.

The person will react with inappropriate emotions if that part is moved, so they avoid engaging it, which leads to stiffness, lack of sensory feedback from this area to the cortex and a lack of cortical awareness (we mentioned this in Chapter 3).

If someone moves that part of the body for the person, the emotional response may well be re-triggered.

Consequences of autonomic association

If the change in pattern persists for a long time, then the body's physiological processes may be kept at an 'artificial' or adapted level. This means that the homeostatic mechanisms may not be as flexible as before, and that long-standing changes in activity may lead to stress through the rest of the body.

Long-term cortisone release consequent to ongoing stress (from chronic pain, for example, or from being in a long-standing 'emotional nightmare' such as a bad marriage, a poor work situation or unemployment) will lead to changes throughout the body, such as premature ageing of tissues and increasingly poor immune response.

The extent of the change and the number of areas involved depend on the level of the original stimulus, how frequently it is repeated and over how long a time period.

Clinical application of the theory

Clinically then, even though the tissue injury might have been to a small, discrete area, it is possible to observe changes throughout the mind/body interaction. Osteopaths learn to assess the palpatory state of the tissues to identify what might be the nature of the tissue reaction. They consider the possible underlying factor within the tissues that maintains their reaction to the injury. In other words they look to see if muscle guarding is protective of an injury or 'protective' of some emotional association. They look to see if the tissue trophism has changed and consider whether this is because of local factors or due to general changes in physiology, for example.

Osteopaths perceive that each different physiological, emotional and somatic outcome (from the processing of pain signals through the integrated connections of the central nervous system) will have a different palpatory outcome for the tissues involved. This type of palpatory assessment forms part of the evaluation criteria within case management.

NEURAL COMMUNICATION

The above example showed some levels of integrated function and connection within the central nervous system. This integration is mediated through the traditionally described divisions of the nervous system:

- the neuromusculoskeletal system;
- the neurovisceral system (the autonomic nervous system);
- the neuroemotional (limbic) system;
- the neuroendocrine–immune system.

They are artificial divisions of the nervous system, but they are still useful when building up a picture of integration.

Note: The concept of communication between parts (visceral, mechanical and emotional) was introduced in earlier chapters when the concept of integrated function was discussed as a primary element to the osteopathic perspective on health and disease. Osteopaths assume that these relationships are not unidirectional, and that problems in the locomotor system could affect visceral function, alter activity in other aspects of the locomotor system or affect emotional or immune responses. As we discuss the arrangement of the nervous system throughout this chapter, we should see that its myriad

links allow this as a theoretical possibility (although researched clinical evidence of this hypothesis is still lacking). However, osteopathic tradition holds that the nervous system can mediate many interesting and clinically important inter-relations that reflect not only effective communication patterns but also ones where communication has become distorted, leading to adapted function that is not physiologically beneficial.

In order to appreciate these ideas further, it is necessary to explore the discrete systems and examine how they might be related.

THE NEUROMUSCULOSKELETAL SYSTEM – SOMATO-SOMATIC REFLEXES

Coordination of movement

Maintaining such things as an appropriate centre of gravity, and a stable platform to ensure effective upper limb and head movement while being able to walk at the same time, clearly demands a high level of coordination. This control is performed through the nervous system.

The neural control of movement is made up of several parts:

- sensing body movement;
- monitoring changes of position and tone;
- interpreting this with the requirements for either static posture or movement;
- initiating signals to effect a response in the motor system;
- effecting a motor action.

Afferent mechanisms

For voluntary movements to be well timed and accurate, they require coordinated tactile, visual and proprioceptive information about the movement in progress. Locomotion should be a stable cycle generated by the sensory links between the musculoskeletal system, the neural system and the environment (Winter *et al.*, 1990). The sensory systems provide an internal representation of the outside world. A major function of this representation is to extract the information necessary to guide the movements that make up our behavioural repertoire.

Littlejohn, the founder of the first school of osteopathy in Britain, felt that all problems started on the sensory side of this whole equation: without adequate sensation, ongoing function is limited and poorly controlled. (This idea will be returned to later.)

Voluntary movement thus depends upon integration of the motor and sensory systems. Sensory information is necessary for the control of movement and is used to correct errors through feedback and feed-forward mechanisms (McCloskey and Prochazka, 1994; Kingham, 1994; Sanes and Shadmehr, 1995; Kalaska, 1994). Any problem or confusion within the sensory side may affect the guidance systems for movement, leading to inefficient muscular activity for the task required.

There are many types of proprioceptor and mechanoreceptor making up the sensory monitors that provide this feedback (Proske *et al.*, 1988) – some of which are listed below.

Aside: Many of these are embedded in the connective tissue surrounding the muscles, and it is thought within osteopathy that alteration in connective tissue state may interfere with this feedback mechanism. The effects of inflammation on connective tissue state (as discussed in the following chapter) may lead to distortion of some of these proprioceptors – hence affecting ongoing feedback.

Efferent mechanisms

In contrast to the sensory (afferent) systems, which transform physical energy into neural information, the motor systems transform neural energy into physical energy by issuing commands that are transmitted by the brain stem and spinal cord to skeletal muscle. The muscles translate this neural information into a contractile force that produces movement.

Movement integration

Most behavioural acts involve all three major functional systems of the brain (the sensory,

motor and motivational systems). Adjustment to an altered pattern of movement may require adaptation at many levels. Whereas the sensory and motor systems are important in performing a movement (such as catching a ball) the stimulus to initiate and complete the behaviour is produced by the motivational system. The motivational or limbic system modulates that motor output to skeletal muscles (Lewthwaite, 1990) and also coordinates the activities of the somatic and autonomic nervous systems.

Motor neurones in the spinal cord are subject to afferent input and descending control. The cerebellum and the basal ganglia have an important role in motor integration: they receive sensory input and modulate the timing and trajectory of movements. These structures are essential for accurately aimed and smoothly executed movements (Forssberg and Hirschfeld, 1994; Vaughan *et al.*, 1996). The central nervous system is arranged so that, in response to a desire for movement, higher centres will send 'down' a set of signals to the spinal cord that initiates activity not in single muscles but in groups of muscles, such that 'whole limb' patterns of movement emerge. Such muscle patterning may be complex, and involve bilateral and other body area muscle groups (Masson *et al.*, 1991).

'Patterns' of movement are laid down in the central nervous system, so that each time you want to move, you don't have to literally think of everything.

Typically, only the initiation and the termination of the sequence are voluntary. Once initiated, the sequence of relatively stereotyped, repetitive movements may continue almost automatically in reflex-like fashion. As we grow, our nervous systems 'learn' – i.e. they are not hard-wired when we are born but develop consequent to the demands we place upon them. Thus the exact arrangement of the patterns of movement labelled, for example, 'walking' may be subtly different for each person (Dietz *et al.*, 1991; Nielsen and Kagamihara, 1992). Each person walks in a slightly different way – which may be due to a short leg, uneven shoes or how they

Course of afferent fibers   Location of motor nuclei

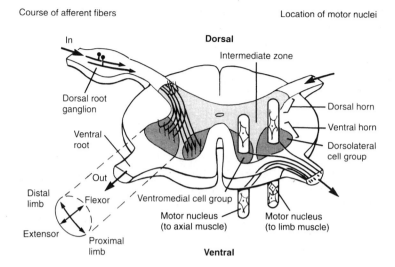

Figure 4.1

The motor nuclei of the spinal cord are grouped functionally in distinct medial and lateral positions. The medial group contains the motor neurones innervating axial muscles of the neck and back. Within the lateral group, the most medial motor neurones innervate distal muscles. Ventrally located motor neurones innervate extensors while dorsal ones innervate flexors. (Reproduced with the permission of Appleton & Large from Principles of Neural Science, 3rd edn, Kandel et al., 1991.)

developed their walking pattern – through mimicry of their parents, for example.

This reinforces the idea that these patterns are not 'hard wired' and may be mutable, a point we will discuss later on.

The complex links between different body parts involved with movement tasks will be extensively explored in subsequent chapters. These are designed to highlight the way different body parts and areas are intercoordinated and explain why dysfunction of one part can lead to dysfunction in another part.

This point is made as osteopaths feel that, to resolve locomotor and biomechanical problems, many areas of the body must be explored in order to achieve long-lasting symptom relief.

This 'global view' of integrated biomechanics (and how musculoskeletal function is integrated with emotional states, for example) is one of the major differences between osteopathic practice and that of many of the other manipulative professions.

Topography in the motor-sensory system

There are medial and lateral motor systems, dealing with the axial skeletal muscles and proximal limb muscles, and the distant limb muscles,

respectively. This is illustrated at a spinal cord level in Figure 4.1.

Motor-sensory components (which bring information about the activity and position of the various structures of the medial and lateral muscle groups/joints) are also split into two groupings:

- **A-afferent**, involving:
  - *the dorsal columns* (dealing with position sense, vibratory sense, two-point discrimination, stereognosis and discriminative touch) via group II (Aß) fibres triggered by pacinian, Meissner and Ruffini receptors;
  - *the spinocerebellar tracts* (dealing with position sense and vibratory sense) via group I (Aα) fibres triggered by muscle spindles and Golgi tendon organs;
- **B-afferent**, involving *the anterolateral system* (dealing with crude touch, pain and thermal sense) via group III and IV (Aδ) fibres and C-fibres, from free/naked nerve endings.

A-afferent systems and B-afferent systems do not remain isolated: they connect at a spinal cord level in the dorsal horn.

Clinical application: gating of pain – A-afferents gate the B-afferent systems

This concept is used in therapeutic manipulation: perform the type of articulation that would normally trigger A-afferent activity (such as rhythmic, gentle articulation of the joint and gentle stretch of the muscles) and this should damp down the level of firing at an interneurone level that is caused by pain signals travelling via the B-afferent system. The pain signals will have triggered a response in the muscles local to the injured part, and will be causing muscle spasm, 'splinting' and reduced joint mobility.

Within the cord, and up through such structures as the thalamus to other higher centres, the medial and lateral motor group cells (axial and lateral muscles respectively) are grouped discretely in long columns. Thus there is a topographical set-up in the thalamus and other higher centres mimicking that within the cord. This means that arm signals can pass very quickly through the thalamus to where the cortex thinks about arm activity, and leg symptoms go to the leg area. However, legs and arms need to communicate, which means that there must be interconnections at some level. As we shall discuss in Chapter 6, this can occur in the spinal cord through the propriospinal system (Mazevet and Pierrot-Deseilligny, 1994) and also by virtue of the fact that there are large numbers of interneurones interconnecting the cell groups of the medial and lateral motor systems throughout the whole central nervous system.

Patterns

As groups of either limb muscles or axial muscles are arranged in close proximity, this makes interconnections between them easy. This close placement between the groups of topographically arranged cells for the medial and lateral motor systems means that the central nervous system can easily control several groups of muscles in an integrated manner, so that, during the desired activity, some muscles are inhibited and some are excited, for example (Crone, 1993).

Patterns are somewhat predetermined as one develops: interneuronal connections are already formed between various muscles groups when we are born. But, as stated earlier, these are then refined as one learns activities (Jones, 1990). Pattern development occurs not only through the spinal cord cell groups but also in higher centres and in the cortex, where emotions, cognition and autonomic functions can be linked into the patterning associations of the muscle groups.

Pattern generation is a sensory driven system
Sensory feedback loops operate continuously (through the motor-sensory structures/pathways listed above) so that the body can refine movement (Young and Marteniuk, 1995; Marder and Calabrese, 1996). If one part is moved a lot, then this triggers extra sensory information, leading to increased synaptic activity and transmitter release, and dendritic formation (throughout the interneurone pool and the cortex, for example), leading to increased cortical representation of various muscles/body parts (Hess and Donoghue, 1994) and increased connections between, say, emotions and autonomic functions, and movement centres.

Plasticity in neural mechanisms allows adaptation of motor patterns
Osteopaths would posit that 're-learning'/adaptation of motor patterns subsequent to demand is a normal function of the neural control of motor activity, but one that might lead to problems.

Littlejohn was quoted earlier as saying that he felt all problems started on the sensory side of the nervous system, and it seems that sensory input is capable of driving change.

The fact that use or disuse of a sensory organ (for example by specific training and execution of repetitive tasks) can lead to significant changes in its area of representation in the developing cortex (Jones, 1990) is intriguing and calls for further investigations aimed at understanding the functional significance and the mechanisms underlying these changes.

But how changeable are these motor patterns? There is evidence that patterns can be changed in response to a variety of factors, including neural injury (and the subsequent altered use; Jankovic, 1994). Could less 'serious' changes such as alteration of tone in one muscle lead to adaptation of patterning responses and subsequent changes in activity and tone in other muscles?

This is a proposition that osteopaths are much interested in.

Sensory barriers to neural communication

Alteration in tone

As appropriate tone and tension is necessary for the structure to be stable, any condition that alters the tone of the muscles leads to instability in the structure during activity. Faults can appear at any level of the above system of control – on the sensory side, the integrative side or the motor side.

There are many pathological processes affecting the neural control of movement (such as cerebrovascular accident, myasthenia gravis, multiple sclerosis, traumatic denervation, Parkinson's disease and many others). These will not be analysed in this book; but what is considered are other reasons for muscle action to be inappropriate or inefficient. These 'less serious' conditions can be placed under the umbrella term of **functional disorders**.

'Functional' implies that the underlying neural tissue is 'normal' but that the information being processed requires adaptation of existing patterns. If one muscle is being active, then it may be necessary for another to be less active or have its action 'graded' to allow the first muscle to perform its activity properly (Koceja and Kamen, 1991). This is standard agonist/antagonist/synergist function (McCollum, 1993). Many muscles are multifunctional – they are required to act in many different situations (Collins, 1995). Hence, after each activity, any muscle must be able to return to some sort of 'neutral' so that it is in the best state to respond to the 'next demand'. This

may not be possible if the muscle has been previously injured, for example. Its length may now be somewhat altered as a result of scarring, and so the natural relationships between it and its fellows are distorted. This may mean that its fellows are 'maintained' in an altered state to ensure that, overall, the body is balanced and most of the rest of its movements can occur as effectively as possible (given the constraints imposed by the injury). Its fellow muscles may be kept at a higher tone, or a lower tone, and may thereafter be less efficient in their ongoing control of joint movement (Collins, 1995; Jankovic, 1994).

The neural mechanisms behind such concepts have been studied in relation to inflammation and nociception, and these should be briefly reviewed to set the stage for this discussion.

Factors required for 'confusion' in neural processing to be a potential outcome

Under normal circumstances, neural processing is well coordinated and appropriate, but such factors as nociception and inflammation may lead to changes in the dorsal horn of the spinal cord (Schaible and Schmidt, 1985; Jeftinija and Urban, 1994; Hanesch et al., 1993) and may involve the long-term plastic changes (potentiation and depression) that we discussed earlier, or affect the receptive field properties of spinal neurones, for example (Grubb et al., 1993; Yaksh, 1993).

If the dorsal horn activity is altered and becomes 'facilitated' then this means that the interneurone pool will react by processing this 'heightened' information throughout the rest of that cord segment and beyond. The cord segment could also become habituated (depressed) and sensitized (another way of saying 'facilitated'; Randic et al., 1993).

This may have a variety of effects. By processing information 'incorrectly' to the ventral horn cells that are going to produce efferent signals to direct a variety of responses to segmentally related tissues, the segmental output may not be finely tuned to the original needs of the tissue that were communicated on the afferent side (to the dorsal horn). For example, inflamed joints may lead to altered segmental activity that changes levels of muscular activity via the efferent output of that cord segment (He *et al.*, 1988; Schaible and Grubb, 1993). Also, it seems that the level of altered response may depend upon the time-course of the original nociceptive/inflammatory event (Schaible and Schmidt, 1988) and that ongoing nociceptive input is not necessary to maintain the altered central processing of such information (Baron and Maier, 1995).

This altered processing may also affect signals passing to higher centres, as ascending signals forming that cord segment may also be adapted as a consequence (Schaible *et al.*, 1987).

Changes on the descending/efferent side

It seems that events such as inflammation and nociception can also lead to eventual adaptation in descending pathways to the ventral horn, leading to altered efferent activity (Cervero *et al.*, 1991; Schaible *et al.*, 1991).

These comments indicate that there are consequences for normal integrated function within neural pathways concerned with/confined to somatic structures when activity in those pathways is altered by nociceptive or inflammatory events.

Osteopaths would also posit that proprioceptive pathways are also involved in the above scenario, but these have not been investigated to the same extent.

Soft tissue 'damage' leading to sensory barriers

Disuse, scarring, trauma to the muscles and ligaments (Lentell *et al.*, 1995), contraction and stiffness in the connective tissues surrounding the muscles and the presence of oedema and inflammation (associated with the above) are all proposed as factors able to compromise sensory feedback by 'bombarding' the afferent mechanisms with information/altered feedback. This is thought to give altered levels of sensory stimulus, leading to such states within the nervous system as facilitation, sensitization, habituation, long-term potentiation and long-term depression, meaning that ongoing processing of information to higher centres is altered (Malenka, 1994).

This may lead to demand for change in existing patterns of action to accommodate the 'new'/'altered' state of the muscles and tissues involved in that situation. If the pattern is changed, the subsequent efferent commands are altered and the body movement will be subtly different as a result (Lewit, 1987).

Clinically, this might mean that the new patterns place slight strain and altered dynamics through the locomotor system, potentially leading to symptoms.

In osteopathic parlance, a good example of this would be the slight change in knee mechanics that occurs after a bad sprain to the ankle joint and surrounding muscular/ligamentous structures. Following the injury there may be laxity in the ankle joint, with slightly abnormal/accessory movements occurring within the joint on subsequent movements. There may be areas of fibrosis and scarring within the soft tissue structure of the joint, further 'adapting' or 'constraining' the function of the joint. This 'new' movement at the ankle means that the tibia and/or fibula may now behave differently during normal movements (walking for example), with their muscles having to be coordinated slightly differently from before, so placing different biomechanical strain at the level of the knee compared to before.

If the altered movement required at the knee now makes it operate (even slightly) outside the limits of its normal functioning range, the knee itself may then become 'distressed' mechanically and suffer some degree of strain, especially if the altered dynamic persists over time. The aberration of movement may not need to be too great in fact, as repetition of a minor distortion of movement may be sufficient to distress the joint. ('Repetitive strain injury' as an entity is now well recognized ergonomically, especially in such situations as the wrist and computer keyboard usage.) This new strain now becomes a potential focus for adaptation in its own right. One could go on, observing the progressive effects of adaptation throughout the whole structure in this way:

The pelvis is likely to become unbalanced, leading to a pelvic tilt of some sort. Then, the whole trunk and upper limb orientation must be coordinated around this 'new sacral base inclination' so that the most effective gait pattern can be re-established.

In this new pattern, there may be different moments of force and amplitude of movement, and different usage of all of the differing components of the rib cage and upper limb. There may also be a demand for differing movement of the intervertebral segments of the upper thoracic spine. Generally speaking, this is a common area of the spine in which to find immobility even without such a chain of events as we have been describing. To place additional movement requirements through this area by asking it to compensate for altered movement elsewhere usually results in a degree of stress and strain to the relevant joint structures. Thus the altered movement patterns can spread through the thorax into the shoulder girdle and upper limb, and eventually through to the head and neck, where a complex set of proprioceptive mechanisms (including the balance mechanisms of the inner ear) ensures that overall postural stability is re-established.

Indeed, when you consider the number of sprains, strains and other irritations that may occur throughout life, one can imagine that each person comes to 'inhabit' a very individual structure indeed, as these each place their own demands for adaptation of the structure and its biomechanics, which must all somehow be balanced out as effectively as possible!

Relationship to practice and clinical decision-making

The clinical outcome of this would be that eventually, a person might present with pain and dysfunction at one site, the cervical spine for example, with no signs of direct injury. The altered postural and locomotor activity that has established the cervical spine distress needs to be assessed, and might be found at a distant site, such as the ankle. This means that one has two choices for treatment: the local changes in the cervical spine soft tissues or those within the lower limb that set off the chain of reactions that led to the cervical distress in the first place. Working on the cervical spine would be working on the adaptations to the more 'primary' injury and would not remove the potential for the symptoms recurring at some point in the future (although the person would gain short-term relief from their symptoms). Working on the more 'primary' injury, the ankle, would remove the 'predisposing' or 'maintaining' factors to the postural and locomotor balance of that person and would resolve the strain at the cervical spine more effectively and over a longer period of time than otherwise. The person should then be left with a much reduced chance of developing the cervical symptoms than if the practitioner had worked only within the cervical spine itself.

As stated, 'patterning' and the inter-relatedness of parts is a major subject of subsequent chapters.

'Effector' (motor) barriers to neural communication

Problems on the efferent side

These should not be forgotten, as they too can interfere with the effective control of locomotion.

Peripheral neuropathy, for example from compression or from trauma, could mean that signals to the motor units become distorted, leading to inappropriate muscle activity, or even no activity if there is sufficient nerve damage. Also, if the muscle is scarred or damaged in some way, it may not be able to act on information, even if this is normal!

Note: The subject of peripheral neuropathy and the factors that can lead to its production are explored in Chapter 9.

Connective tissue barriers

Connective tissue consequences and potential relevance for ongoing function

Immobility/altered movement means that the connective tissue sheaths of the muscles, and the capsular and ligamentous components of the body, will now be adapted to this altered movement pattern. This can have consequences on the efferent side, as it might affect muscle function. The connective tissue itself will change and remodel according to altered movement patterns, with fibroblasts laying down collagen in new directions, for example. The subsequent connective tissue 'stiffening' that this leads to will then act as a restraint to further motion, as this can bind muscle fibres together and reduce contractile efficiency. This may well affect proprioceptive feedback, and creates a connective tissue component to biomechanical inefficiency, which now also needs to be overcome if movement patterns and function are to return to normal. Stretching and articulation will help to release connective tissue tension so that active contraction by the person becomes more possible.

Summary of this section

The aims of this section were to illustrate the neural control of movement, how problems might arise within those control mechanisms and what might be the potential clinical outcomes. There are other discrete systems, which we will now continue to discuss.

THE NEUROVISCERAL SYSTEM (THE AUTONOMIC NERVOUS SYSTEM) – VISCERO-VISCERAL, VISCERO-SOMATIC AND SOMATO-VISCERAL REFLEXES

The neurovisceral system is unique in that one of its components, the digestive tract, has its own nervous system, the enteric nervous system, which can function to a degree without reference to the rest of the central nervous system. The central nervous system, via the autonomic nervous system, serves to adapt gut function to the needs of the whole individual in given circumstances and under different situations.

The general arrangement of the autonomic nervous system is shown in Figure 4.2.

The **sympathetic nervous system (SNS)** innervates:

- fascia/connective tissue;
- smooth muscle of the vasculature throughout the body;
- smooth muscle of hair follicles;
- secretory cells in the sweat glands of the skin;
- smooth muscle of the organs;
- cardiac muscle;
- nodal tissue;
- glandular organs of the thoracic, abdominal, pelvic and perineal viscera.

The **parasympathetic nervous system (PSNS)** innervates visceral organs and blood vessels in the following areas:

- head and neck;
- thorax;
- abdomen;
- pelvis.

Together, the divisions of the autonomic nervous system then influence the activity of:

- vasculature and fascia;
- organs of the head;
- organs of the neck;
- organs of the thoracoabdomino-pelvic cavity;
- spleen;
- thymus;
- bone marrow;
- lymph nodes.

Note: All the discussion of the functions of connective tissue and the extracellular matrix (ECM) within the preceding chapter (and their interactions with blood flow, immunity and cell function) should now be considered as a more complex dynamic as the actions of the ECM itself can sometimes be regulated by neural activity.

The autonomic nervous system (ANS) is not just an efferent system. There are many afferent fibres as well (often called the visceral afferent system). This means that there is a lot of two-way neural communication possible between the divisions of the autonomic nervous system, and one should consider that they work in concert to con-

Figure 4.2

General organization of the autonomic nervous system. CNS = central nervous system; PNS = peripheral nervous system. (Redrawn with permission from American Osteopathic Association, Foundations for Osteopathic Medicine, Lippincott Williams & Wilkins 1997.)

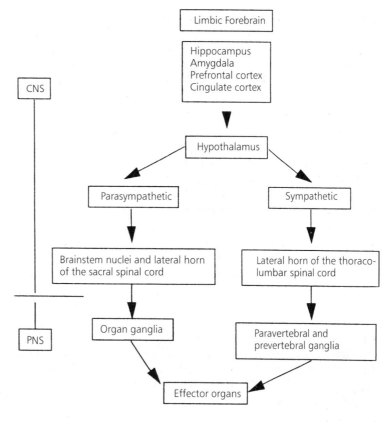

trol function in their respective target tissues. (It is interesting to note, though, that only the sympathetic division of the ANS generally modulates somatic tissues.)

The ANS is interesting for osteopaths in that not only does it play a role in regulating the internal environment of the body but it has many links with the musculoskeletal system, which we will discuss in a moment. It is also interesting in that the SNS innervates all the vasculature within the body: altering levels of activity within the SNS will alter levels of vessel tone and vasomotion. This can have corollaries for tissue perfusion, and hence function, and is one of the factors that explains the effects that sympathetic activity can have for regulation of the internal environment of the body.

Additionally, the ANS is interesting for osteopaths as they perceive that many disease processes within the body may arise through a disturbance in the balance and integration of func-

tion between the SNS and the PSNS. In terms of treatment for and intervention in a variety of circulatory and visceral diseases/dysfunction, though, the ANS is mainly interesting in so far as osteopaths can affect its activity through manipulating/mobilizing various soft tissue components of the body. For example, irritation within the small intestine might be affecting visceral afferent activity – leading to a general adaptation of intestinal activity. This could be altered by massaging the intestinal wall, reducing spasm and irritation and 'normalizing' afferent input/feedback. This idea is not particularly novel.

However, osteopaths also postulate that, by massaging somatic structures that are segmentally related to the relevant section of the intestine, this too will adapt visceral neural activity and function. This idea would seem incredible to many. There may be some theoretical foundation for this deeply held concept within osteopathy, though, and for this reason one needs to consider the links between the visceral and somatic nervous systems.

Leaving aside for a moment the question of exactly how manual procedures applied to the musculoskeletal system may be able to influence visceral nervous activity, the general concept within osteopathic philosophy is that working on various parts of the body will affect the activity of the autonomic nervous system.

When osteopaths consider disease processes and dysfunctions within the body they look at what is occurring within the autonomic nervous system and try to see if there is too much SNS activity, or too much PSNS activity, for example.

In sinusitis, for instance, is there too much mucus production? In intestinal problems is there too little or too much intestinal motility (peristalsis)? In circulatory disorders, is there too much vasoconstriction in the somatic periphery, or is there too much within the intestinal vascular bed, which is affecting the overall control and regulation of blood volume? In cases of headache, is there a local vasoconstriction leading to ischaemic pain? In reproductive system function, is there too little glandular activity, or inappropriate peristaltic activity within the fallopian tubes? Or, is there imbalance in the endocrine system, with one organ either working too much or too little? Or is there sufficient lymphatic drainage and motility within a particular region to aid immunity and tissue health? And so on.

In this type of analysis, one is not looking solely for recognized pathological processes but exploring situations where there is seemingly 'no obvious cause' for the dysfunction. Osteopaths would consider a situation where the autonomic control of an organ/system has become distorted as constituting a category of 'disease' in its own right, and one which could also complicate the existence of 'traditional' disease processes.

So, osteopaths consider that there are ANS components to many disease processes/pathophysiological conditions. They consider that normalizing the autonomic function would help those disease processes diminish and help the body redress the pathophysiological conditions within the tissues. They consider that drugs and surgery may not be the only ways to help this process, and that these interventions may be aided by regulating the autonomic function by other means (physical manipulations of some sort).

When osteopaths reflect on disease processes, these are some of the things that they consider, and when they look at the functions of the ANS, they try to assess whether SNS or PSNS activity is inappropriate (while remembering that there might be problems on both sides, rather than just within one branch alone). They then look to the pathways/passage of fibres through the body between the central nervous system and the organ/tissue involved, and then to which parts of the spinal cord or brain regulate the particular aspect of autonomic control that is 'faltering'. They do this because they consider that there may be many points along the neural pathway that could be processing 'distorted neural feedback' and might affect either the functioning of the peripheral fibres/plexi/ganglia of the autonomic nervous system or the central processing of visceral information (within the spinal cord or brain).

There are two main ways that the musculoskeletal system might be able to interfere with autonomic function:

- by inducing some sort of peripheral neuropathy;
- by inducing some sort of 'confusion' within neural processing within the autonomic nervous system, through adapting function at the dorsal horn of the spinal cord and within higher processing centres.

Peripheral neuropathy

The stellate ganglion (inferior cervical ganglion), for example, is sited just anterior to the head of the first rib and is tightly packed in among various structures within the thoracic inlet area. Biomechanical problems of the first rib, clavicle, scalenes and so on might constrict the dynamics of this area sufficiently to irritate/compromise function within this collection of autonomic (sympathetic) fibres. All neural tissue needs effective circulation, and fascial/connective tissue torsion acting around nerve tissue may affect the vasa nervorum and so lead to local irritation and ischaemia of that neural tissue. This is the same mechanism that arises within the intervertebral foramen, which affects somatic nerve roots and leads to various clinical presentations of paraesthesia, anaesthesia and motor weakness.

The clinical presentation of autonomic 'peripheral neuropathy' is not so well explored within orthodox science, but could lead to a variety of presentations. Irritation of the stellate ganglion may lead to Horner's syndrome, for example.

Another example could be of chronic vagal stimulation by mechanical disturbance of the jugular foramen or upper cervical spine, leading to a variety of intestinal disorders (Tougas *et al.*, 1992).

Peripheral neuropathy in general is discussed in Chapter 9, as there is a fluid component in this aspect of neural dysfunction, introduced above.

'Confusion' in neural processing

The discussion earlier in the chapter concerning the factors required for confusion in neural processing to be a potential outcome is very relevant here.

That discussion related the idea that nociceptive and inflammatory signals arising in the periphery (on the afferent side) could alter cord activity and lead to sensitization, habituation, long-term potentiation or long-term depression within the interneurone pool and synaptic junctions, through to higher centres and on to the efferent side. All of this leads to adapted neural processing, so that efferent output is adapted in a way that may, in the long term, adversely affect end-tissue function.

Within the visceral system, there are many viscero-visceral reflexes operating, and we need to appreciate that, if an organ has become irritated for some reason (perhaps through infection, damage, dietary imbalance or mechanical torsion of some sort, e.g. adhesion or muscular contrac-

tion), then this gives altered afferent input to the cord and higher centres. Sufficient distortion of such signals, through prolonged inflammation and nociceptive activity, leads to adapted visceral function on the efferent side.

Examples of this might be a gastric ulcer leading to a change in stomach peristalsis, a change in cardiac or pyloric sphincter coordination, and possible reflux or 'dumping' into the duodenum. Now, the oesophagus and the small intestine will have to adapt function as a result. This leads to possible inefficiency in these parts, creating more and more symptoms as a result. Another example could be bladder inflammation leading to reflex dyssynergia within the urethra and external urethral sphincter, distorting the control of micturition, giving frequency, urgency and incontinence. Another example could be ovarian cysts leading to activity in the hypothalamic–pituitary axis, perhaps leading to thyroid or adrenal dysfunction. Another example could be lung irritation leading to altered respiratory efficiency, promoting upper respiratory tract adaptation and altered breathing patterns, perhaps leading to ear, nose and throat dysfunction.

All of these things would be mediated through the viscero-visceral reflexes within the ANS (both divisions) as they become distorted through altered afferent feedback. Altered central processing has been noted in a number of visceral hyperalgesia and other visceral disorders (Mayer and Gebhart, 1994; Giamberardino *et al.*, 1997; Mayer and Raybould, 1990). The discussion of soft tissue factors in the section on the neuromusculoskeletal system is relevant here also, as changes in smooth muscle contracture, local visceral inflammation and changes in the connective tissue components of the organs (within them, and also external to them, like the peritoneum and pleura) would all maintain and prolong this adapted afferent feedback. The aim during case management would be to reduce smooth muscle contraction and spasm, improve elasticity within the connective tissue components and reduce inflammation by promoting more effective tissue drainage and circulation through various manual manoeuvres.

These things would all constitute visceral barriers to neural communication. In 'removing' (reducing) them during treatment, one is trying to restore a more normal communication between the two aspects of the ANS – the SNS and the PSNS. Overactivity in one component could be 'compensating' for underactivity in the other, and both components would need exploration and management to effect resolution.

Somatic barriers to visceral–neural communication

Interestingly, according to osteopathic hypotheses, if the interneurone pool is sufficiently distorted, then any tissue sending a signal to that segment may 'tip the segment' into a state of confusion such that any adverse afferent signal gives a distorted efferent response. In other words, inflammation or irritation within the somatic tissues could lead to an adapted visceral efferent signal (or *vice versa*). This constitutes a somato-visceral reflex, or a viscero-somatic reflex, giving visceral barriers to somatic function and somatic barriers to visceral function.

This novel concept is discussed in more detail in the following section.

Visceral and somatic (musculoskeletal) inter-relations

It seems that there is much evidence for a variety of interactions between somatic and visceral systems (Alarcon and Cervero, 1990).

The most classically recognized clinical syndrome arising out of this interconnection is the phenomenon of referred pain: where the dysfunction within the viscera is projected on to a part of the somatic body, through segmentally based neurological links. This is not the only link/effect that osteopaths consider.

In the preceding chapter, some discussion was made of the reasons why visceral and somatic components of the nervous system must communicate. In reviewing the connections between the visceral and somatic nervous systems it may be possible to demonstrate the idea that neural communication between the two could become disturbed/distorted, with potentially clinically significant outcomes.

Convergence between visceral and somatic signals

It now appears that in most areas of the spinal cord practically every interneurone that receives inputs from a visceral nociceptor also receives input from a somatic source. It also appears that almost 80% of interneurones that receive inputs from somatic structures also receive visceral inputs. There is at present no evidence for any ascending pathways that transmit only visceral sensory signals from the spinal cord to the brain.

American Osteopathic Association, 1997

An important point was made earlier: the somatic (A- and B-afferent systems) and the visceral system (b-fibre system) use the same cells in the dorsal horn to synapse on to in order to pass their information to higher centres (Hobbs *et al.*, 1992).

For example, the two systems use wide-dynamic range cells that sit in the interneurone pool (in particular laminae) of the spinal cord where both systems are trying to make contact. (Laminae I, V, VI and VII contain both visceral and somatic cells and laminae I and V have a considerable overlap of visceral and somatic inputs; De Groat, 1994.) The wide dynamic cell has to interpret the origin of the signals so that it can pass on the information appropriately. Figure 4.3 shows the laminae of the dorsal horn and the termination of somatic and visceral afferents. Figure 4.4 shows the termination of nociceptive neurones into the laminae and Figure 4.5 shows the convergence of visceral and somatic input to the dorsal horn.

The interpretation of the origin of the signal is clearly vital if appropriate processing of the information is to occur, so giving an appropriate response.

Remember that we are discussing sensitization and habituation, long-term potentiation and

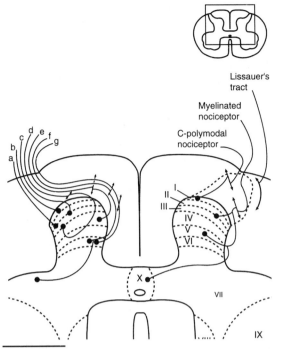

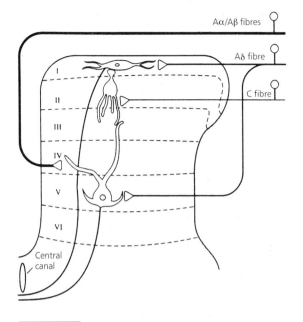

Figure 4.3

Terminal patterns of primary afferent collaterals in transverse plane of spinal cord. **Left**. a = g represent primary afferent terminations of axons not associated with nociception. The arrows indicate that the parent axon bifurcates and ascends and descends the spinal cord for one to seven segments and gives off collaterals along this course.
Right. Nociceptor afferents from both somatic and visceral structures. Laminae are labelled on the right and outlined by dotted lines. (Reproduced with the permission of S. Karger AG from The Initial Processing of Pain and Its Descending Control, Light, 1992 in American Osteopathic Association, 1997.)

Figure 4.4

The afferent fibres of nociceptors terminate on projection neurones in the dorsal horn of the spinal cord. Projection neurones in lamina I receive direct input from myelinated (Aδ fibre) nociceptors and indirect input from unmyelinated (C-fibre) nociceptors via stalk cell interneurones in lamina II. Lamina V neurones are predominantly of the wide dynamic range type. They receive low-threshold input from large-diameter myelinated fibres (Aα) of mechanoreceptors as well as both direct and indirect input from nociceptive afferents (Aδ and C). In this figure the lamina V neurone sends a dendrite up through lamina IV, where it is contacted by the terminal of an Aα primary afferent. A lamina V cell dendrite in lamina III is contacted by the axon terminal of a lamina II interneurone. (Reproduced with permission from American Osteopathic Association, Foundations of Osteopathic Medicine, Lippincott Williams & Wilkins, 1997, after Fields, 1987.)

long-term depression throughout the spinal cord, interneurone pool and links to higher centres. Thus there is potential for confusion on the afferent side if this signal recognition becomes faulty.

This can create segmentally mediated reactions if signalling mechanisms become altered/'confused'.

Referred pain is one example (and is illustrated in Figure 4.5). This is where the interpretation of the original signal is thought to originate from somatic tissues rather than visceral ones (Garrison, 1992).

However, the 'confusion' at this level may lead to further effects throughout the rest of the spinal cord segment, and also within higher centres, leading to other expressions of altered efferent activity than referred pain.

Inputs from each area of the body and from descending brain areas interact on a highly overlapping and integrated neural network in the spinal interneurones. Afferent inputs from any source influence both visceral or somatic structures. For normal functioning of organs, muscles, fluid motion, and other body activities, these complex and interacting networks within the nervous system must act in concert. Should one area of the neural network respond either more or less

Figure 4.5

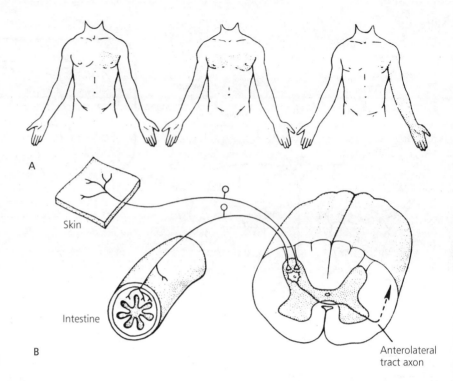

Signals from nociceptors in the viscera can be felt as pain elsewhere in the body. The source of the pain can be readily predicted from the site of referred pain. **A.** Areas of deep referred pain in myocardial infarction and angina. (Reproduced with permission from Teodori and Galletti, 1962.) **B.** Convergence of visceral and somatic afferents may account for referred pain, According to this hypothesis, afferent fibres from nociceptors in the viscera and afferents from specific areas of the periphery converge on the same projection neurones in the dorsal horn. The brain has no way of knowing the actual source of the noxious stimulus and mistakenly identifies the sensation with the peripheral structure. (Reproduced with permission from American Osteopathic Association, Foundations of Osteopathic Medicine, Lippincott Williams & Wilkins, 1997, after Fields, 1987.)

than normal, the finely tuned balance necessary for normal and optimal physiological function will be disturbed. Not only must the control mechanisms from the brain be normal for proper reflex function, but the networks of neurones that make up the reflexes must also be acting normally.

American Osteopathic Association, 1997, page 145

This text carries on to say:

There are descending influences on the activity of both somatic and visceral reflex pathways. In many of the reflex loops driven by both visceral and somatic inputs, there is a strong effect of descending pathways on the long-lasting excitability of the reflex outflows. Likewise, the long-lasting descending influences can be inhibitory as well, resulting in lowered somatic or autonomic outflows.

American Osteopathic Association, 1997, page 141

Both the visceral and somatic ventral horn cells are networked together, and altering the level of activity within a segment, either from higher centres or from signals that arose from within other parts of that segment, will affect the output of both these groups of cells. Any segmental output can be either heightened or damped down.

Consequences

The implication is that, under nociceptive/inflammatory conditions in the periphery, neural processing will become adapted, and begin to affect activity in a part of the central nervous system that would not normally be influenced by a non-inflammatory signal arising from the same tissue/part.

Visceral afferent signals may provoke somatic responses (Gillette *et al.*, 1994), which, as well as giving the referred pain phenomenon mentioned earlier, also gives a response into the skeletal musculature surrounding the disturbed organ, so 'splinting' it and protecting it. The converse also seems to be possible: that somatic activity and afferent signals may provoke a visceral response. Additionally, under such circumstances regular visceral segmental reflex loops and somatic loops may not operate correctly, further compounding feedback and function.

In other words, anything that normally receives an output from that segment may become disturbed through excessive stimulation or inhibition from any structure that gives afferent signals to that segment (whether across the segment from the dorsal horn or via higher centre pathways), when that structure is somehow irritated.

The concept that somatic activity (under irritated circumstances) can cause visceral dysfunction is not recognized as a clinical entity within the orthodox systems of science and medicine, but it is a fundamental concept within osteopathic principles and practice (Van Buskirk, 1979).

Additionally, as we shall discuss in more detail later, osteopaths propose that resolving the somatic distress and improving somatic function will, through altering somatic afferent activity (though manual treatment), help to 're-set' the neural function, leading to a resolution/improvement in visceral function (American Academy of Osteopathy, 1979, 1993). This idea that manipulation of the body tissues can somehow 'drive' the activity of the cord segments and central nervous system is considered highly controversial in orthodox circles.

This discussion leads us to a concept of a functionally 'unstable' cord segment.

The 'unstable' spinal cord segment

The neural events thus described arise because, for whatever reason, the normal levels of activity within the spinal cord segment become adapted, working at either too high a level or too low a level, leading to inappropriate efferent activity of that segment. Normally, the clinical consequences of this are more obvious if the cord segment is 'facilitated' or 'heightened' in its activity, giving too much pain, contraction or vasoconstriction (and so ischaemia), for example. If the cord activity is 'damped down' and 'habituated', then, although there may be decreased sensitivity to pain and some loss of tone within muscular structures, it is less likely that the person will present saying they cannot feel pain, and so on.

Supporting evidence

Various studies have monitored the effects on visceral function of a variety of nociceptive events within somatic tissues. There has been a long history of exploration within osteopathic literature of such integration.

It is useful to remind readers here that, when originally conceived and practised (from the late 1870s onwards), osteopathy was primarily concerned with the management of medical disorders.

All the early texts of osteopathic practice are concerned with the management through physical manipulations of a wide variety of medical conditions from fevers to obstetric cases, gallbladder disease, infections and many, many others. Back pain and problems associated with musculoskeletal system dysfunction (such as various biomechanical sprains and strains and sports injuries) seemed to feature very little in these works. Throughout this century books and articles have continued to be written linking osteopathic practice with medical conditions rather than just musculoskeletal ones.

Although it is fair to say that most osteopaths seem more interested in the daily challenges of clinical practice, some research has been undertaken to appreciate the possible underlying mechanisms within such clinical interventions (although virtually no clinical trials have been carried out in a clinical setting of the outcomes of osteopathic manipulations for such medical conditions).

Irvin Korr

Much early work was done by Irvin Korr, an American physiologist who was closely allied to the osteopathic profession. His work was designed to investigate the potential therapeutic relationship between the physical manipulations that osteopaths carried out in a variety of clinical situations and for a variety of clinical conditions. Korr's work has been extensive, and he has made a fundamental contribution to the osteopathic profession.

In *The Collected Works of Irvin K. Korr* (American Academy of Osteopathy, 1979), Michael Patterson outlined the scientific contribution of Irvin Korr. Patterson discussed several of Korr's papers and reviewed many of the original concepts that Korr described:

> The second paper: 'The neural basis of the osteopathic lesion' is one of the most important of Korr's works in the profession. Here he put forth the ideas of the 'neurological lens' and 'the facilitated segment'. This major theory of regional excitation of the spinal cord serving as an abnormal area of overactivity, being driven by both external and internal sources of stimulation and focusing this activity into abnormal patterns of skeletal and visceral activity, was a conceptual breakthrough....
>
> The major impact of this work was the explicit demonstration, through various means, of the existence of abnormal activity patterns within the autonomic nervous system in apparently normal as well as diseased humans, and the correlation of some abnormal autonomic patterns with musculoskeletal abnormalities. Throughout this period, Korr wrote on the interactions which were to him evident between the autonomic and skeletal portions of the nervous system, the implications of abnormal autonomic activity for health and disease, and the long-term effects of overactivation of any portion of the nervous system on innervated structures.
>
> American Academy of Osteopathy, 1979, pages 11–12

Patterson goes on to remind us of some of Korr's other work – he was a major contributor to scientific understanding of the neurotrophic function of nerves:

> Long standing in the field of neurophysiology that the only effect of nerves on their target tissues was the release of neurotransmitter substances to excite the organ to activity....

> Using specially developed techniques and procedures, Korr found strong evidence for the delivery of protein substances transsynaptically from the hypoglossal nerve to tongue muscle fibres. This work, published in Science in 1967, was the first evidence that nerves continuously provide substances other than transmitters to the organs they innervate.
>
> American Academy of Osteopathy, 1979, pages 11–12

Some of Korr's publication titles are listed here as an indication of the extent of his work, and contribution to osteopathic understanding (American Academy of Osteopathy, 1979):

- *The Emerging Concept of the Osteopathic Lesion* (1948)
- *The Concept of Facilitation and its Origins* (1955)
- *The Somatic Approach to the Disease Process* (1951)
- *The Sympathetic Nervous System as Mediator Between the Somatic and Supportive Process* (1970)
- *The Segmental Nervous System as a Mediator and Organizer of Disease Processes* (1970)
- *The Neurotrophic Function of Nerves and their Mechanisms* (1972)
- *The Spinal Cord as Organizer of Disease Processes: Some Preliminary Perspectives* (1976).

Some of Korr's work has now been surpassed – for example he originally postulated the role of proprioceptors in the facilitated segment, whereas nowadays the influence of nociceptive stimuli is recognized to be a more accurate contributor to spinal facilitation. However, this fact does not diminish his unique contribution.

Louisa Burns

Even before Korr began his research, there was a tradition of investigation of spinal reflexes, their expression within the paraspinal tissues and the movement consequences for the interspinal articulations. During the 1930s, work was also carried out by Louisa Burns, DO, an osteopath who explored the effects of spinal restrictions on the paravertebral tissues and articular components of the spine. She noted many changes within these tissues, such as trophic change, changes in the vascular beds of the tissues, levels of tissue oedema and levels of contracture in the muscular structures. Attempts were made to explore the effects of particular spinal restrictions on various viscera.

This work represented some of the earliest attempts to correlate palpatory findings with histological changes in tissues and hence physiological consequences of altered spinal movement. Her work has inspired many osteopaths to further this study (Denslow, 1972).

Littlejohn and Fryette

These authors (Littlejohn being the founder of osteopathy in Britain and Fryette an early student (and practitioner) of osteopathy) made extensive studies into the nature of spinal restrictions, and into articular relations and interactions that could be found (principally) within the spinal and pelvic articulations of the body, contributing to the reflex phenomenon thought to be consequent to/aetiological to neural reflex disturbance between the visceral and somatic nervous systems.

Within this they looked strongly at the mechanical relations between parts of the spine and pelvis (and limbs), and this may have led to the idea that they concentrated on biomechanics rather than on the physiological effects *per se*. However, anyone who has read much of Littlejohn's work will note that he is constantly referring to the effects of such restrictions upon the physiological and homeostatic function of the internal environment of the body.

Understandably enough, because of this intense focus on articular mechanics, it seems unsurprising that osteopathy became to be seen as a system of biomechanics concerned with painful conditions of the spinal articulations and the structural integration of the body.

Denslow, Patterson and Van Buskirk

Other work has been carried out by Denslow, (American Academy of Osteopathy, 1993). Patterson (1976) and Van Buskirk (American Academy of Osteopathy, 1979), who have also made an attempt to correlate prior work and to discuss the clinical implications. (Note: Patterson has also done much work concerning the effects of facilitation within the somatic nervous system).

Denslow in particular was a pioneer in osteopathic research; his work in fact stimulated Korr's interest in the osteopathic theory of structure–function relationships and integration of function.

Much of Denslow's work was to explore the electromyographic correlates of palpatory findings, looking at such things as: the reflex activity in the spinal extensors; the central excitatory state associated with postural abnormalities; quantitative studies of chronic facilitation in human motor neurone pools; neuromuscular reflexes in response to gravity; spinal reflex thresholds as related to medical stresses and ageing; and much more (American Academy of Osteopathy, 1993).

Sato

More recent work has expanded upon these osteopathic concepts, and does indeed seem to indicate that there are significant inter-relations between the visceral and somatic nervous systems that can become active under certain circumstances (such as in the presence of inflammation). Nociceptive stimuli within the somatic field give rise to abnormal visceral activity: reflexes that may underlie the hypothetical clinical relevance of manipulation of the physical body to help resolve visceral disturbances.

Sato's publications include:

- The somatosympathetic reflexes: their physiological and clinical significance. In: *The Research Status of Spinal Manipulative Therapy* (ed. M. Goldstein), National Institutes of Health, Washington, DC, 1975, pp. 163–172.

- 'Somato-vesical reflexes in chronic spinal cats' (Sato *et al.*, 1983)
- 'Sympathetic nervous system response' (Sato and Swenson, 1984)
- 'The reflex effects of spinal somatic nerve stimulation' (Sato, 1997).

Other works by other authors include:

- 'Somatovisceral reflexes' (Cole, 1951)
- 'Somatovisceral reflexes' (Cole, 1953)
- 'Visceral and spinal components of viscero-somatic interactions' (Cervero, 1992)
- 'The somatic component in visceral disease' (Grainger, 1958).
- 'The physiological basis of the osteopathic concept of visceral disease' (Dove, 1961).

(Note: these last two are contemporary reviews of the literature of their time.)

Criticism of these works

One paper (Nansel and Szlazak, 1995) has looked at the rationale for the management of visceral disease through spinal manipulation (based upon the concept of spinal articular restrictions being an aetiological factor in those visceral diseases), and argues that the reflexes involved are not associated with true visceral disease. The authors felt that in fact the somatic structures might be referring pain to the visceral sites, thus mimicking visceral disease, and that this is what is affected through the spinal manipulation, not a resolution of true visceral disease.

However, this paper does not discuss the potential ramifications of altered neurotrophic function on the integrity of both the end-target tissue and the neural cell involved, nor any potential effect from altering cellular level structure and function of those tissues as a result. These may be important contributory factors to compromising cellular reactivity and immunity, which may help to predispose to pathological processes. Also, this paper does not discuss the potential role in disease processes of alteration of the vascular tree/capillary bed activity in the target tissue, which might become adapted through the influence of altered autonomic activity from the cord segment(s) involved. Nor does it consider the outcomes of alteration in mucosal secretions that could also be an effect of adapted efferent signals from the cord. Such concepts are important ones to reflect upon when discussing the potential role of the neural changes we have been discussing in models of tissue health and disease/pathology. Pain, albeit it an important consideration, is not the only factor to investigate when exploring these phenomena.

Exploring the potential outcomes at a segmental level in more detail

Depending on the level of activity that enters the spinal cord, segmental interneuronal activity can be altered, and segmental reflex actions, and signalling to higher centres, are distorted. In higher centres, information can also become reinforced or confused, and eventually, higher centre influence can exert a descending influence on segmental cord activity, with the whole thing summating at a few cord levels, affecting dramatically the output of that cord segment and the function of all associated peripheral tissues.

Structures receiving an efferent supply from any cord segment

These include skeletal muscle, blood vessels (in both somatic and visceral structures), sweat glands and other epithelial structures, smooth muscle and visceral/endocrine glands (according to segmental level).

So, when the segment becomes distorted, changes are created in associated tissues, such as vasoconstriction, increased tone in skeletal muscle (and consequent restriction of articular mobility), increased visceral smooth muscle contractility, altered glandular action, and so on.

Other segmental effects that are not mediated through the ventral horn (i.e. not through efferent fibres)

In addition to the effects throughout the interneurone pool, and via higher centres to the ventral horn and efferent fibres, afferent information that affects the neural processing within the dorsal horn seems to be capable of inducing anterograde signals (back down the afferent fibre) back to the tissue where the noxious stimulus originated from (Bagust *et al.*, 1993; Rees *et al.*, 1994, 1996).

Such events are called dorsal root reflexes, and represent a type of 'backfiring' of the primary afferent fibre from the spinal cord (Shefner *et al.*, 1992).

As changes in the dorsal horn start to occur, the dorsal horn triggers the sensory fibres to release various transmitters (via antegrade transport) back down to the tissues they have come from. The substances that are released are potent mediators of inflammation, and include Substance P. This release has the effect of inducing an inflammatory response in the tissues on the afferent side of the equation. This phenomenon is thought to be related to the phenomenon of neurogenic inflammation.

This so-called 'neurogenic inflammation' may be responsible for a whole variety of visceral 'diseases' and dysfunctions, ranging from asthma (Kowalski *et al.*, 1989; Ozerdem and Tozeren, 1995; Barnes, 1986; Shelhamer *et al.*, 1995) to ulcerative colitis (Keranen *et al.*, 1995), irritable bowel syndrome (Accarino *et al.*, 1995) and interstitial cystitis (Elbadawi, 1997).

Neurogenic inflammation: hypothetical consideration

If there is a problem/injury in the somatic tissues of a certain level of the spine, for example, then, if these trigger altered dorsal horn activity (because of inflammation/nociception), the dorsal horn might trigger not only somatic cell bodies to release inflammatory mediators back down the sensory nerves (to the somatic tissues) but also (via shared connections) visceral cell bodies to send inflammatory mediators down their sensory fibres, provoking an inflammatory response in the related organ – which was not required at all. There may be another 'somatic cause' for visceral inflammatory conditions.

(This mechanism may also work the other way, inducing spinal articular structures to become inflamed and irritated (as a consequence of visceral disease) when they have not been directly injured.)

Note: The concept of neurogenic switching, where a stimulus at one site can lead to inflammation at a distant site, is recognized and may contribute to the events described above. Neurogenic switching is proposed to result when a sensory impulse from a site of activation is rerouted via the central nervous system to a distant location to produce neurogenic inflammation at the second location (Meggs, 1993).

Hypothetical management

Anything that might lead to better processing of information at a cord (or higher level) might reduce these neural consequences. Normalizing tissue mobility and local tissue circulation and signalling may help to 'normalize' signals that are entering the cord, and so gradually allow the neural systems to shift back to normal. This may mean that there is a role for the manipulation of peripheral tissues in resolving neural distortion phenomena that are involved or implicated in various disease or pathophysiological conditions (in whatever tissue type or body system).

What's in a name?

This whole range of neurological factors was originally called by osteopaths the osteopathic lesion. The term 'osteopathic lesion' has now fallen out of favour: it was felt that the use of the word 'osteopathic' was not necessarily valid as it is not only osteopaths who could palpate and work with such a phenomenon. The term 'somatic dysfunction' was then coined as a description of the events involved.

However, to the author this still seems an inappropriate term as it seems to focus the attention on the somatic components of the problem, leading to a concentration of management of the somatic tissues in distress rather than, as should be the case, management of all the segmentally related tissues – visceral, fascial, vascular and somatic – that are related through their neural interconnections. Management of this phenomenon should include all factors involved.

So, at the moment, there is still no term that is satisfactory! In the text it will be referred to as 'a lesion', but this too is unsatisfactory as it implies something different to those outside the profession.

In historical reflection the state of the spinal cord segment involved in this phenomenon was thought to be 'facilitated', as the changes seemed to create a state of heightened activity within that segment, so that whatever tissue received a signal/output from the ventral horn of that segment would be somehow 'bombarded' by too many signals, many of them 'inappropriate' to the needs of that tissue, and so dysfunction of that tissue would ensue. As has already been discussed, thresholds would be lowered within the cord, allowing increased excitation or inhibition (according to the architecture of the cells/synapses/interneurones within the segment), thus altering output.

In the light of current understanding, though, the states of habituation and long-term depression may also be important clinical entities involved with this phenomenon. In fact, the author feels that the depressed habituated state of the cord may be involved in some of the 'chronic' findings within the lesion complex, as outlined below. This phenomenon/these altered states can be palpated and recognized within the tissues of the body.

As we shall see, these changes induced (among other things) movement restrictions in the articular structures of the spinal column. However, a simple restriction of movement within these articulations is not indicative of the presence of an osteopathic lesion in the absence of the other accompanying features. Not all spinal restrictions are involved in the type of neural 'confusion' or 'discoordination' that are thought to be capable of affecting physiological and homeostatic dysfunction through induced changes in the nervous system.

Within the lesion complex/phenomenon, there are classically a number of changes thought to occur, mediated by this changed output:

- skin changes;
- vascular changes ('vasomotion');
- muscular changes;
- end-organ changes ('visceromotion');
- altered sweat gland activity;
- altered neurotrophism.

Thus there would be altered activity within the sclerotome, viscerotome, myotome, dermatome associated with that segment. These changes would be able to be palpated but, depending upon how long the changes had been manifest at a tissue level, the palpatory changes would also be different. The changes induce such things as altered tone of the muscles, altered tension of the skin, changes in vascular activity (leading to oedema in some instances, ischaemia in others) and altered visceral activity. In the way that a peripheral neuropathy (from a disc herniation in the spinal canal, for example) induces a recognizable syndrome of changes, such as myopathy and sensory changes, so the facilitated segment expresses a syndrome of changes that can be palpated; these changes lead to a variety of symptoms such as pain, altered muscle function and coordination, altered vascular activity (affecting the chemical environment of the interstitium), differing tone and pliability of the connective tissue of the area (even down to the level of the extracellular matrix) and changes in visceral function (such as altered glandular secretion, changes in peristalsis and motility of the smooth muscles, and altered mucosal secretion/other functions of the viscera affected). The site of all these changes would depend upon which segment of the spinal cord had become affected.

There could therefore be acute or chronic conditions, depending on the time course of the changes within that segment.

The acute response

These changes manifest as increased activity in the muscles served by that segment; which at the level of the spinal intervertebral column leads to an articular restriction of the associated apophyseal joints. Here the range of motion would be decreased from normal, may be painful and, as one passively attempted to move the joint to its end of range, the muscles would be very 'reactive' and 'kick back' (the muscles being somewhat in spasm in response to the movement challenge). The skin would be more 'bound down', in other words there would be increased resistance to physical stretching of the skin in this area – the connective tissue within would be somehow tighter/contracted. There would be increased sweating of the skin overlying the site of the related spinal articular restriction, and there would also be heat and oedema present in the skin, due to changes in vascularity and local microcirculation.

The chronic response

Here the skin would be progressively 'bound down' and immobile over its underlying tissues; there would be no redness or heat; there would be no oedema (or very little) and the tissues would feel less hydrated, more inelastic and generally less reactive. The motion of the articular segment would be reduced, but there would be no accompanying spasms of the muscles; instead a chronically contracted/adherent state of the muscles would be present. The tissues would feel thinner, more fibrous and less healthy in general.

When such palpatory findings are recognized at a spinal level, then close attention would be paid to the presenting symptoms and case history of the patient, to see if there were any correlations. In other words, the practitioner would be looking for indications of dysfunction in a segmentally related organ. So, if there was some sort of visceral disease or dysfunction present, this would be related to the 'lesioned' segment of the spine – clearly this segment would be bombarding that organ with all sorts of inappropriate signals, altering the vascular activity within that organ, affecting the activity of the smooth muscles within it, and generally disrupting its local homeostasis. Very often the organ would be thought to be ischaemic, and so suffer from hypoxia, inducing pain and discomfort. The saving grace in this situation would be the reversibility of the situation, if it had not been there for too long. If the changes persisted,

though, it would be more and more likely that the health and immunity of the tissue would be detrimentally affected, making it less resistant to disease and more likely to suffer dysfunction.

To reverse all this activity, it is necessary to direct a new set of different signals at the affected segment of the spinal cord, in order to somehow 're-set' the threshold of the segment and induce a normal level of activity within it. Releasing the articular restrictions, by a variety of manipulative techniques, is thought to achieve this, and so spinal treatment would be 'prescribed' for the visceral disease. However, the more chronic the changes palpated, the less reversible the situation is thought to be – and the more treatments would be needed to make any inroads into the spinal articulation before it could start sending different signals back into the cord segment again, eventually re-normalizing cord function, and hence reducing whatever symptoms were arising from this. Of course, in chronic situations, the tissue being affected by the segment's facilitation would also be undergoing long-term tissue adaptation, and so even if the spine could be made more mobile there would be a limit to how much the tissue could respond to new signals coming from the cord anyway. Thus, therapeutically, long-standing conditions are harder to achieve a clinical success with.

The presence of the lesion complex in the absence of clinical manifestation of visceral (or somatic) disease

It is the case that, in the presence of this neural phenomenon and accompanying palpatory changes at one or more spinal articular segments, the visceral changes may not (yet) be so great as to result in pronounced visceral symptomatology.

The changes are thought to be precursors to dysfunction within the tissues. In this context the palpatory changes could be diagnostic indicators of subclinical dysfunction, which, if left unchecked, could at a later time manifest itself in a recognizable clinical pattern. This point has very important implications for screening programmes, if proved valid through repeated research.

This also means that there may be some focal irritation or dysfunction within the viscera, for example, that is sending some irritative signal to the spine and so is causing some local irritation to manifest itself within the spinal articulation without there being overt clinical signs of visceral dysfunction. The visceral condition could still be palpated and identified, though, and, unless this component is explored, then someone just manipulating the spine to resolve those local changes and restrictions usually finds that the restrictions do not stay resolved for long. This amounts to a case of treating the effects of the disturbance and not the cause.

In this mind set, the spinal column could be thought of as a sort of keyboard, which one could play – releasing various keys (joints) and improving function of the tissues/organs related to those keys – or as a mirror, each articulation acting as a reflection of the state of whatever organ/tissue sends signals to that segment. In this way the spinal column could be used as a diagnostic tool, picking up reactions to changing function on the organs perhaps even before frank visceral symptoms and signs manifested themselves. Whichever way it was viewed the spinal column was acting as a window on the internal environment of the body.

A point not to be overlooked here is that these phenomena relate not only to visceral disease and dysfunction but to the intercoordination of all tissue events. This means that a lesioned segment could be disturbing effective intercommunication between all tissues, including one part of the somatic body and another, as discussed earlier. In subsequent chapters we shall see that many movement patterns within the somatic field depend on effective neural communication and coordination between parts and that, if this is distorted in any way, then biomechanical control will become compromised. This can manifest itself in an enormous variety of locomotor and biomechanical irritations, sprains, strains and painful presentations.

These form a very large part of osteopathic practice, and the full range of neural consequences of 'lesioned' segments should not be forgotten. The neuroemotional and neuroendocrine–immune systems that are about to be discussed are also a part of this phenomenon.

THE NEUROENDOCRINE–IMMUNE SYSTEM

Although the endocrine system can clearly be implicated within the relationships discussed above, there is a special relationship between the nervous system, the endocrine system and the immune system that can adapt many body functions on a large scale and not just an organ-specific level. As shall be seen, the emotions can also feed into this relationship, adding another dimension to the factors governing homeostasis and health. (In the next section we will make reference to interactions between the emotions and the musculoskeletal system, which have further relevance for clinical practice.)

Professor Frank Willard

In considering the neuroendocrine–immune network the profession owes a great debt of gratitude to Professor Frank Willard of the New England College of Osteopathic Medicine, Maine. He has done much to integrate current understanding of neurophysiological mechanisms that are applicable to the osteopathic philosophy, and has greatly improved the profession's appreciation of the interactions within body systems. He has also done much work on integrating the various studies on nociception and acute and chronic inflammation that underpin many pain presentations within clinical practice. In addition he is renowned for his excellent anatomical dissections and presentations, which enable osteopaths (and others) to understand the deep level of knowledge that is required when trying to interpret clinical findings in the light of neurophysiological understanding.

The discussions below are based on his work in the field of neuroendocrine–immunology. They

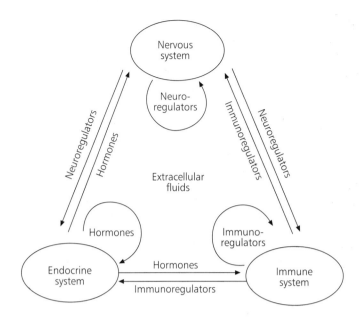

Figure 4.6

Complex neural, endocrine and immune communication networks in the extracellular spaces. (Reproduced with permission from American Osteopathic Association, Foundations of Osteopathic Medicine, Lippincott Williams & Wilkins, 1997.)

are brief and limited because of confines of space, and should not be considered to comprise the totality of possible discussion on these points.

In a book entitled *Physiotherapy in Mental Health*, Professor Willard states:

> *The protective homeostatic activities of the neuroendocrine–immune network are responsive to two major types of sensory information, neural and immune. The peripheral nervous system is capable of detecting changes in various forms of energy surrounding and within the body, such as mechanical, chemical and light energy. In response to such stimuli, these sensory neurones release a coded signal of neurotransmitters in the central nervous system to initiate protective reflexes. Similarly, white blood cells (immune cells) sense changes in the antigen body map and, in response, release a coded signal composed of immunoregulators such as interleukins, a family of small peptide messenger molecules. These immunoregulators coordinate the activity of immune cells, as well as other cells to initiate protective immune responses. Both the neural and immune sensory signals*

> *lead to alterations in body chemistry as well as behaviour and cognition. These changes in bodily functions represent significant features of the general adaptive response.*
>
> Willard, 1995

Interactions of the neuroendocrine-immune system/network are shown in Figure 4.6.

Each of these three systems produces messenger molecules called neuroregulators, immunoregulators and hormones, respectively. Not only do these messengers influence cells in their own systems, but they also have effects on cells in other systems. Thus, the three systems truly function as a single, coordinated whole.

The general adaptive syndrome

The general adaptive syndrome, or stress response, is a phenomenon first detailed by Hans Selye (1978).

Professor Willard goes on to say that:

> *Once a general adaptive response has begun in response to stressors, activity in the central nervous system shifts into a state of increasing arousal, vigilance, and awareness, termed behavioural adaptation.*

Simultaneously, the physiological pathways of adaptation such as gluconeogenesis, the breakdown of complex compounds to form glucose, and the mobilization of energy stores for escape and wound repair processes are activated. Also simultaneously, non-adaptive pathways such as those involved in digestion and reproduction are suppressed. Ultimately, an overall damping of immune system functions occurs as well as a short-term desensitization of the neural system, termed antinociceptive response. These responses prevent massive overreaction of the body's defences to the stressor(s). While in the short term these adaptive responses are very beneficial to the survival of the individual, if excessively prolonged the same adaptive responses can themselves prove to be detrimental to the body.

Willard, 1995

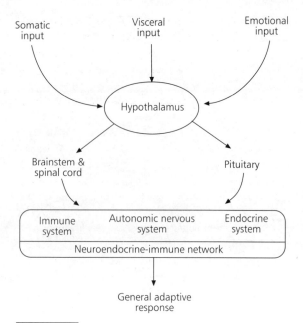

Figure 4.7

The response of the neuroendocrine–immune network to signals emanating from somatic, visceral or emotional dysfunction.
(Reproduced with the permission of Butterworth Heinemann Publishers from Physiotherapy in Mental Health: A Practical Approach (Eds Everett et al.), Willard, 1995.)

Figure 4.7 shows the general adaptive response being mediated through several structures.

Precise regulation of the general adaptive response is necessary to maintain the normal health of the individual. Prolonged exposure to inescapable stress, be it emotional (including the impact of social environment characteristics; Taylor *et al.*, 1997), mechanical (somatic injury) or visceral (visceral injury or disease), damages the feedback control systems designed to monitor the activity of the general adaptive response.

As stated, the general adaptive response has implications for function within many body systems. The extensive effects of the general adaptive response will not be discussed here, but a few points are included as an illustration.

Activation of the hypothalamic–pituitary axis through the general adaptive response engages the sympathetic division of the autonomic nervous system. Corticotrophin-releasing hormone is produced by neurones in the hypothalamus that also project axons into the brain stem, suggesting a possible direct neural control of the brain stem autonomic nervous system by the hypophysiotrophic neurones (neurones that regulate the endocrine functions of the anterior

pituitary gland). Physiologically, the increased activity in the sympathetic nervous system that results from this is expressed as increased heart rate, blood pressure and total oxygen consumption, with decreased gastric function.

The immune system is affected in a number of ways, through the innervation of lymphoid tissue (Felten and Felten, 1987, 1988; Felten *et al.*, 1992) and the effects of stress on immune cell distribution. For example, immune cell trafficking is crucial to the performance of the surveillance as well as effector functions of the immune system. Because immune cells travel between tissues through the blood stream, the numbers and proportions of leukocytes in the circulation provide an important representation of the state of leukocyte distribution in the body. Stress-induced changes in plasma corticosterone (an effect of the general adaptive response) lead to a significant decrease in numbers and percentages of lymphocytes, an increase in neutrophils and a greater reduction in B-cells and monocytes than T-cells. Such a redistribution/alteration of immune components may significantly affect the ability of the immune system to respond to potential or ongoing immune challenge (Dhabhar *et al.*, 1995).

Cognition and memory are affected also. Prolonged exposure to stress leads to loss of neurones, particularly in the hippocampus. Recent evidence suggests that the glucocorticoid- and stress-related cognitive impairments involving declarative memory are probably related to the changes they effect in the hippocampus, whereas stress-induced catecholamine effects on emotionally laden memories are postulated to involve structures such as the amygdala (McEwen and Sapolsky, 1995).

Brain function in general is affected, through the lifelong interplay between genes and the environment. This interplay is instrumental in shaping the structure and function of the body in general, and these interactions apply to the brain as a plastic and ever-changing organ of the body. Hormones are key regulators of gene expression throughout the body, and the actions of hormones on the brain are instrumental in shaping sex differences and in determining the effects of stress on brain function, including brain ageing (McEwen, 1997). This means that the very stressors that are working through the brain to generate an adaptive response will affect the brain itself and those neural tissues that are partaking in that process. This means that the brain gradually becomes less efficient at regulating the general adaptive response as exposure to the various stressors continue.

The altered levels of hormonal activity that regulate gene expression throughout the body mean that the general adaptive response affects all tissues and their products over time. This means that the general adaptive response works with the intrinsic genetic susceptibility to determine the progression towards declining health (McEwen, 1997).

Thus there is a price for adaptation.

A new term has been coined to illustrate the shifting focus of homeostatic function from effective homeostasis towards declining health and illness. This term is **allostatic load**.

Allostatic load is the cumulative physiological toll exacted on the body over time by efforts to adapt to life experiences, disease and injury. Homeostasis is thought to be shifted towards new parameters of function that are more detrimental to health than before. The more stressors, and the longer they persist, the greater the allostatic load and the greater the shift of homeostasis towards disregulation and declining health (Seeman, 1997).

This concept ties in very neatly with the osteopathic perspectives on health and disease that were discussed in Chapters 1 and 2 (where the inter-relatedness of parts was discussed, as was the concept of entropy and increasing randomness within body function) and with the mind–body interactions behind the holistic aspects of osteopathy (Sternberg and Gold, 1997).

The clinical relevance of allostatic load to osteopaths is that one must look for all components within the person's body and environment that are acting as stressors, and work to remove or reduce as many of these factors as possible. This may mean reducing and treating many minor aches, pains and problems within the musculoskeletal system; it may mean discussing diet and fluid intake with the patient (or suggesting they see a nutritionist) to ensure adequate nutrition is being maintained; it may mean reflecting on the environmental situation of the person concerned – identifying factors that the patient may be aware of, or may not have considered as stressors to their general health, well being and ability to recover and heal. Note: these may be factors that neither the osteopath nor the individual can affect but, where possible, these are addressed (perhaps through referral to a psychologist or counsellor, by moving house or changing job and so on).

Thus the integration of mind, body and spirit comes together in a scientific and physiological concept of allostatic load, which can be appreciated by all branches of the healthcare system.

THE NEUROEMOTIONAL SYSTEM

As stated before, there is also a relationship between the musculoskeletal system and the emotions. It is worth mentioning the relationship in detail, as there are different representations arising from this interaction compared to those that arise from the emotional relationship to allostatic load discussed above.

This emotional and musculoskeletal interaction is also mediated through the nervous system, and is expressed in several different ways. As discussed before, the whole way that we live our lives and express our actions, thoughts and innermost feelings is through the musculoskeletal system. Because of this it is not surprising that there should be an especial relation between the musculoskeletal system and the emotions (Keleman, 1985). Looking at people and observing their expressions and body language often gives many indications of inner feelings and emotional states.

In an earlier discussion (on the neural control of movement), reference was made to the many components of the higher centres within the brain that contribute to muscular activity. There are many inter-relations between different parts of the brain that concern emotion (Kandel *et al.*, 1991). Figure 4.8 illustrates these.

The limbic system (including the parahippocampal gyrus, the cingulate gyrus and the subcallosal gyrus) has many links with the hypothalamus, and through that to the activity of many body systems (via the endocrine and the visceral systems). The relation between these two areas and the amygdala (which is involved in learning, particularly those tasks that require coordination from different sensory modalities) and the cortex provides a pathway that ensures the influence of emotion on many body activities and on the state of the muscular system.

Emotional memory is laid down through these different areas of the brain and creates a diverse pattern of memory throughout the nervous system. It seems that any stimulus, such as smell or touch or pain, that matches such memory patterns may trigger recall of the emotion that originally laid down that memory (Fuster, 1995).

These links also ensure that there is a very potent link between touch, emotions and the physiological processes within the body.

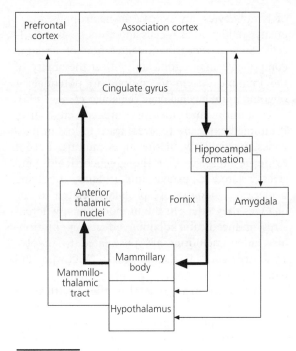

Figure 4.8

A proposed neural circuit for emotion. The circuit in the original proposal is indicated by thick lines; more recently described connections are shown by thin lines. (Reproduced with the permission of Appleton & Lange from Principles of Neural Science, *3rd edn, Kandel et al., 1991.)*

Both of these phenomena (emotional memory and the influences of touch) are incorporated into many therapeutic practices, including osteopathy.

Clinical application

Some parts of the profession are highlighting the potential powerful influence of the emotions upon the state of the muscular system (Nathan, 1995; Latey, 1996; Grainger, 1967). In cases where one is trying to resolve problems associated with altered muscular activity and biomechanical function, one of the major 'holding' or maintaining factors for that pattern of muscular dysfunction lies within the emotional 'problems' or reactions of the person involved.

Therapeutically, one can help the person recognize the (emotional) origin of their problem by educating them to recognize the pattern of muscular tension within them. Releasing muscular tension, and tension within the fascia and connective tissues of the body, may, through feeding back via the links mentioned above, trigger a release of some deeply felt and often 'buried' emotion, so contributing to its resolution.

So-called 'somato-emotional release' techniques have been gaining prominence within parts of the profession and in other manipulative therapies, highlighting another growing aspect of therapeutic intervention available to people in need. John Upledger has been a strong exponent of this type of therapeutic intervention.

Recognizing this component within people is perhaps not as difficult as one might imagine. Certainly, standard observation of the person as a human being, listening to them speak, reflecting on how soft tissue tensions change as the person discusses events, and so on, gives many clues. Also, the 'quality' of the tension within those soft tissues can give many clues, even when the person has not verbalized any particular emotional problem openly.

Palpatory qualities to emotional states in tissues
Each practitioner must build up their own subjective description of what the tissue states mean to them clinically, whether this is to do with the degree of actual injury or some sort of emotional problem. Experience and careful reflection on the nature of tissue reactions and responses to manipulations are an important part of maturing as a professional, and by their very nature are descriptive terms unique to the individual practitioner. Because of their subjective nature they can be difficult to analyse in an orthodox sense, but this should not detract from their importance within a clinical setting.

Some examples from the author's own experience, expressed in diagrammatic form, are given in Figures 4.9, 4.10 and 4.11.

The sort of reflection shown in these illustrations can help one decide if releasing the tissues would lead to a positive response or create some sort of additional stress if the person is not yet ready to 'let go' of the emotional factors involved. As in all clinical situations, respecting

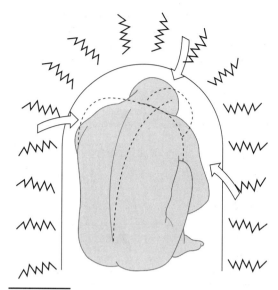

Figure 4.9

Palpatory responses – avoiding change. The arrows indicate that, if touch is attempted, the person recoils and 'shrinks' even more into themselves, as indicated by the dotted outline. The surrounding shell represents a shield that repels touch and keeps anything from invading the person within. The shield reacts angrily when touched.

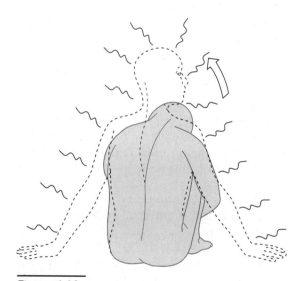

Figure 4.10

Palpatory responses – considering change. The arrow indicates that the person is open to some sort of change, by 'opening up' out of their curled (inward) position when touched. The lines emanating from them indicate that the protective shield is less strong and touch is not actively repelled. The tissues can be touched and may be persuaded to change. Change is not easy, but it is not actively resisted.

Figure 4.11

Palpatory responses – actively changing. The lines indicate that there is very little resistance in the tissues as they are touched. The person is not afraid, and there is no real shield/barrier to stop touch. When touched, the tissues are waiting to connect. They actively respond to the help – there is an immediate positive response. Change just needs a little encouragement in the right direction, which, once initiated, carries on under its own momentum.

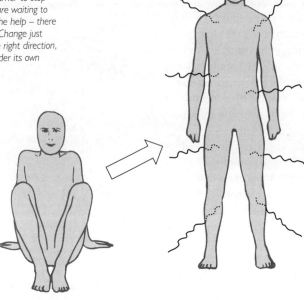

the person and the reactions their tissues demonstrate is vital, and recognizing when properly trained counselling practitioners should be the prime carers is very important to avoid inappropriate work with emotional issues.

As I have said, such comments reflect one individual interpretation and other osteopaths or practitioners in this field would have other comments and observations to make that would be equally, if not more, effective in introducing this aspect of osteopathic work.

'Body types – emotional types' and the way people respond to physical treatment

In a slightly different context, levels of activity in the nervous system seem to influence the way people behave and the way their bodies react to different types of touch and therapeutic manipulative procedures.

It seems that, although there is normally a balanced and integrated relationship within the different components of the autonomic nervous system (the sympathetic and parasympathetic

components), one of these might predominate in overall activity.

Again, observing people, one can see examples of certain types, such as:

- the stressed and overworked executive or busy mother, who is constantly in a state of poor health and lowered immunity;
- the laid back and easy-going young person;
- the tired and delicate older person;
- the fit and healthy athlete.

Each of these people would have internal systems at different states of activity and responsiveness. The stressed person may have a more active sympathetic system, and the laid-back person may have a more predominant parasympathetic system, leading to different expressions of vitality, physiology, strength and 'robustness'.

Of course, there are many other reasons for different levels of strength and robustness (such as degenerative change, disease and so on), which will mean that one cannot treat all people in the

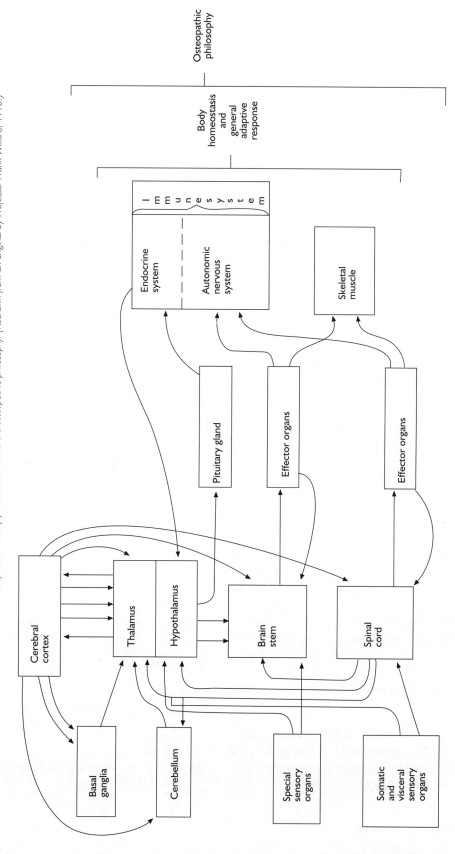

Figure 4.12

The range of interactions within the nervous system as a whole. The neural network illustrated here should work in concert and any 'confusion' in function created by barriers throughout the body will have an effect throughout the web. The outcomes of such reactions may not be wholly predictable. This is the osteopathic philosophy. (Redrawn from an original by Professor Frank Willard, 1996.)

Note: Basal ganglion loop and cerebellum loop can, via thalamus, regulate cortex, which can moderate central axis, e.g. thalamus, hypothalamus, brainstem and spinal cord.

same way. However, levels of reactiveness within the nervous system that could express themselves in the above 'body-emotional types' lead to the concept that different people must be treated in different ways in order to ensure a positive therapeutic outcome.

> There are many different styles of manipulative procedure used in osteopathy, and many different styles of overall management, which need to be chosen with care to suit the person who has presented for help.

Some patients do not like more direct manipulations such as high-velocity thrust techniques, while others do not feel that the more gentle techniques (such as the functional technique and those that make use of the involuntary mechanisms – terms that will be described later) have done anything for them, and think that the more direct techniques are required to achieve success.

Some techniques are therefore more 'soothing', and others more 'stimulatory' and, when choosing them, one must evaluate what state the person is in before applying them. This means evaluating the physical state of the tissues, with respect to such things as degree of soft tissue injury or degenerative change, but also with respect to what the person can cope with. Distressed and overtired people may not respond well to direct and strong techniques. Young people or children might be frightened by them. Some strong and direct, positive people may be wary of more gentle or indirect techniques, where the immediate benefits are not obvious or only emerge after time – they may not feel 'treated' by these manoeuvres. Also some people will react adversely to some types of treatment, creating more distress and pain, and others will not be helped by treatment that is not direct enough.

There are many examples one could give along these lines but, in summary, recognizing the state of the tissues and all the underlying ramifications is a fundamental component of the osteopathic approach.

SUMMARY

Ramifications of confusion throughout the whole nervous system – Chinese whispers

When all the above considerations have been put together, one can see that the potential ramifications of signalling distortion within the nervous system are complex, diverse, and very probably mostly unpredictable (at least, given current understanding).

Figure 4.12 maps out a variety of interconnections and networking relationships within the nervous system that could lead to a whole variety of consequences if the web of their intercommunication is distorted.

The following chapters bring us back into a discussion of biomechanics and inter-relations between parts with respect to movement. Hopefully, while these next chapters are digested, the reader can still keep in mind the concepts introduced within this one.

REFERENCES

Accarino, A. M., Azpiroz, F. and Malagelada, J. (1995) Selective dysfunction of mechanosensitive intestinal afferents in irritable bowel syndrome. *Gastroenterology*, **108**, 636–643.

Alarcon, G. and Cervero, F. (1990) The effects of visceral stimulation of A and C visceral afferent fibres on the excitability of viscerosomatic neurones in the thoracic spinal cord of the cat. *Brain Research*, **509**, 24–30.

American Academy of Osteopathy (1979) *The Collected Works of Irvin M. Korr*, American Academy of Osteopathy, Indianapolis, IN.

American Academy of Osteopathy (1993) *1993 Year Book*, American Academy of Osteopathy, Indianapolis, IN.

American Osteopathic Association (1997) *Foundations for Osteopathic Medicine*, Williams & Wilkins, Baltimore, MD.

Bagust, J., Chen, Y. and Kerkut, G. A. (1993) Spread of the dorsal root reflex in an isolated preparation of hamster spinal cord. *Experimental Physiology*, **78**, 799–809.

Barnes, P. J. (1986) Asthma as an axon reflex. *Lancet*, i, 242–245.

Baron, R. and Maier, C. (1995) Painful neuropathy: C-nociceptor activity may not be necessary to maintain central mechanisms accounting for dynamic mechanical allodynia. *Clinical Journal of Pain*, **11**, 63–69.

Cervero, F. (1992) Visceral and spinal components of viscero-somatic interactions. In: *The Central Connection: Somatovisceral/Viscerosomatic Interaction* (eds M. M. Patterson and J. N. Howell), American Academy of Osteopathy, Indianapolis, IN, pp. 77–86.

Cervero, F., Schaible, H. G. and Schmidt, R. F. (1991) Tonic descending inhibition of spinal cord neurones driven by joint afferents in normal cats and in cats with an inflamed knee joint. *Experimental Brain Research*, **83**, 675–678.

Cole, W. V. (1951) Somaticovisceral reflexes. A preliminary report of the experimental aspect of somaticovisceral reflexes immediately following electrical stimulation and a minor vertebral strain. *Journal of the American Osteopathic Association*, **50**, 67–73.

Cole, W. V. (1953) Somaticovisceral reflexes. The effects of spinal fixation at the thoracolumbar junction on certain visceral structures. *Journal of the American Osteopathic Association*, **52**, 74–82.

Collins, J. J. (1995) The redundant nature of locomotor optimization laws. *Journal of Biomechanics*, **28**, 251–267.

Crone, C. (1993) Reciprocal inhibition in man. *Danish Medical Bulletin*, **40**, 571–581.

De Groat, W. C. (1994) *Nociceptors and the Neuroendocrine-immune Connection*, American Academy of Osteopathy, Indianapolis, IN.

Denslow, J. S. (1972) Neural basis of the somatic component in health and disease and its clinical management. *Journal of the American Osteopathic Association*, **72**, 149–156.

Derryberry, D. and Tucker, D. M. (1990) The adaptive base of the neural hierarchy: elemental motivational controls on network function. *Nebraska Symposium on Motivation*, **38**, 289–342.

Dhabhar, F. S., Miller, A. H., McEwen, B. S. and Spencer, R. L. (1995) Effects of stress on immune cell distribution. Dynamics and hormonal mechanisms. *Journal of Immunology*, **154**, 5511–5527.

Dietz, V., Trippel, M., Discher, M. and Horstmann, G. A. (1991) Compensation of human stance perturbations: selection of the appropriate electromyographic pattern. *Neuroscience Letters*, **126**, 71–74.

Dove, C. (1961) The physiological basis of the osteopathic concept of visceral disease. *Journal and Proceedings of the Osteopathic Association of Great Britain*, **1**, 1–23.

Elbadawi, A. (1997) Interstitial cystitis: a critique of current concepts with a new proposal for pathologic diagnosis and pathogenesis. *Urology*, **49**, 14–40.

Felten, D. L. and Felten, S. Y. (1987) Immune interactions with specific neural structures. *Brain, Behavior, and Immunity*, **1**, 279–283.

Felten, D. L. and Felten, S. Y. (1988) Sympathetic noradrenergic innervation of immune organs. *Brain, Behavior, and Immunity*, **2**, 293–300.

Felten, S. Y., Felten, D. L., Bellinger, D. L. and Olschowka, J. A. (1992) Noradrenergic and peptidergic innervation of lymphoid organs. *Chemical Immunology*, **52**, 25–48.

Forssberg, H. and Hirschfeld, H. (1994) Postural adjustments in sitting humans following external perturbations: muscle activity and kinematics. *Experimental Brain Research*, **97**, 515–527.

Fuster, J. M. (1995) Memory in the cortex of the primate. *Biological Research*, **28**, 59–72.

Garrison, D. W. (1992) Viscerosomatic convergence onto feline spinal neurones from oesophagus, heart and somatic fields: effects of inflammation. *Pain*, **49**, 373–382.

Giamberardino, M. A., Valente, R., Affaitati, G. and Vecchiet, L. (1997) Central neuronal changes in recurrent visceral pain. *International Journal of Clinical Pharmacological Research*, **17**, 63–66.

Gillette, R. G., Kramis, R. C. and Roberts, W. J. (1994) Sympathetic activation of cat spinal neurones responsive to noxious stimulation of deep tissues in the low back. *Pain*, **56**, 31–42.

Grainger, H. G. (1958) The somatic component in visceral disease. *Academy of Applied Osteopathy Year Book*, 25–32.

Grainger, H. G. (1967) Psychic stress and the tonic muscle spindle. *Academy of Applied Osteopathy Year Book*, 68–74.

Grobstein, P. (1994) Variability in brain behaviour. In: *Encyclopaedia of Human Behaviour* (ed. V. S. Ramachandran), Academic Press, London.

Grubb, B. D., Stiller, R. U. and Schaible, H. G. (1993) Dynamic changes in the receptive field properties of spinal cord neurons with ankle input in rats with chronic unilateral inflammation in the ankle region. *Experimental Brain Research*, **92**, 441–452.

Hanesch, U., Pfrommer, U., Grubb, B. D. and Schaible, H. G. (1993) Acute and chronic phases of unilateral inflammation in rat's ankle are associated with an increase in the proportion of calcitonin gene-related peptide-immunoreactive dorsal root ganglion cells. *European Journal of Neuroscience*, 5,154–161.

He, X., Proske, U., Schaible, H. G. and Schmidt, R. F. (1988) Acute inflammation of the knee joint in the cat alters responses of flexor motoneurons to leg movements. *Journal of Neurophysiology*, 59, 326–340.

Hess, G. and Donoghue, J. P. (1994) Long-term potentiation of horizontal connections provides a mechanism to reorganize cortical motor maps. *Journal of Neurophysiology*, 71, 2543–2547.

Hobbs, S. F., Chandler, M. J., Bolser, D. C. and Foreman, R. D. (1992) Segmental organization of visceral and somatic input onto C3–T6 spinothalamic tract cells of the monkey. *Journal of Neurophysiology*, 68, 1575–1588.

Jankovic, J. (1994) Post-traumatic movement disorders: central and peripheral mechanisms. *Neurology*, 44, 2006–2014.

Jeftinija, S. and Urban, L. (1994) Repetitive stimulation induced potentiation of excitatory transmission in the rat dorsal horn: an in vitro study. *Journal of Neurophysiology*, 71, 216–228.

Jones, E. G. (1990) The role of afferent activity in the maintenance of primate neocortical function. *Journal of Experimental Biology*, 153, 155–176.

Kalaska, J. F. (1994) Central neural mechanisms of touch and proprioception. *Canadian Journal of Physiology and Pharmacology*, 72, 542–545.

Kandel, E. R., Schwartz, J. H. and Jessel, T. M. (1991) *Principles of Neural Science*, 3rd edn. Prentice Hall, Englewood Cliffs, New Jersey.

Katz, P. S. (1996) Neurones, networks, and motor behaviour. *Neuron*, 16, 245–253.

Keleman, S. (1985) *Emotional Anatomy*, Centre Press, Berkeley, CA.

Keranen, U., Kiviluoto, T., Jarvinen, H. *et al.* (1995) Changes in substance P-immunoreactive innervation of human colon associated with ulcerative colitis. *Digestive Diseases and Sciences*, 40, 2250–2258.

Kingham, D. J. (1994) On the general theory of neural circuitry. *Medical Hypotheses*, 42, 291–298.

Koceja, D. M. and Kamen, G. (1991) Interactions in human quadriceps-triceps surae motoneuron pathways. *Experimental Brain Research*, 86, 433–439.

Kowalski, M. L., Didier, A. and Kaliner, M. A. (1989) Neurogenic inflammation in the airways. l. Neurogenic stimulation induces plasma protein extravasation into the rat airway lumen. *American Review of Respiratory Disease*, 140, 101–109.

Latey, P. (1996) Feelings, muscles and movement. *Journal of Bodywork and Movement Therapies*, 1, 44–52.

Lentell, G., Baas, B., Lopez, D. *et al.* (1995) The contributions of proprioceptive deficits, muscle function, and anatomic laxity to functional instability of the ankle. *Journal of Orthopaedic and Sports Physical Therapy*, 21, 206–215.

Lewit, K. (1987) Chain reactions in disturbed function of the motor system. *Manual Medicine*, 3, 27–29.

Lewthwaite, R. (1990) Motivational considerations in physical activity involvement. *Physical Therapy*, 70, 808–819.

Lund, J. P., Donga, R., Widmer, C. G. and Stohler, C. S. (1991) The pain-adaptation model: a discussion of the relationship between chronic musculoskeletal pain and motor activity. *Canadian Journal of Physiology and Pharmacology*, 69, 683–694.

McCloskey, D. I. and Prochazka, A. (1994) The role of sensory information in the guidance of voluntary movement: reflections on a symposium held at the 22nd annual meeting of the Society for Neuroscience. *Somatosensory and Motor Research*, 11, 69–76.

McCollum, G. (1993) Reciprocal inhibition, synergies, and movements. *Journal of Theoretical Biology*, 165, 291–311.

McEwen, B. S. (1997) Hormones as regulators of brain development: life-long effects related to health and disease. *Acta Paediatrica (Supplement)*, 422, 41–44.

McEwen, B. S. and Sapolsky, R. M. (1995) Stress and cognitive function. *Current Opinions in Neurobiology*, 81, 205–216.

Malenka, R. C. (1994) Synaptic plasticity. Mucking up movements. *Nature*, 372, 218–219.

Marder, E. and Calabrese, R. L. (1996) Principles of rhythmic motor pattern generation. *Physiological Reviews*, 76, 687–717.

Masson, R. L. Jr, Sparkes, M. L. and Ritz, L. A. (1991) Descending projections to the rat sacrocaudal spinal cord. *Journal of Comparative Neurology*, 307,120–130.

Mayer, E. A. and Gebhart, G. F. (1994) Basic and clinical aspects of visceral hyperalgesia. *Gastroenterology*, 107, 271–293.

Mayer, E. A. and Raybould, H. E. (1990) Role of visceral afferent mechanisms in functional bowel disorders. *Gastroenterology*, 99,1688–1704.

Mazevet, D. and Pierrot-Deseilligny, E. (1994) Pattern of descending excitation of presumed propriospinal neurones at the onset of voluntary movement in humans. *Acta Physiologica Scandinavica*, 150, 27–38.

Meggs, W. J. (1993) Neurogenic inflammation and sensitivity to environmental chemicals. *Environmental Health Perspectives*, 101, 234–238.

Nansel, D. and Szlazak, M. (1995) Somatic dysfunction and the phenomenon of visceral disease simulation: a probable explanation for the apparent effectiveness of somatic therapy in patients presumed to be suffering from true visceral disease. *Journal of Manipulative and Physiological Therapeutics*, 18, 379–397.

Nathan, B. (1995) Philosophical notes on osteopathic theory: part III. Non-procedural touching and the relationship between touch and emotion. *British Osteopathic Journal*, 17, 30–34.

Nielsen, J. and Kagamihara, Y. (1992) The regulation of disynaptic reciprocal Ia inhibition during co-contraction of antagonistic muscles in man. *Journal of Physiology*, 456, 373–391.

Ozerdem, B. and Tozeren, A. (1995) Physical response of collagen gels to tensile strain. *Journal of Biomechanical Engineering*, 117, 397–401.

Patterson, M. M. (1976) A model mechanism for spinal segmental facilitation. *Journal of the American Osteopathic Association*, 76, 17–25.

Proske, U., Schaible, H. G. and Schmidt, R. F. (1988) Joint receptors and kinaesthesia. *Experimental Brain Research*, 72, 219–224.

Randic, M., Jiang, M. C. and Cerne, R. (1993) Long-term potentiation and long-term depression of primary afferent neurotransmission in the rat spinal cord. *Journal of Neuroscience*, 13, 5228–5241.

Rees, H., Sluka, K. N., Westlund, K. N. and Willis, W. D. (1994) Do dorsal root reflexes augment peripheral inflammation? *NeuroReport*, 5, 821–824.

Rees, H., Sluka, K. N., Lu, Y. *et al.* (1996) Dorsal root reflexes in articular afferents occur bilaterally in a chronic model of arthritis in cats. *Journal of Neurophysiology*, 76, 4190–4193.

Sanes, J. N. and Shadmehr, R. (1995) Sense of muscular effort and somesthetic afferent information in humans. *Canadian Journal of Physiology and Pharmacology*, 73, 223–233.

Sato, A. (1997) The reflex effects of spinal somatic nerve stimulation on visceral function. *Journal of Manipulative and Physiological Therapeutics*, 15, 57–61.

Sato, A. and Swenson, D. C. (1984) Sympathetic nervous system response to mechanical stress of the spinal column in rats. *Journal of Manipulative and Physiological Therapeutics*, 7,141–147.

Sato, A., Sato, R. F., Schmidt, R. F. and Torigata, Y. (1983) Somato-vesical reflexes in chronic spinal cats. *Journal of the Autonomic Nervous System*, 7, 351–362.

Schaible, H. G. and Grubb, B. D. (1993) Afferent and spinal mechanisms of joint pain. *Pain*, 55, 5–54.

Schaible, H. G. and Schmidt, R. F. (1985) Effects of an experimental arthritis on the sensory properties of fine articular afferent units. *Journal of Neurophysiology*, 54,1109–1122.

Schaible, H. G. and Schmidt, R. F. (1988) Time course of mechanosensitivity changes in articular afferents during a developing experimental arthritis. *Journal of Neurophysiology*, 60, 2180–2195.

Schaible, H. G., Schmidt, R. F. and Willis, W. D. (1987) Enhancement of the responses of ascending tract cells in the cat spinal cord by acute inflammation of the knee joint. *Experimental Brain Research*, 66, 489–499.

Schaible, H. G., Neugebauer, V., Cervero, F. and Schmidt, R. F. (1991) Changes in tonic descending inhibition of spinal neurons with articular input during the development of acute arthritis in the cat. *Journal of Neurophysiology*, 66, 1021–1032.

Seeman, T. E. (1997) Price of adaptation – allostatic load and its health consequences. MacArthur studies of successful ageing. *Archives of Internal Medicine*, 157, 2259–2268.

Selye, H. (1978) *The Stress of Life*, McGraw-Hill, New York.

Shefner, J. M., Buchthal, F. and Krarup, C. (1992) Recurrent potentials in human peripheral sensory nerve: possible evidence of primary afferent depolarization of the spinal cord. *Muscle and Nerve*, 15, 1354–1363.

Shelhamer, J. H., Levine, S. J., Wu, T. *et al.* (1995) NIH conference. Airway inflammation. *Annals of Internal Medicine*, 123, 288–304.

Sternberg, E. M. and Gold, P. W. (1997) The mind–body interaction in disease. *Scientific American*, **Special Issue**, 8–15.

Taylor, S. E., Repetti, R. L. and Seeman, T. (1997) Health psychology: what is an unhealthy environment and how does it get under the skin? *Annual Review of Psychology*, 48, 411–447.

Tougas, G., Fitzpatrick, D., Hudoba, P. *et al.* (1992) Effects of chronic left vagal stimulation on visceral function in man. *PACE*, 15, 1588–1596.

Van Buskirk, R. L. (1979) Nociceptive reflexes and the somatic dysfunction: a model. *Journal of the American Osteopathic Association*, 90, 792–794.

Vaughan, J., Rosenbaum, D. A., Diedrich, F. J. and Moore, C. M. (1996) Cooperative selection of movements: the optimal selection model. *Psychological Research*, 58, 254–273.

Wallace, K. G. (1992) The pathophysiology of pain. *Critical Care Nursing Quarterly*, 15, 1–13.

Willard, F. H. (1995) Neuroendocrine-immune network, nociceptive stress and the general adaptive response. In: *Physiotherapy in Mental Health: A Practical Approach* (eds T. Everett, M. Dennis and E. Rickells), Butterworth/Heinemann, London, pp. 103–126.

Winter, D. A., Patla, A. E. and Frank, J. S. (1990) Assessment of balance control in humans. *Medical Progress through Technology*, 16, 31–51.

Yaksh, T. L. (1993) The spinal pharmacology of facilitation of afferent processing evoked by high-threshold afferent input of the postinjury pain state. *Current Opinion in Neurology and Neurosurgery*, 6, 250–256.

Young, R. P. and Marteniuk, R. G. (1995) Changes in inter-joint relationships of muscle movements and powers accompanying the acquisition of a multi-articular kicking task. *Journal of Biomechanics*, 28, 701–713.

5 BODY STRUCTURE, MOTION AND FUNCTION

The previous chapters included a lot of detail on communicating networks, and this chapter now 'opens out' the perspective and begins to consider the musculoskeletal system in general.

One of the main themes of this chapter is to get the reader to appreciate the diverse structure–function relations of the musculoskeletal system, and to realize the number of different challenges that exist to normal function within the musculoskeletal system. This sets the stage for a discussion of the multitude of possible effects that could arise from musculoskeletal system dysfunction. It begins to illustrate the diversity of mechanical barriers that can arise within the human form.

To explain the potential challenges and barriers to communication that the musculoskeletal system poses, we must first have an overview of 'normal' function within the musculoskeletal system, to appreciate what challenges there are to its function and therefore to the integrity of the internal environment.

Only when one can consider the overall movement challenges that the body faces can one begin to appreciate how they might summate to give the effects that were described in the preceding chapters, and how one might have to work on the whole body in order to resolve movement problems in one part (so resolving the physiological consequences of that restriction).

This chapter should also help to illustrate some of the palpatory perceptions used within osteopathy, and the ideas that osteopaths hold with respect to tissue quality and movement.

THE MUSCULOSKELETAL SYSTEM: HOW IT IS STRUCTURED, HOW IT MOVES, WHAT ITS FUNCTIONS ARE AND HOW THESE CAN BE CHALLENGED

The differing parts of the musculoskeletal system need to be coordinated to cope with the diverse needs of humans as locomotive entities. The biomechanical arrangement of the human form has many demands placed upon it: it has to take part in and withstand many different activities. It has many different roles, which means that it is influential to many aspects of function within the human form.

The roles of the musculoskeletal system

What is life?
Without getting too bogged down(!) life is often said to be perpetual, and that we exist to reproduce

ourselves. Attempting to answer why life needs to be ongoing/renewed is beyond this book, but given that there is some purpose to it, we can see that our reproductive mechanisms must be healthy to ensure that the human race is perpetuated.

As each of us is just one sex, and it takes a coupling of two different sexes to produce offspring, we need to be able to move to where someone of our opposite sex is to be found. For this we need a locomotor system. Thus locomotion is of prime importance to reproduction.

However, the musculoskeletal system is involved in more than reproduction: it is involved with many and varied activities.

The musculoskeletal system is involved with carrying out life itself.

The musculoskeletal system is involved with:

- **Locomotion.** This in itself means we can move to where there is food, collect it and eat it. It means we can move to where our mates are and perform acts of reproduction, and it means that we can carry out a multitude of daily tasks necessary to support and care for ourselves.
- **Defence.** This means we can protect ourselves and our family.
- **Communication.** We need our musculoskeletal system to communicate, whether physically, emotionally or verbally. We cannot do any of these things properly without our musculoskeletal systems. Anyone that looks at us observes us through the actions of our musculoskeletal system and often has to compare what we are saying or doing with our bodies as opposed to our voices to get a true picture of what we are 'saying' (Morris, 1978).

The essence of these statements is that **the somatic component is the final common pathway by which we carry out our lives** (which is perhaps backed up by considering that the corticospinal tract is the largest descending fibre tract from the brain; Kandel *et al.*, 1991).

- **Support.** In addition to the above, the musculoskeletal system performs one more function: that of support (in an architectural sense). All of the organs and systems that make up the organism need to be contained, supported and protected. Even if these organ functions are in themselves 'supportive' in a physiological as opposed to a physical sense, they need to be contained so that no damage can come to them (and hence to the organism as a whole) and they need to be easily carried about, so that the organism can carry out whatever activities it needs or wants to do.

The primacy of the musculoskeletal system

It is because of all of the above that certain opinions were formed by an American physiologist, Irvin Korr, who has a very long-standing association with the osteopathic profession: '[t]hat the musculoskeletal system is the primary machine of life' and that 'the musculoskeletal system's role far exceeds that of providing the framework and support' (American Academy of Osteopathy, 1979).

To understand these functions, the architectural arrangement of the human form needs to be appreciated.

THE ARCHITECTURAL ARRANGEMENT OF THE HUMAN FORM

To use spiritual concepts for a moment: man has often been said to have been created in the image of God, and therefore to be perfectly designed. Some osteopaths (and many others) feel that the study of the architectural arrangement of the human form is a very significant thing spiritually, and would have much to say about symbolism within anatomy in such a context (Nuttgens, 1983; Mann, 1993).

This aside, the profession generally acknowledges the significance of the fact that the body has been constructed in such a way that it (and the spirit/soul that resides within it) can 'go through life' without 'falling apart at the seams', and any departure from this form (through altered biomechanics) will have far-reaching effects.

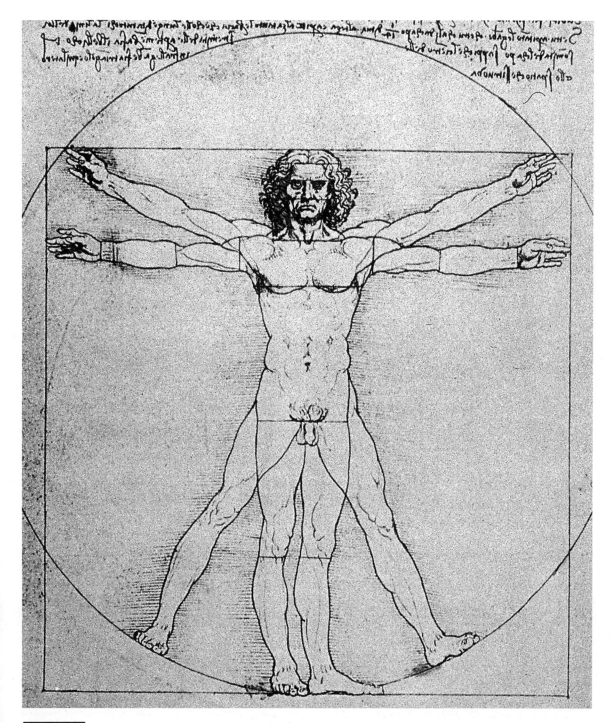

Figure 5.1

Proportions of the human figure, as drawn by Leonardo da Vinci (1452– 1519). The circumference of the circle is the same as the perimeter of the square, thereby 'squaring the circle'. The human body is the place where the synthesis of earth (square) and heaven (circle) occurs.

Humans are considered to be in dynamic equilibrium and to have a form that may have an ideal arrangement and balance, as shown in Figure 5.1, but is often unbalanced and in chaos.

Thus the nature of the arrangement of the human form – its architecture and how it moves – is central to osteopathic philosophy.

From the ideal to the actual

Without being irreverent to God, He/She does not have to live on earth and deal with all its attendant 'challenges', such as gravity and the daily toil of life's tasks. Therefore the human form is in reality a compromise between the ideal and the actual. The fact that the structure has to be multifunctional means that, for each separate individual function arising from the same structure, the form of the structure may not be ideal. In this way, structure places some constraints/limits on function.

This indicates a reciprocal relationship between structure and function, which is an important theme within osteopathy.

Posture and locomotion: an osteopath's view of biomechanics

From the moment we are conceived, our individual bodies develop, grow and emerge with slight variations in structural arrangement, so that when we embark upon our own individual lives after birth (or even before it), we do not all 'start with the same blank slate'. Therefore, how one person's structure will continue to develop to perform certain biomechanical tasks will be subtly different from another person. We do all seem to be able to make the best of things in most instances, though, as illustrated by the following quote: 'A conclusion that seems inescapable is that each of us learns to integrate the numerous variables that nature has bestowed upon our individual neuromusculoskeletal systems into a smoothly functioning whole' (Inman *et al.*, 1981).

Posture and locomotion possibilities arise in part from the nature of the architectural arrangement of the human form. Adaptations to structure and posture may limit their adaptability to locomotion and the activities where we rely upon our musculoskeletal systems for effective function/expression.

Architectural support in the human form

The human form is a composite structure of parts. Having evolved over the millennia from single-celled structures, we now have much more complex bodies and structures designed to meet our needs compared to these early forms.

Early forms of life – unicellular structures – are a bit like a bubble, which is very stable structurally (all forces pushing out are balanced by forces pulling in). Humans have various moveable appendages, requiring an adaptation of internal structure to provide support while allowing movement, and preserving stability while still incorporating a balance between external and internal forces. Clearly, even in the human form, all forces need to be counterbalanced to ensure stable function.

In our evolved 'human' shape, the architecture of support is provided by an internal framework that supports and interconnects the different sections. In the human body, this internal framework is provided by the connective tissues of the body. The connective tissue system aids the support of the body by its ability to 'spread load' and 'provide stability'. Connective tissue structures range from bones through large fascial sheaths and planes to cellular-level components such as the extracellular matrix and the cytoskeleton; and all these things hold the body together from the inside.

In addition to what has already been discussed, the actions and interactions of connective tissues are complex, but vital to appreciate for an understanding of osteopathic principles in practice.

The role of connective tissues has in fact been recognized by osteopaths for a long time (Cathie, 1974a, b) but is only now beginning to be incorporated within models for analysing the biomechanics of the human form, for example by relating the structure of the human form to tensegrity structures.

Architecturally, structures that are strung together from the inside as opposed to being

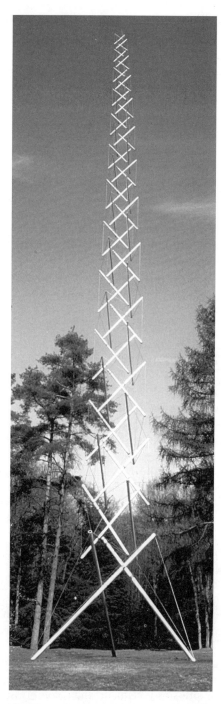

Figure 5.2

Tensegrity structure. Neville Tower II (1969) Aluminium & Stainless Steel 30 × 6 × 6 m. Collection: Kröller Müller Museum, Otterlo, Holland. Photo: Kröller Müller Museum.

'piled up' like a stack of bricks fall under the umbrella term of **tensegrity structures**. Figure 5.2 shows a tensegrity structure.

As shall be described, the human body is a form of tensegrity structure (Robbie, 1977) and viewing the body in this way is of great value to osteopaths as it provides an understanding for much of what we observe, and has many ramifications in the way we examine and treat people.

(Note: This may be the first time some osteopaths have viewed the body in this way and it is hoped that it will clarify and not confuse their views of biomechanics!).

TENSEGRITY

The following discussion should bring home the curious nature of tensegrity structures: that they are held together by components that are trying to pull the structure apart! Human beings have previously been studied as 'compressional' structures when it comes to biomechanics (as in the pile of bricks mentioned above), which has often caused quite a few conundrums, because it is not clear in such an arrangement how the tissues of the body withstand the compressive forces supposedly acting upon them. Reviewing the relevance of tensegrity concepts to human biomechanics might go some way to solving such conundrums.

Synergy in tensegrity structures

When tensional and compressional materials are used together in a truly complementary way, they form structures that can bear loads far exceeding estimates based on traditional structural analysis. Tensegrity structures often appear delicate but are surprisingly strong and resilient. When tensional and compressional elements are used together this is called **synergy**. Synergy in a structure also means (oddly, perhaps) that the behaviour of the whole is unpredicted by the behaviour of its parts when considered separately. When one part of a tensegrity structure moves, the reaction to this is not isolated but permeates through the whole of the rest of the structure virtually simultaneously (Salvadori, 1980).

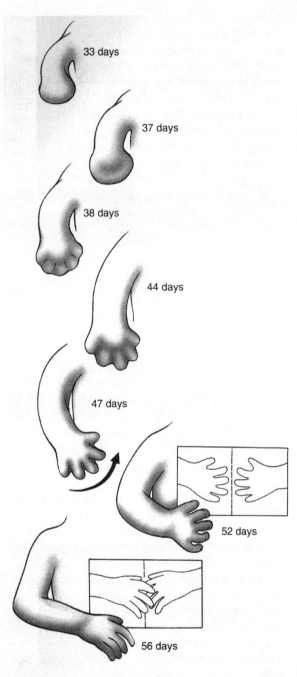

Figure 5.3

The development of the upper and lower limb buds occurs between the fifth and the eighth week of intrauterine life. The limb buds push outwards from the body cell and elongate into recognizable limbs. (Reproduced with the permission of Churchill Livingstone, from Human Embryology, Larson, 1993.)

To appreciate this, consider another example of a tensegrity structure: a spider's web. Pull on one part of the web and the rest moves: a spider sitting anywhere can sense immediately 'where' its meal has arrived! (This is an analogy that will be returned to during a discussion of examination and treatment techniques used by osteopaths, later in the book.)

This inter-relatedness caused by synergy is one reason why the current methods of studying biomechanics, which look at isolated segments of the body, are somewhat flawed, as they are not complex enough to account for all components.

Tension and compression components in the human form

To appreciate the nature/form of tensional and compressional components within the human framework, let us look at the way the body forms during embryology.

As a limb (for example) grows, the bones (in the form of cartilaginous precursors) are laid down first. The bones literally 'push out' the shell of the embryo so that the limb buds expand laterally from the core structure of the embryo. This is illustrated in Figure 5.3, and Figure 5.4 shows the changes within the limb buds that form bones and joints.

Embryologically, bone grows outwards, i.e. it expands into the mesenchymal tissue within the limb. Bone acts as a stiffener to the structure – and therefore is analogous to the compressional rods in a tensegrity structure. In fact, the choice of the word 'compressional' can be misleading, as, although these elements are certainly compressed along their length, it is also equally important to state that they provide an expansive force along their length – i.e. they 'push outwards', as stated earlier. Bone is therefore not built simply to withstand compressional force, but to act as a reinforcer to other, softer, tissues. So, 'stiffeners' is a much better term to apply to the compressional elements than 'compressional'!

Developmentally, although there are cartilaginous precursors to bone, the 'adult' structure of the 'bony' components (i.e. ossification) of the limb actually forms last (indeed ossification of some

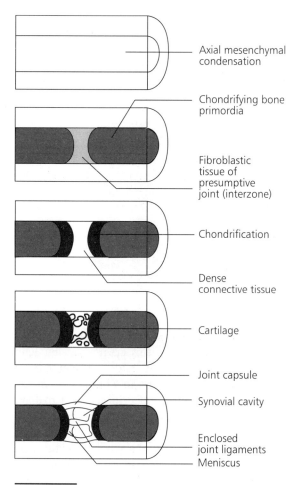

- Axial mesenchymal condensation
- Chondrifying bone primordia
- Fibroblastic tissue of presumptive joint (interzone)
- Chondrification
- Dense connective tissue
- Cartilage
- Joint capsule
- Synovial cavity
- Enclosed joint ligaments
- Meniscus

Figure 5.4

Formation of joints. Cartilage, ligaments and capsular elements of the joints develop from the interzone regions of the axial mesenchymal condensations that form the long bones of the limbs. (Reproduced with the permission of Churchill Livingstone, from Human Embryology, *Larson, 1993.)*

bones is not complete until many years after birth). The relevance of this point to growth and clinical practice will be discussed later in this chapter.

The muscles, accompanied by or encased in fascial/connective tissue 'bags' or 'sleeves', migrate from the proximal part of the limb and become attached to various parts of the bony precursors. The muscles and fascial structures elongate by passive stretching caused by the continued expansion of the 'bones'.

In this way these soft tissue elements (including the developing neurovascular bundle) can act as restraints to limb expansion. The muscles and fascial sheaths are therefore a type of tensional component within the structure, in the adult as well as the embryo.

Cursorily skipping past further embryological discussion at this stage, one can use this concept of bones as stiffeners within soft tissue membranes to give an illustration of how man stands up. (Note: This is the analogy that was 'borrowed' and used in the preceding chapter.)

Tensegrity illustration of how a man stands up

Take one flat, baggy, soft man (like a deflated balloon). Now, start inserting rods in him, like the poles in a tent. These rods (bones) fix on to points on certain membranes inside the floppy man. There are no external guy ropes for this tent-man, only the internal ones formed by the membranes as they are pulled taut by the insertion of the bones. Gradually, as all the bones are in place, the man is beginning to stand. If you lengthen the bones enough, i.e. make them 'push out' more, they will straighten out the membrane of the man and make it tense. This tenseness will then reciprocally help the bones stay orientated in the right direction by pulling against the bone like a guy rope. Thus the membranes always pull against their points of attachments (like muscles and fascia on to bone) and so they have to be able to resist this constant pull. The bones, under the influence of the compression acting along their length, have to resist internal buckling and so have to be relatively dense. These ideas are shown in Figure 5.5.

Examples of this tension–compression balance occur throughout the human form; two examples are shown in Figures 5.6 and 5.7, which give schematic views of the shoulder girdle and the hip joint respectively.

Returning to our 'man': if the membranes are elastic, then the whole arrangement is very springy and able to withstand tremendous external pressures acting on the whole of the structure while only a little bit of that force is applicable to each individual part (as all force is simultaneously spread through the whole structure, wherever it

Figure 5.5

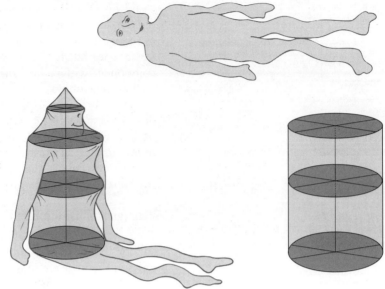

The 'rubber-tent' man. **A.** Imagine a deflated rubber man, lying flat on the ground. **B.** Now imagine a series of rods being inserted within the rubber skin of the man. These rods push out the skin so that the man begins to stand. Instead of being inflated by air, the shape of the man is formed by the rubber membrane being pushed taut by internal rods. **C.** Inside the trunk, limbs and head a series of horizontal membranes within the rubber skin of the man help to divide the man into compartments. These are expanded by the insertion of the rods that are helping the man to stand upright.

is applied from). Elastic membranes make for a very 'resilient' structure. The membranes are in fact made up of muscles, ligaments, tendons and connective tissues

So, our tent-man is a stable, shock-absorbing structure, but he can't move!

It is interesting to note that muscles are not used as the main structural membranes of the body: the connective tissues are. This is because if these muscles were to contract they would pull on the bones (stiffeners) and, as soon as one part was tensed, this would make the structure as a whole tighter. In this way movement becomes more and more impossible the more muscles are contracted to try to create it. (Tense muscles make you immobile: a fact that probably doesn't surprise many!)

Muscles and joints

How can this inertia be overcome? The simplest way to achieve this is to section the compressional rods. Remember that in a standard tensegrity structure the 'bones' would be trying not to buckle. Placing a joint in the bone is the same as creating a break in the compressional rod. Now the bone is free to buckle, the 'stranglehold' of the muscle is 'broken' and movement follows.

The conundrum caused by having joints

Clearly, the movement this creates is a bit haphazard: adding a joint adds an element of instability to the structure, in which the joint can be viewed as a 'weak link'. Joints need to have limits placed upon them, and their 'available movement' and 'play' need to be stabilized, if they are not to weaken the whole structure too fundamentally. Joint capsules and ligaments help to splint the joint, while the muscles create movement by acting in different planes to the membranes/fascial sheaths of the body.

In truth, muscles can also act as stabilizers to joint function, but are not designed to do so over protracted periods of time, whereas the membranous/fascial sheaths **are** designed to do this. Muscle actions are complex and diverse, often act over more than one joint, and work both as stabilizers and prime movers, depending on the action required and the plane in which they are working.

Increasing the number of movement possibilities required from a limb or part means increasing the number of joints within that part and consequently the potential instability caused by having many joints.

Obviously any instability created by moving any one joint has to be counterbalanced by

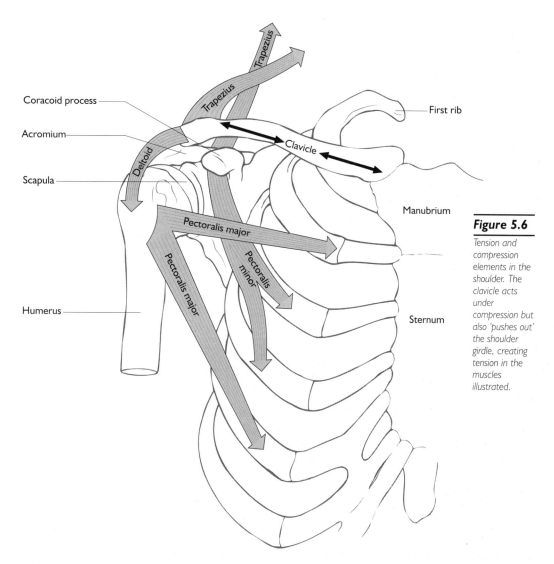

Figure 5.6

Tension and compression elements in the shoulder. The clavicle acts under compression but also 'pushes out' the shoulder girdle, creating tension in the muscles illustrated.

activity in other parts of the tensegrity structure. To cope with this, many muscles work in concert, and on more than one joint at a time. As stated above, some muscles will tense one part of the limb/body area, ensuring its stability, while other muscles move a particular individual joint.

Multisectional rods
The greater the number of joints in an original compressional rod and the greater the number of movement possibilities that are required, the more finely balanced this interplay of the component parts needs to be.

The spine is the largest multisectional rod in the body, and it has very many muscles acting on its component parts. Small locally acting muscles around two adjacent structures will affect one section of the rod, but in doing so can also affect the movement of all the rest of it. This is shown in Figure 5.8.

Also, some of the muscles acting on the spine, such as the scalenes acting on the cervical spine and the psoas on the lumbar spine, do so in a direction that can compress it. The spine is curved, and in this situation the scalenes and psoas act a bit like a bowstring to a bow: they buckle the

Figure 5.7

Tension and compression elements in the hip. The femoral neck acts under compression but also 'pushes out' the hip girdle musculature, creating tension in the muscles illustrated.

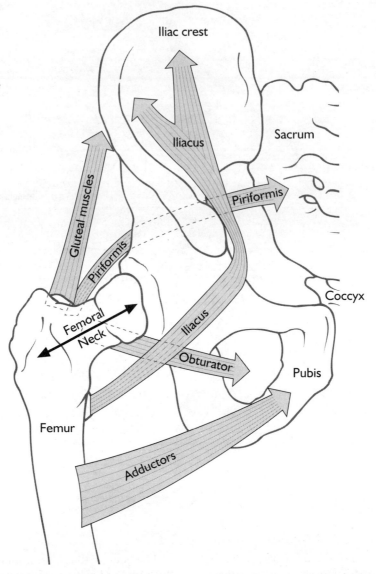

structure. This is counteracted in the bow by the spring in the bow arms. In the spine it is counteracted by the action of other muscles, such as the locally acting erector spinae muscles or the integrated action of the various abdominal/trunk muscles. Therefore there is a balancing act between all the different muscles acting on the spine.

Viewing the whole body as a set of interconnected multisectional rods

Looking at the whole body, the spine is balanced on two other multisectional rods (the legs), via the pelvis; and the spine also has two multisectional rods (the arms) hanging off it, and the multicomponent rib cage. All these parts are inter-related and the effects of movement in one part can be quite diverse. In real life, then, the human form is potentially not the most stable tensegrity structure that could be envisaged – indicating that the control mechanisms for muscle action need to be complex (Johansson and Magnusson, 1991).

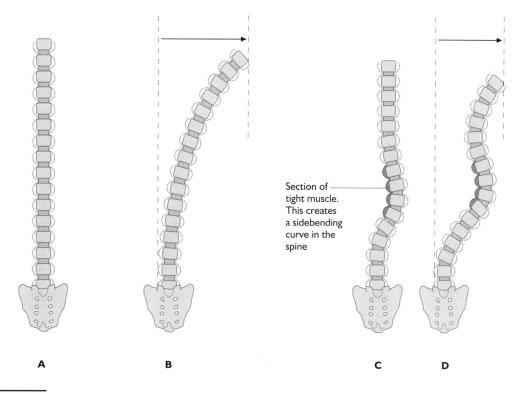

Section of
tight muscle.
This creates
a sidebending
curve in the
spine

A   **B**   **C**   **D**

Figure 5.8

*Multisectioned rods. When a multisectioned rod (**A**) is sidebent, as in **B**., there is a degree of lateral deviation from the midline. If there is a section of tension in a multisectioned rod, a small area of sidebending is created (**C**). Now, when this rod is sidebent, as in **D**., there is a smaller lateral deviation from the midline. In other words, a curve in a section of the spine limits the overall range of movement.*

These control mechanisms (mediated within the nervous system) were discussed in Chapter 4. However, the connective tissues (fascia, tendons, ligaments and so on) also help to bind structures together and coordinate movement patterns, and as such need some introduction.

Connective tissue function in relation to locomotion

Connective tissues bind us together and form supportive sheets and membranes within us, as previously hinted at. Connective tissue is physically important to the body in many different ways. (The physiological importance of connective tissues was discussed in Chapter 4.)

The mechanical/physical functions of connective tissues are:

- absorption
- support and leverage
- synergy.

Absorption

Connective tissues do not initiate movement within the body but tend to absorb movement and, as they are pliable and elastic, can help to dissipate any irregularities that slightly uneven muscle activity creates. Thus the state of the connective tissue is crucial as a 'damping down' structure to awkward movement.

Note: Muscles can also absorb forces but they use energy to do so. Fascial planes and ligaments are inherently elastic (because of their histological arrangement) and they do not require energy to provide support or absorb forces. This is clearly much more efficient for the body as a whole than resorting to using muscles.

However, if the muscle or its fascial sheath is too tight or inelastic, then the structure does not have the same capacity to absorb shock and force. Hence in a 'stiff' person, whose tissues are not regularly stretched out and so kept elastic, muscle and soft tissue tearing and rupture is more likely than in some very supple and pliable individual. Poorly 'damped-down' forces often lead to such things as muscle tears and other soft tissue injuries.

Support and leverage

Connective tissues/fascia can form specific anatomical structures such as the 'rectus sheath' and the 'thoracolumbar fascia', which support the rectus abdominis and the erector spinae muscles, respectively, and in doing so help the actions of these muscles by giving them something to 'push/lever' against. In order to appreciate the 'balancing act' that fascia/connective sheaths can perform, we need to complete our picture of how the human body is stacked up and arranged.

The previous analogy used in the discussions on tensegrity was that man was made up from membranes, with stiffeners (bones), somewhat like a tent with its poles. If we consider our tent man to be three-dimensional, with many different membranous (fascial) sheets being interconnected, and all of this being stiffened out at some strategic places, then we end up with many pockets and enclosed spaces throughout our man.

These pockets are not empty, and if we fill up some of the spaces with various soft and relatively incompressible structures (such as organs) and the rest with fluid, we have in effect 'inflated' our man by filling him up and *voilà*! – he stands! This is illustrated in Figure 5.9.

Fluid-filled spaces and support

As indicated in Figure 5.9, all these 'fluidic' parts provide a degree of 'pushing out' to counteract compressive or 'collapsing' forces within the structure. This makes the man very much more

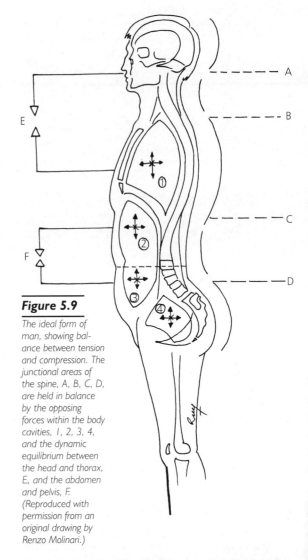

Figure 5.9

The ideal form of man, showing balance between tension and compression. The junctional areas of the spine, A, B, C, D, are held in balance by the opposing forces within the body cavities, 1, 2, 3, 4, and the dynamic equilibrium between the head and thorax, E, and the abdomen and pelvis, F. (Reproduced with permission from an original drawing by Renzo Molinari.)

stable as a structure, and able to withstand many forces. Having these relatively incompressible structures/areas to 'push against' adds tension to the fascial structures and means that they can be much more effective in providing greater leverage for the muscular system to act against without being damaged.

The way the abdomen helps posture and minimizes forces in the lumbar spine is a good example of this. The diaphragm and the abdominal muscles, aided by the pelvic floor muscles, can 'push against' the abdominal viscera, which are relatively incompressible. This causes a counter pressure against which the abdominal muscles can create tension in the thoracolumbar fascia, providing controlled leverage for the erector spinae muscles and at the same time forming a binding, stabilizing sheath for the vertebral column, to prevent the forces used during erector spinae contraction from levering the joints apart.

Clinical application
Clearly, any weakness in the fascial sheaths, abdominal muscles, diaphragm or pelvic floor muscles reduces the cooperative relationship between these structures, meaning that a good compressive force cannot be uniformly directed to the abdominal contents, so that the required stabilizing counter pressure is not set up, thus reducing the effectiveness of the stabilizing erector spinae sheath. This results in stress and strain to the lumbar vertebral articulations and surrounding soft tissues.

Conversely, if the thoracolumbar fascial sheaths are too tight, then the erector spinae muscles and multifidus could suffer a type of compartment syndrome – where, as they bunch up during contraction, they cut off their own blood supply. In this scenario, too much pressure builds up in the fascial sheath, which is in effect too small/won't expand to accommodate the bunched up muscle. This results in muscle ischaemia, pain and dysfunction.

Synergy (interconnection between parts)
In standard tensegrity structures, the tensional and the compressional components are individual structures that are sectioned together. One can easily dismantle the structure into its component parts. Synergy was described as relating to the interconnectedness of parts – movement in one area is immediately transferable to another area.

Synergy in humans is aided by the fact that there is often a fine line between where connective tissue structures such as tendons and ligaments (the tensional components) end and where bone (the compressional component) begins, adding to the whole concept of interconnectedness.

If one takes hold of one part of the body and moves it, this motion will be dissipated through the structure. Watching and feeling how this movement is transmitted gives a good indication of the elasticity and pliability within body parts both local to and quite distant from the point of contact. If an area of the body is restricted in some way, this can be appreciated from a distant point of contact as it alters the way that the induced motion is transmitted. The person initiating the motion can detect this (as it feels different from 'normal'/'expected' movement) and it gives them clinically significant information as to the state of the structure of that body. In other words, an assessment of the structural integrity of the person can be 'tested' by movement evaluation from an isolated part of the body (although osteopaths generally test several parts, so gaining as good a three-dimensional picture of integrity or dysfunction as possible).

Such ideas are the basis of many evaluatory techniques and also some therapeutic manipulations used by osteopaths. These will be discussed in more detail in a later chapter.

When connective tissues were discussed before, it was in their capacity as elements of the extracellular matrix and the cytoskeleton. The role of these tissue matrices was discussed with respect to fluid dynamics, cellular health and immunity, and signalling mechanisms. What was not discussed was the idea that movement itself can adapt and alter the structure of the ECM, so potentially adapting the physiological processes carried out by those components.

As already stated, the idea that structure and function are interlinked is central to osteopathic belief systems. The connective tissue systems of the body are incredible in their capacity to adapt their internal structure and thus their functional capability. This has many clinical corollaries, which we will attempt to uncover. First, though, we need to take one more look at how humans stand up, and how the arrangement of the human form helps us to stand upright, and function as an integral whole.

HUMANS AND GRAVITY

The architectural arrangement of the human form is specially adapted so that it can act as a springy, sensitive system acting under tensegrity principles. In this way man can function with strain and stress evenly distributed through all parts of the body, without accumulating at any one point of the locomotor system, or indeed in any other part of the body.

One of the greatest forces acting on the human framework is that of gravity, and were it not for the interlinking system of bones, ligaments and connective tissue structures, coupled with the relatively incompressible fluid- and organ-filled cavities of the body, then humans would not counter gravitation stress very well. All of these factors stabilize the human form, enabling us to stand upright and also allowing for the support of the spinal vertebral column to be efficient. This is shown in Figure 5.9, which shows the dynamic interaction of forces through the body. Within this system, the vertebral column is evenly supported and can function as a spring through the coupling action of its curves with the tissues of the rest of the body.

Around the external aspects of the body several structures combine as tensional components, spreading load: the thoracolumbar fascia, the erector spinae muscles, the nuchal ligament, the prevertebral fascia, the manubriosternum, the abdominal muscles, the iliotibial tract, the plantar fascia of the foot, the Achilles tendon of the calf, the hamstring muscles and gluteal muscles, through to the ligamentous arrangement of the pelvis, through to the thoracolumbar fascia.

Internally, the prevertebral fascia links to the deep fascia of the neck, and through the internal mediastinal fascia (supporting the heart and lungs) to the diaphragm. From here the peritoneum of the viscera, and the psoas muscles, dissipate forces through to the pelvic girdle and the hip joints, and so out again into the external system of support in the legs. Within the thorax, the relatively negative forces of the lungs are balanced by the external tensional components acting around the thorax, and balanced out by the 'pushing out' or relatively incompressible forces acting in and around the heart. Within the abdomen, the relatively positive pressures of the abdominal viscera will 'push out' the abdominal walls and engage the external tensional components of the rectus sheath and thus the thoracolumbar fascia, which aids the posterior supportive mechanisms.

Again, internally, the membranes within the cranium and spinal column, the dura and meninges, act as another tensional system of tissues balancing out forces acting within this innermost part of our being.

Spinal support

All these forces acting together support the body and its internal structures and make up the whole picture of support for the spinal vertebral column. Spinal biomechanics cannot be explored without reference to these other factors, and this view of whole-body support and integral functioning represents a major contribution from the osteopathic profession to the rest of the community.

The spine, then, acts as a springing system of interacting curves, within a framework of external tensional components and internally acting tension and compression dynamics (Levin, 1995).

Gravitational forces are balanced out only if the whole body acts in concert. If for any reason (injury, illness, surgery, emotional distress, fatigue and so on) the postural dynamics of the body are altered, then the finely balanced tensegrity forces will begin to fail. If all parts of the body do not work in synergy, then stress and strain will not be evenly distributed and extra strain on the connective tissue components results. Altered load-bearing follows as biomechanical balance shifts, and increasing muscular workload is required to try to maintain some sort of balance and as effective a motion pattern as possible. All of this can eventually lead to symptoms, both within the musculoskeletal system and in the internal organs of the body (as cavity dynamics are also adapted). This latter point will be taken up in Chapter 9.

With regard to symptoms in the musculo-skeletal system, these can be many and varied. Also, the important point to remember is that the area of dysfunction that sets off the chain of events of postural decompensation is usually not where the person eventually suffers the symptoms of this consequence. The problems can start anywhere and end anywhere. This is the nature of tensegrity structures, and underpins the osteopathic concept of whole-body examination and management for whatever symptom. You simply cannot have dysfunction in isolated parts and believe the effects will only be local.

Myofascial strain

One of the manifestations of this postural decompensation, as already indicated, will be **myofascial strain** throughout the body (Kuchera, 1995). This leads to muscular strain and incoordination, and to connective tissue strain (through its non-linear and viscoelastic responses to load). These changes lead to widespread **somatic dysfunction**, which is a term originally coined by osteopaths for the asymmetry, restricted motion and tissue texture changes palpable in certain pathophysiological states. The term has been adopted by orthopaedic physicians and is now recognized in the International Classification of Disease as a codable diagnosis by region of the body.

Myofascial dysfunction/strain, including myofascial trigger points, is a specific form of somatic dysfunction with subjective pain and recordable weakness and autonomic and vascular-lymphatic characteristics. Treatment of myofascial strain can be by general body manipulations or by the treatment of various trigger points located within the dysfunctional tissues. Trigger-point treatment is now a widespread therapeutic intervention throughout the manipulative and orthodox professions.

Trigger-point treatment will not be covered here but it is useful to consider the wider implications (i.e. throughout the whole body) of connective tissue responses to changes in biomechanics and movement, which can lead to distress in all body parts and tissues through the extensive fascial planes of the body and the extracellular and intracellular components supporting all our tissues.

How movement may change connective tissue structure

To appreciate the effects of physical force on the connective tissues, the role of fibroblasts needs to be reviewed.

Fibroblasts

Fibroblasts interact and work with all connective tissues of the body, from the extracellular matrix to bone formation and remodelling. Fibroblasts make sure that the structure of the tissue is suitable to its needs.

The action of body movement on connective tissues and fibroblast activity is very interesting and offers a route whereby altered body movement may affect cellular level activity. Also, it provides a mechanism through which osteopathic manipulation may have powerful and direct effects.

Fibroblasts were mentioned in Chapter 3 but the implications of their ability to alter structure in response to physical loads and injury (inflammation) have not yet been explored. Regardless of whether they are aware of it at the time, anyone who manipulates a tissue is communicating directly with fibroblasts and is having a direct effect on cellular activity!

Tensile/physical forces and fibroblast activity

For further discussion of this subject see Pender and McCulloch, 1991; Baskin *et al.*, 1993a, b; Alberts *et al.*, 1994; Lodish, 1995.

We have described how the ECM and cell junctions must adapt to strain – it is the fibroblasts that detect stretch and strain, and that lay down collagen in differing amounts, rendering the tissue either 'more stretchy' or 'less stretchy' in various directions. If a fibroblast detects motion in three dimensions, then it will lay down collagen to resist stretch and movement in these planes. This means the collagen is laid down in an irregular arrangement. This gives strength in all directions but no one direction more than another. It also gives the tissue uniform elasticity.

If a tissue is only moved in a certain way, or strain applied to it acts most of the time in just one or two directions, then the fibroblasts react accordingly and lay down collagen that will resist movement in those directions. The collagen fibres will be aligned in parallel, and the tissue will become very 'inelastic' in that orientation. Fibroblasts orientate collagen according to applied mechanical stress.

If the tissue needed to become fully pliable again, then the fibroblasts would need to be re-stimulated. This would require a constant new pull acting on the tissue to stimulate the fibroblasts to lay down new collagen in new directions to allow a more three-dimensional motion than before.

Disease processes and injury also direct fibroblasts to act differently and lay down extra/new collagen. Inflammation (which we will discuss below) is often the trigger for this (Smith *et al.*, 1997).

Tissue compliance

Through the above mechanisms fibroblasts direct the natural compliance and elasticity of a tissue.

Compliance in a tissue is a measure of the state of the ECM and its potential influence on all the cell functions, mechanisms and fluid dynamics we discussed above. The clinical importance of this statement cannot be overestimated.

PALPATION OF TISSUES TO DETECT THEIR PHYSIOLOGICAL EFFICIENCY

Osteopathic palpation should be a reflection of the underlying state of the tissues and an interpretation of their capacity for function. When examining someone osteopaths look for movement possibilities within tissues, and any disturbance of normal motion within a tissue. The following discussion on palpation and interpretation of findings needs to be kept in mind for the

section on inflammation below, as inflammation also affects the palpatory state of tissues.

Clinical perspective on palpatory findings

Interpreting findings

If osteopaths find areas of stiffness within tissues, they look at the biomechanical arrangement of that area of the body and consider how it is co-ordinated with whole-body movement. If the body is not being used effectively, and in multiple directions and patterns, then it is unlikely that all the tissues of its component parts are being sufficiently stretched. Therefore, it is likely that this non-engagement of the tissues (and their ECMs) will maintain stiffness within the tissue (as the fibroblast has no stimulus for change).

Relevance for the patient

However, the converse is true: if a person wants to move their body in a new way and has not done this for a while, then the 'directional stiffness' that is 'preset' within their tissues will not allow them to do so. This means that they can overstrain their insufficiently elastic tissues if the movement is forced, and that they should gradually 'work on their fibroblasts' by doing smaller repetitive stretches in the desired direction to help 'convert' the connective tissues to allow motion and suppleness in that plane of action.

The effects of trauma and long-standing movement problems

The patterns of movement restriction within the body are called 'lesion patterns' in osteopathic parlance. 'Lesion patterns' are the gross expressions of connective tissue adaptation and are therefore external representations of the fibroblast map of our internal structure.

'Lesion patterns', once established, can often 'freeze' you in time, so that if you want to move subsequently you can't do so in the same way as before. A 'lesion' is often some sort of trauma that has shocked the body in some way, or injured it (causing post inflammatory stiffness that we will mention below), or caused a muscle reaction that then remains adapted, or left pain or fearful emotional associations that have the effect of making the person avoid movement of that part. 'Lesions' can be many things, but each time they engage the connective tissue structures and so adapt our structure and function capabilities.

The effect of them is that some areas of the body are moved less than they should be (and often other areas then have to move more, to compensate). In this way, some parts become chronically fixed and some become relatively unstable, simply through remodelling of connective tissue structures.

This gives a pattern of restriction that is a unique history of the trials and tribulations suffered by that person.

Relevance for the practitioner

On examining a body, then, the osteopath can reflect on the patterns and extent of tissue compliance and relate this to the traumas, injuries, body postures and ergonomic factors in the person's lifestyle, to work out (a) how the tensions might have come along in the first place and (b) how much of the body they might need to work on to restore overall biomechanical efficiency.

The state of the tissue compliance dictates whether this will take a long time or a short time and helps to indicate what type of manipulative procedure would be the most effective. For example, in chronic lesion patterns, stretching and other soft tissue techniques might be more successful than high-velocity thrust manipulations (which seem to have a more neurally mediated effect).

This does not represent all the palpatory repertoire of osteopaths, but at least gives an example.

INFLAMMATION

Inflammation also has an effect on ECM compliance and fibroblast activity (Smith *et al.*, 1997). It is a complex phenomenon and one that is not completely understood. There are a whole range of inflammatory mediators whose function is not clear, and new subtleties and interactions are being discovered all the time.

Inflammation is one of the most fundamental defence reactions of the body, and is basically non-specific – you get a similar response in reaction to a whole variety of traumas, insults and irritating/infective agents.

There are two main types of inflammatory response, acute and chronic, which have subtle but important distinguishing features (Cawson *et al.*, 1982). The following is a selective description of inflammation, to help with the general theme of the chapter. Readers should look elsewhere for a complete analysis of the subject.

Acute inflammation

Acute inflammation is characterized by vasodilation, increased vascular permeability, increased heat production, increased tenderness and swelling. This response is mediated by various substances, such as prostaglandins, bradykinin, vasoactive amines and cytokines (including interleukins, interferons and growth factors). These trigger a variety of responses, and the damaged tissue fills up with fluid, to bring in as many immunological factors as possible; the area is sealed off (by fibroblast activity) and the tissue is gradually healed. Thereafter all responses should revert to normal and leave the tissue much as it was before.

However, the effect of acute inflammation on fibroblasts is important as this controls the level of tissue fibrosis in response to the insult and can provoke tissue scarring if required.

Chronic inflammation

This may be a sequel to acute inflammation or it may appear without a preceding acute phase. It is characterized by less tenderness, less or more localized swelling (which tends to be firmer than in acute inflammation) and less heat. It is much less dramatic to observe but no less powerful in effect. Indeed, the sequelae of chronic inflammation can be quite devastating to tissue function.

Whereas acute inflammation is characterized by an exudative phase and a cellular phase (where the neutrophil is the typical active cell), chronic inflammation is largely a cellular response in which the lymphocyte, the plasma cell, the macrophage and the fibroblast predominate.

Complications of chronic inflammation

The chronic inflammatory response can be thought of as a 'no-win' contest between the causal stimulus and the protective response. The persistent nature of the inflammatory response results in slow tissue destruction or distortion despite the body's attempts at fibroblastic repair. Indeed it is these 'poorly directed' attempts by the fibroblast that lead to a stiff, resistant, 'overcrowded' and distorted ECM web, which makes normal cellular function difficult and impedes both fluid dynamics and immune cell mobility. All these consequences lead to poor tissue health and function, which can become increasingly clinically significant.

Palpation and manipulation of inflamed tissues

Testing tissue pliability, examining for heat, tenderness and swelling and looking for areas of altered compliance tissue reactivity and fibrosis are all part of an osteopath's normal routine (as they are for many other practitioners).

Physically mobilizing the tissues and the surrounding structures may lead to a re-adaptation of the extracellular matrix and the general connective tissue throughout the area (or at the very least to re-establishment of some of the inherent elasticity and pliability of these elements) and have a beneficial effect upon the mobility of fluid through the area. Clinically, wherever there is chronic inflammation there are recognizable palpatory changes such as oedema and reduced elasticity and pliability of the tissues. A few moments of manipulation, stretch and massage is often enough to disperse this fluid, increase the mobility of the tissue and seemingly normalize the tone of the muscular structures, leading to a reduction in symptoms and improvement of subsequent

function in the structure involved. However, long-term reorganization of such tissues can take many weeks and months of mobilization by the practitioner, and stretching and exercise by the patient concerned. The person literally needs to relearn a more effective movement pattern – one that engages the stiff tissues and keeps stimulating the fibroblasts to readapt the tissue structure.

In cases of chronic tissue pathology or tendency to recurrent bacterial infection, it may well be useful to mobilize the affected tissues with the aim of restoring more effective immune function therein, thus helping the body's own self-healing and regulatory mechanisms to deal with the pathology/chronic infection. As mentioned before, care needs to be taken in such cases, and there could be some strong relative contraindications. Only a sound knowledge of pathological mechanisms and tissue physiology will enable a safe intervention by the practitioner to be given. It is a wise practitioner who knows when not to treat.

Acutely inflamed tissue is mobilized quite differently from chronically inflamed tissue. Acutely inflamed tissue needs gentle techniques to subtly disperse fluids, and gentle rhythmic motion to reduce pain and relax muscle 'guarding'/spasm. Chronically inflamed tissue requires a slightly more active process whereby the tissues are stretched and mobilized more directly with the aim of improving tissue (and ECM) mobility. Muscular action needs to be stimulated, to get the area mobilized through active movement of the patient and to trigger a better neural control over the area.

Note: Chronically inflamed areas are often moved less, which of course leads to increasing connective tissue stiffness. However, it also leads to a decrease in proprioceptive afferent signals passing to the cord and central nervous system. This leads to a long-term adaptation of neural control, in that the brain first learns not to use that part (because of the pain or irritation) and then, because it hasn't moved it for so long, 'forgets about it' and reorganizes the patterning control to 'dis-include' that part in any ongoing movement.

The above is a very loose description of a poorly understood mechanism. However, the adaptive and relearning processes that go on through rehabilitation are gradually being investigated and the need for retraining of the nervous system through changing activity in the periphery (by manipulation and patient-performed active exercises) is gaining increasing acceptance.

Other clinical perspectives on inflammation, oedematous states and neural consequences are given later in the book.

SUMMARY SO FAR

The arrangement and architectural form of the human body has been discussed both to illustrate the need for dynamic controls of motion and to illustrate how motion passes through all tissues of the body in a synergistic/simultaneous way. The movement passing through the tissues plays a role in maintaining the structural make-up of that tissue, and if the structure should change (as a result of immobility on some part of the structure, disease or traumatic episodes) then it can limit ongoing motion and effective physiology/immunity within those tissues.

BONES: FORMATION AND REMODELLING

It is not just the extracellular matrix that can adapt in this way, though. Bones can also re-model, and this has interesting consequences for biomechanics and locomotion, especially when one reflects on growth within the human form.

Details of the embryology of musculoskeletal formation were briefly given earlier, as an aid to the discussion of the human body as a tensegrity structure. It is clear that bodies change dramatically in shape and size as we grow rapidly from babies, to infants, to children and to adults. Even as adults, although the external forms of bones, for example, do not change much, the individual component parts of bone are being continually turned over and our bones continue to 'grow'/'live' while being continuously subjected

to diverse physical forces. There are some very interesting clinical correlations to this, which it would be opportune to discuss here.

One might think that the structure of bones is very fixed, that they are quite unchangeable in structure unless you happen to fracture one and that bone can resist force with no alteration to its own physical structure. However, living bone is much more malleable and plastic than one might suspect from looking at preserved specimens.

On dissection it can be practically impossible to dissect a ligament away from the bone to which it is attached without damaging the bone and taking the periosteum with it. Because of the merging of connective tissue into bone, forces acting through the ligament will be immediately transferred to the bone, and it has to be able to resist them.

Bone is simply a 'continuation' of ligaments, tendons and fascia that have become 'stiffened' in response to load.

Bone formation

In mammalian evolution, the shapes of the bones have evolved in response to the tensions and pulls acting on them from soft tissue structures. In balanced efficient movement, the pulls on the bones are ones that the bone has been structured to withstand (Lovejoy, 1988).

When we previously discussed posture and locomotion, and the architectural arrangement of the human form, we used a tensegrity analogy and illustrated this with a floppy 'tent' man who was 'stiffened' by rods to make him taut and so stand up. If the man/structure as a whole is balanced, then the diversity of pulls acting through the soft tissue ('tensional components') on to the bones ('stiffeners'/'rods') is equal and the bones will remain 'stable'.

To appreciate the potential effects of soft tissue forces on bone, one must revisit embryology and consider the stages of growth at which bones ossify, before their shape becomes 'set'.

Embryology
We previously mentioned that bones form as soft cartilaginous structures that gradually expanded

against a variety of forces created, for example, by the passive resistance in muscles inserting on to the bones. The cartilaginous 'bones' expand and gradually begin to ossify.

In the limbs at birth, for example, the diaphyses or shafts of the limb bones (consisting of a bone collar and a trabecular core) are completely ossified, whereas the ends of the bones (called the epiphyses) are still cartilaginous. After birth, secondary ossification centres develop in the epiphyses, which gradually ossify. Ossification does not happen universally in all bones at the same time, nor in all parts of the same bone at the same time, with some bones (or parts thereof) remaining cartilaginous until at least 20 years of age.

This growth arrangement clearly does not stop the moment you are born – the adult skeleton has grown and changed considerably in shape and size compared to that of the neonate. As the bones continue to develop, a layer of cartilage called the epiphyseal cartilage plate (growth plate) persists between the epiphysis and the growing end of the diaphysis. Continued proliferation of the chondrocytes in this growth plate allows both lengthening of the diaphysis and emergence of the final adult shape of the bones.

Such changing shapes include the neck of the femur, the skull, the angulation of the spheno-basilar junction, the curves in the spine and the rotation/longitudinal torsion of the long limb bones.

During growth of the musculoskeletal system, muscles and tendons are stretched and these pressures and deformations in the muscular system tissues influence the subsequent development of bones. The interdependence between muscle and bone formation is therefore tied to the interaction of forces generated and imposed upon the complete complement of well-integrated tissues that comprise the musculoskeletal system (Carter et al., 1991).

During this growing and moulding phase, uneven, unbalanced or slightly disrupted biomechanics throughout the body and lower limb may eventually lead to a moderate adaptation of the final architectural structure of the bones, which could lead to the articular surfaces being oriented in a less than optimum direction, as they are close to the growth plate, the area most prone to distortion.

Osteopathic perspective

Many children have muscular tensions and tight/tense areas of fascia within their bodies, even when very young. Muscles could 'limit' or hold back this expansion if they were too tight or did not elongate at the right rate. Trying to grow evenly through all this tension must place some constraints on normal bone expansion. Even if the shape of articular facets is subsequently only slightly modified, or the length of limb bones is not quite symmetrical, then this is thought to have significant repercussions on biomechanical forces later in life.

Paediatric osteopathy

Osteopaths specializing in paediatric osteopathy (the care of children) feel that this type of consideration is particularly important in the growing skull. Problems of poor expansion within the skull (after the normal moulding and folding of the skull plates during birth and their attempted re-expansion after delivery) are thought to be particularly important to resolve, as they could potentially contribute to many neurological and developmental problems, both in the neonatal period and later in life (Magoun, 1976).

Sutherland, an American osteopath, coined the analogy of the body being like a twig that bends: a twig that is flexible enough to bend is more resilient than one that is rigid and therefore brittle. Freedom from tension at a connective tissue level ensures that the body is flexible, can bend (like the twig) and so escape stress and strain as it grows (Sutherland, 1990).

Even in adulthood, such analogies are not irrelevant.

Bone remodelling

Throughout the life of a bone remodelling is a normal process, and adaptation to imposed stress may help the bone develop an effective internal architecture that can resist and absorb a variety of strains.

Stresses developed in the mid-shafts of most long bones are primarily the result of bending, often engendered by axial forces transmitted about the bone's longitudinal curvature. The consistency of bending-induced skeletal strain over a range of physical activity and the associated expense of increased strain magnitude that this form of loading incurs suggest that functional strain patterns developed through bending may be a desirable architectural objective of most long bones. Alteration of a bone's normal functional strain distribution, therefore, is probably a key factor underlying adaptive remodelling in response to changes in mechanical loading (Biewener, 1991).

Stress overload on bone remodelling mechanisms

If too much stress is applied to a bone, it will break, or a tendon insertion will be avulsed from its bony attachment (often taking a section of periosteum away with it). These traumas must then be resolved/healed as effectively as possible.

In order to understand the osteopathic perspective on this, one needs to remember that bones are little more than fascial bags filled up with stiffening material, to which other structures insert. Readers are referred back to Figure 5.4.

Soft tissue tension creates torsion in the fascial bag of the bone, which determines the shape into which it can 'set'. The general arrangement of muscular attachments and other fascial structures external to the bone but attaching to it means that the whole bone is encased in a large sleeve of tissue, which helps to dissipate force. However, tendon insertion points represent a point of high stress to the bone and, even under normal movement, microtraction forces are established between the tendon and the periosteum. This triggers piezoelectric forces (a property that bone shares with other crystalline structures), which somehow polarize the cells responsible for osteolysis and bone deposition so that the bone structure is reorganized in a

manner that resists the predominant mechanical stresses (Scott and Korostoff, 1990). This remodelling also occurs within the associated connective tissues of the tendon, i.e. the inserting point of the tendon also undergoes adaptation and restructuring.

'Tennis elbow'/'periostitis'

If the microtraction forces are too great, then inflammation develops, leading to periostitis and irritation of the tendon adjacent to the insertion. In this situation, the more pull there is on the structure the greater the inflammation and the greater the bony remodelling (and consequent temporary weakening).

Management strategies

Locally applied steroids to reduce inflammation may help symptomatically but will not reduce the stress acting on the periosteum. Only reducing the pull from the musculotendinous structure will do that. Hence, working on the biomechanical balance of the limb, by reducing tension in the muscle as well as perhaps some habit retraining of the way the person uses that part of their body, will gradually allow the bone to complete its remodelling process, build up a strong periosteum and lead to a resolution of the inflammation and pain.

Fractures

If a bone is fractured, then it is the job of the fascial bag/sleeve (coupled with the 'jacket' of surrounding muscle) to help to guide the different sections of the fractured bone into an appropriate alignment, so that, as the bone heals, the original shape of the bone can be remodelled.

Ensuring that soft tissue tensions around the fracture site and forces acting upon the fascial 'bag' enclosing the bones are minimized should help reformation of the bone to be as optimal as possible. Even if the fracture site must be supported (by plaster cast for example) for a few weeks, once this is removed, work can still be undertaken to ensure that soft tissue tension does not compromise the final callus resolution and bone realignment.

Management strategies

Many orthopaedic practitioners would feel that this is quite an unlikely idea but, even within orthodox traumatology, the concept of totally immobilizing fracture sites is becoming outdated. The idea that one should allow minimal movement so that the body can realign the bone gently and without constraint, while ensuring local circulation is not compromised, is now gaining recognition – which osteopaths go along with.

Osteopaths would not suggest that no support of a fracture is necessary but that balancing soft tissue forces around the fracture site is beneficial to the healing process.

'Awkwardly' healed bone may have consequences for the orientation of the articular surfaces of the bone, and hence articular biomechanics, and also for the mechanical properties of the bone itself (see below).

Other strains on bones

Many strains acting on bones are not so severe as to produce fracture, but can still have noticeable effects (especially over time).

Research has indicated that loads far less than bone fracture-strain (about 25 000 microstrain) can lead to a type of remodelling or drifting of bony architecture, and that strains at lesser levels (above 3000 microstrain) also increase bone damage and the remodelling that normally repairs it (Frost, 1994).

What type of activity produces these levels of strain? During normal activity, studies have revealed that canine peak strain values, for example, have been put at around 200–400 microstrain (Szivek *et al.*, 1994a) while equine peak strain values are in the region of 3000–4500 microstrain (Nunamaker *et al.*, 1990); so, if body mass has anything to do with it, man ought to be somewhere in between. This means that, during slightly changed biomechanical function or during slightly load-bearing situations, strain levels in man might be sufficient to cause bone remodelling.

Degenerative conditions of bones/articulations

Indeed, weight cannot be the only factor in the equation, as in another study bone remodelling

was identified in rabbits simply by changing the way they held their heads over time (Yu, 1993). In this study, they changed the stresses and strains on the rabbit's necks by maintaining an altered head position. The longer the strain was applied and the greater the strain, the more evident the morphological changes in the cervical vertebrae, akin to spondylosis. There were also changes in the surrounding soft tissues, and the authors felt that this was applicable to the human situation, where abnormalities of the soft tissues around the spine would play an important part in the development of cervical spondylosis, and considered that morphological changes in the cervical column are the basis for the biomechanical pathogenesis of cervical spondylosis.

Management strategies

So, in terms of prevention, preservation of balanced locomotion and biomechanics may over time ensure that degenerative change is delayed or offset. Additionally, if it has already developed to some degree, could continued work on the biomechanics induce any form of reversal in the condition/or at the least stop it developing further? Degeneration in this instance would be viewed not as a fixed state but as a 'snapshot in time' of the bone's response to stress.

(This concept actually turns the way that clinicians traditionally view degenerative change on its head. Degeneration is not a 'weight-bearing problem' *per se*: it is to do with perverted pulls and movement. Weight must play a role, but may not be the major component.)

Bone as a springy structure

Bones may not bend much, but bend they do. This elastic property, especially in the softer bones of children, has importance for the shock-absorbing capacity of bone. Bone needs to be able to absorb shock, as this helps to reduce strain on articular surfaces, and this has been demonstrated within the lumbar spine, for example, where bone compliance in lumbar vertebra is relevant to the motion of the lumbar spine (Shirazi-Adl, 1994). Absorbing the shock created during movement is a role of various connective tissue structures of the body that has already been introduced.

One can palpate (with a bit of practice) the elastic recoil properties of bones, particularly the long bones, which are easier to handle/bend.

Various conditions seem to create tension within the bone – healed fracture sites, implants (Page et al., 1993) and degenerative change, but also accumulative soft tissue tension as a result of altered biomechanics/locomotion.

Chronic myofascial strain acting on the bone leads to constriction at a periosteal level, which may interfere slightly with the remodelling processes discussed above, leading to an exaggeration of bone remodelling at the site of the myofascial constriction. Altered load bearing forces can also affect trabecular bone, causing it to remodel (Goldstein et al., 1991). This would lead to denser bone at that point. In fact, even in normal situations, different parts of bone will have different internal structures and mechanical properties based upon their load-bearing responsibilities (Dalstra et al., 1993).

In effect the bones become too 'stiff' and inelastic at these points. This is akin to the developmental strains imposed on bones by muscles and soft tissues (Carter et al., 1991), discussed above. Up to this point, physiologists **might** agree.

Intraosseous strain

Osteopaths would say that such an increase in density would alter the whole dynamic of the bone, affecting its natural spring and resilience and ultimately contributing to articular stress and soft tissue strain. This is where osteopaths and orthodox practitioners tend to part company.

The concept of intraosseous strain seems to be a concept peculiar to osteopaths and a few other manipulative professions, and one that anatomists, physiologists and medics have some trouble rationalizing. It is a phenomenon that can occur not only in relation to fractures but within healthy bone that is exposed to a degree of mechanical stress (although there does seem some supportive evidence for this: mechanical loading can cause microfracture within individual

trabeculae, where the bone has to continually remodel during exposure to cyclical loading – Guo et al., 1994).

Management strategies

The osteopathic perspective would be to reduce the soft tissue tension and to release right through all the layers of soft tissue constriction, through to the bone itself. Feeling through the soft tissues, one can appreciate the torsion and tension of the bone itself and work to release it, using a variety of techniques. Having done so the bone should be more malleable and, as it should now be more 'shock-absorbing' in its 'springier' state, lead to less articular stress.

This is a difficult technique to demonstrate (on X-ray, for example), as one is clearly not going to alter the gross shape of the bone, just its internal dynamics. Therapeutically, though, osteopaths would argue that it is a worthy concept.

REMODELLING PHENOMENA IN OTHER CONNECTIVE TISSUE STRUCTURES

Capsules and tendons

The cartilaginous surfaces of joints, the soft tissues around them – the capsule and tendons, for example – and the pulley/tendon couplings throughout the body are all specially designed for the specific loading characteristics in their area (Benjamin et al., 1993, 1995).

If forces change, then so too can the structure of these tissues. Joint capsules adapt to forces acting upon them by becoming more fibrocartilaginous and less elastic, for example (Szivek et al., 1994b). Such changes can also occur during simple immobilization (and can be reversed by remobilization; Schollmeier et al., 1996).

Gliding tendons also adapt. For example, in the supraspinatus and biceps brachii tendons there is a normal functional adaptation at the point of stress where the tendons glide over their 'pulley' (McNeilly et al., 1996). This adaptation leads to fibrocartilage deposition and avascular tissue. This area can then be prone to rupture, especially if there is unphysiological tensile stress placed on the gliding tendon, as in some sports (Tillmann and Koch, 1995; Koch and Tillmann, 1995). In this type of case, altered orientation of the upper limb consequent to altered bio-mechanics may play such a role both in sports and even under normal circumstances, providing a potential point of friction, 'weakness' and eventual symptomatology.

Joint cartilage

Cartilage is avascular as well as aneural. This means that cartilage cells depend on mechanical factors to control their function and to provide transport of nutrients and metabolites (Macirowski et al., 1994). Chondrocytes, a type of fibroblast, are found within cartilage and are responsible for remodelling of cartilage components in response to mechanical loading. The internal structure of cartilage gives it viscoelastic properties, so that it can deform and 'creep back' into shape during different mechanical loading (Buschmann et al., 1995). The structure of cartilage gives it poroviscoelastic properties. This means that, as it comes under pressure, it thickens and blocks fluid transfer through the cartilage, which helps to maintain joint fluid pressures (Setton et al., 1993) – which in itself helps reduce cartilage stress, as we shall see below.

Thus cartilage has many responses to adapt to strain (Krane and Goldring, 1990). Interestingly, changes that occur to the cartilage during simple immobilization can be reversed during remobi-lization, whereas those caused by joint instability cannot (Muller et al., 1994). However, immobi-lization of an immature joint may cause cartilage changes that may affect the future development of articular cartilage in such a way that very slow recovery or permanent alteration is induced (Kiviranta et al., 1994). Overall, though, main-taining efficient biomechanical load throughout the body may help limit cartilage damage, or even improve its capacity for recovery after damage.

Synovial fluid

Synovial fluid has viscoelastic properties and, although it allows lubrication, when joints come under load the synovial fluid becomes thicker between the two approaching contact points of the cartilaginous joint surfaces and forms a stable gel (thus delaying the approach of these surfaces; Hlavacek, 1993). Synovial fluid is therefore a very dynamic substance, and its structure changes not only in movement but in a lot of different pathological states. Pathological states such as degenerative joint disease, rheumatoid arthritis, mixed connective tissue disease and pseudogout all lead to increased synovial fluid viscosity (Gomez and Thurston, 1993).

This increase in viscosity is associated with an increase in hyaluronan content in these disease states (Praest et al., 1997), but is also found in simple immobilized joints. The increased hyaluronan levels in immobilized joints are thought to be deleterious for the joint tissues and can lead to osteoarthritic changes (Konttinen et al., 1991). Keeping joints mobile should keep the viscosity of synovial fluid at optimal levels and help maintain joint tissue health.

Intervertebral discs

The dynamics of the intervertebral disc are very important for overall biomechanical efficiency within the spine. But, how does the disc actually work – is the nucleus pulposus a solid or a fluid? This in fact depends upon what it is 'being asked to do'. It behaves like a fluid under transient stress but more like a viscoelastic solid under more dynamic loading conditions (Iatridis et al., 1996). Also, there is a considerable variation in the regional tensile properties of the anulus (Ebara et al., 1996). These regional variations lead to naturally differing biomechanical be-haviour throughout the disc (Best et al., 1994).

If the disc is subjected to injury or consistently altered biomechanical activity, then its structure will begin to adapt, through fibrous remodelling, and so the regional variation in dynamics of the disc will be disrupted, which will alter the dynamics and function of the disc as a whole

(Acaroglu *et al.*, 1995). This will then feed back into spinal motion patterns, and further alter biomechanical behaviour – leading to a vicious circle of degenerative cause and effect.

SUMMARY

This chapter has discussed a variety of activities within the musculoskeletal system and its component parts. It has given some indication of the potential problems involving movement, structure and function that can arise from disturbed function, from an osteopathic perspective.

The following chapters look at the interrelatedness of parts within the musculoskeletal system in more detail, to reinforce the concepts in integration and cause and effect within dysfunction that we have introduced.

REFERENCES

Acaroglu, E. R., Iatridis, J. C., Setton, L. A. *et al.* (1995) Degeneration and aging affect the tensile behavior of human lumbar anulus fibrosus. *Spine*, **20**, 2690–2701.

Alberts, B., Bray, D., Lewis, J. *et al.* (1994) *Molecular Biology of the Cell*, 3rd edn, Garland Publishing, New York.

American Academy of Osteopathy (1979) *The Collected Works of Irvin M. Korr*, American Academy of Osteopathy, Indianapolis, IN.

Baskin, L., Howard, P. S. and Macarak, E. (1993a) Effect of mechanical forces on extracellular matrix synthesis by bovine urethral fibroblasts in vitro. *Journal of Urology*, **150**, 637–641.

Baskin, L., Howard, P. S. and Macarak, E. (1993b) Effect of physical forces on bladder smooth muscle and urothelium. *Journal of Urology*, **150**, 601–607.

Benjamin, M., Ralphs, J. R., Newell, R. L. and Evans, E. J. (1993) Loss of the fibrocartilaginous lining of the intertubercular sulcus associated with rupture of the tendon of the long head of biceps brachii. *Journal of Anatomy*, **182**, 281–285.

Benjamin, M., Qin, S. and Ralphs, J. R. (1995) Fibrocartilage associated with human tendons and their pulleys. *Journal of Anatomy*, **187**, 625–633.

Best, B. A., Guilak, F., Setton, L. A. *et al.* (1994) Compressive mechanical properties of the human anulus fibrosus and their relationship to biochemical composition. *Spine*, **19**, 212–221.

Biewener, A. A. (1991) Musculoskeletal design in relation to body size. *Journal of Biomechanics*, **24**(Suppl. 1), 19–29.

Buschmann, M. D., Gluzband, Y. A., Grodzinsky, A. J. and Hunziker, E. B. (1995) Mechanical compression modulates matrix biosynthesis in chondrocyte/agarose culture. *Journal of Cell Science*, **108**, 1497–1508.

Carter, D. R., Wong, M. and Orr, T. E. (1991) Musculoskeletal ontogeny, phylogeny, and functional adaptation. *Journal of Biomechanics*, **24**(Suppl. 1), 3–16.

Cathie, D. (1974a) Considerations of fascia and its relation to disease of the musculoskeletal system. *American Academy of Osteopathy Year Book*, 85–88.

Cathie, D. (1974b) The fascia of the body in relation to function and manipulative therapy. *American Academy of Osteopathy Year Book*, 81–84.

Cawson, R. A., McCracken, A. W. and Marcus, P. B. (1982) *Pathologic Mechanisms and Human Disease*, C. V. Mosby, St Louis, MO.

Dalstra, M., Huiskes, R., Odgaard, A. and Van Erning, L. (1993) Mechanical and textural properties of pelvic trabecular bone. *Journal of Biomechanics*, **26**, 523–535.

Ebara, S., Iatridis, J. C., Setton, L. A. *et al.* (1996) Tensile properties of nondegenerate human lumbar anulus fibrosus. *Spine*, **21**, 452–461.

Frost, H. M. (1994) Wolff's Law and bone's structural adaptations to mechanical usage: an overview for clinicians. *Angle Orthodontist*, **64**, 175–188.

Goldstein, S. A., Matthews, L. S., Kuhn, J. L. and Hollister, S. J. (1991) Trabecular bone remodelling: an experimental model. *Journal of Biomechanics*, **24**, 135–150.

Gomez, J. E. and Thurston, G. B. (1993) Comparisons of the oscillatory shear viscoelasticity and composition of pathological synovial fluids. *Biorheology*, **30**, 409–427.

Guo, X. E., McMahon, T. A., Keaveny, T. M. *et al.* (1994) Finite element modelling of damage accumulation in trabecular bone under cyclic loading. *Journal of Biomechanics*, **27**, 145–155.

Hlavacek, M. (1993) The role of synovial fluid filtration by cartilage in lubrication of synovial joints – I. Mixture model of synovial fluid. *Journal of Biomechanics*, **26**, 1145–1150.

Iatridis, J. C., Weidenbaum, M., Setton, L. A. and Mow, V. C. (1996) Is the nucleus pulposus a solid or a fluid? Mechanical behaviors of the nucleus pulposus of the human intervertebral disc. *Spine*, **21**, 1174–1184.

Inman, V. T., Ralston, H. J. and Todd, F. (1981) *Human Walking*, Williams & Wilkins, Baltimore, MD, pp. 22–117.

Johansson, R. and Magnusson, M. (1991) Human postural dynamics. *Biomedical Engineering*, **18**, 413–437.

Kandel, E. R., Schwartz, J. H. and Jessel, T. M. (1991) *Principles of Neural Science*, 3rd edn. Prentice Hall, Englewood Cliffs, NJ.

Kiviranta, I., Tammi, M., Jurvelin, J. *et al.* (1994) Articular cartilage thickness and glycosaminoglycan distribution in the young canine knee joint after remobilisation of the immobilised limb. *Journal of Orthopaedic Research*, **12**, 161–167.

Koch, S. and Tillmann, B. (1995) The distal tendon of the biceps brachii. Structure and clinical correlations. *Anatomischer Anzeiger*, **177**, 467–474.

Konttinen, Y. T., Michelsson, J. E., Gronblad, M. *et al.* (1991) Plasma hyaluronan levels in rabbit immobilisation osteoarthritis: effect of remobilisation. *Scandinavian Journal of Rheumatology*, **20**, 392–396.

Krane, S. M. and Goldring, M. B. (1990) Clinical implications of cartilage metabolism in arthritis. *European Journal of Rheumatology and Inflammation*, **10**, 4–9.

Kuchera, M. L. (1995) Gravitational stress, musculoligamentous strain, and postural alignment. *Spine*, **9**, 463–490.

Larson, W. J. (1993) *Human Embryology*, Churchill Livingstone, New York.

Levin, S. M. (1995) The importance of soft tissues for structural support of the body. *Spine*, **9**, 357–363.

Lodish, H. (1995) *Molecular Cell Biology*, W. H. Freeman, New York.

Lovejoy, C. O. (1988) Evolution of human walking. *Scientific American*, **259**, 118–125.

Macirowski, T., Tepic, S. and Mann, R. W. (1994) Cartilage stresses in the human hip joint. *Journal of Biomechanical Engineering*, **116**, 10–18.

McNeilly, C. M., Banes, A. J., Benjamin, M. and Ralphs, J. R. (1996) Tendon cells in vivo form a three dimensional network of cell processes linked by gap junctions. *Journal of Anatomy*, **189**, 593–600.

Magoun, H. I. (1976) *Osteopathy in the Cranial Field*, 3rd edn. Journal Printing Company, Kirksville, MO.

Mann, A. T. (1993) *Sacred Architecture*, Element, Shaftesbury, Dorset.

Morris, D. (1978) *Manwatching. A Field Guide to Human Behaviour*, Triad/Panther Books, St Albans.

Muller, F. J., Setton, L. A., Manicourt, D. H. *et al.* (1994) Centrifugal and biochemical comparison of proteoglycan aggregates from articular cartilage in experimental joint disuse and joint instability. *Journal of Orthopaedic Research*, **12**, 498–508.

Nunamaker, D. M., Butterweck, D. M. and Provost, M. T. (1990) Fatigue fractures in thoroughbred racehorses: relationships with age, peak bone strain, and training. *Journal of Orthopaedic Research*, **8**, 604–611.

Nuttgens, P. (1983) *The Story of Architecture*, Phaidon Press, London.

Page, A. E., Allan, C., Jasty, M. *et al.* (1993) Determination of loading parameters in the canine hip in vivo. *Journal of Biomechanics*, **26**, 571–579.

Pender, N. and McCulloch, C. A. (1991) Quantitation of actin polymerization in two human fibroblast sub-types responding to mechanical stretching. *Journal of Cell Science*, **100**, 187–193.

Praest, B. M., Greiling, H. and Kock, R. (1997) Assay of synovial fluid parameters: hyaluronan concentration as a potential marker for joint diseases. *Clinica Chimica Acta*, **266**, 117–128.

Robbie, D. L. (1977) Tensional forces in the human body. *Orthopaedic Review*, **6**, 45–48.

Salvadori, M. (1980) *How Buildings Stand Up*, W. W. Norton & Co, New York.

Schollmeier, G., Sarkar, K, Fukuhara, K. and Uhthoff, H. K. (1996) Structural and functional changes in the canine shoulder after cessation of immobilisation. *Clinical Orthopaedics and Related Research*, **323**, 310–315.

Scott, G. C. and Korostoff, E. (1990) Oscillatory and step response electromechanical phenomena in human and bovine bone. *Journal of Biomechanics*, **23**, 127–143.

Setton, L. A., Zhu, W. and Mow, V. C. (1993) The biphasic poroviscoelastic behavior of articular cartilage: role of the surface zone in governing the compressive behavior. *Journal of Biomechanics*, **26**, 581–592.

Shirazi-Adl, A. (1994) Analysis of role of bone compliance on mechanics of a lumbar motion segment. *Journal of Biomechanical Engineering*, **116**, 408–412.

Smith, R. S., Smith, T. J., Blieden, T. M. and Phipps, R. P. (1997) Fibroblasts as sentinel cells. Synthesis of chemokines and regulation of inflammation. *American Journal of Pathology*, **151**, 317–322.

Sutherland, W. G. (1990) *Teachings in the Science of Osteopathy*, Rudra Press, Cambridge, MA.

Szivek, J. A., Johnson, E. M., Magee, F. P. *et al.* (1994a) Bone remodeling and in vivo strain analysis of intact and implanted greyhound proximal femora. *Journal of Investigative Surgery*, **7**, 213–233.

Szivek, J. A., Magee, F. P., Hanson, T. and Hedley, A. K. (1994b) Strain redistribution in the canine femur resulting from hip implants of different stiffnesses. *Journal of Investigative Surgery*, 7, 95–110.

Tillmann, B. and Koch, S. (1995) [Functional adaptation processes of gliding tendons]. *Sportverletzung und Sportschaden*, 9, 44–50.

Yu, J. K. (1993) [The relationship between experimental changes in the stress–strain distribution and the tissues structural abnormalities of the cervical column]. *Chung-Hua Wai Ko Tsa Chih [Chinese Journal of Surgery]*, **31**, 456–459.

6 IDEAS WITHIN OSTEOPATHY: THE SPINE

THE APPROACH TAKEN IN THIS CHAPTER

One of the main aims of this chapter is to introduce models of biomechanics within the spine as used by osteopaths over time.

The anatomy of the vertebral column and soft tissue components will not be analysed in detail, nor will pain presentation patterns be discussed at this stage. Load-bearing characteristics and intervertebral disc mechanics will also not be analysed. This might seem a strange omission in a chapter on spinal biomechanics. However, it must be understood that, although osteopaths may come to similar conclusions about how damaged an area has become, can reflect on the local tissue changes in the various structures in and around the spinal column and can correlate these to various categories of rheumatological or orthopaedic disease/dysfunction, it is what they choose to do with the spine to alleviate the problem that makes osteopathic practice different from the world of orthopaedics and orthodox biomechanics.

Studies of biomechanics, anatomy, ergonomics and so on provide a strong foundation for manipulative practices, but osteopathy is more than a set of basic sciences.

If one was simply to recount current medical perspectives on the subtleties of soft tissue articular dynamics and the integrated neural control of posture movement and locomotion, one would have learned much, but perhaps not about osteopathy. Of course, osteopathy uses all those things and could not be practised in the modern age without them. But in themselves they do not describe osteopathy; it is the use that osteopaths make of such information that leads to osteopathic practice. This point cannot be stressed strongly enough, and any osteopath who can only relate his/her work in terms of technique applied with an understanding of basic science but without an idea of underlying principles will perhaps have lost something very potent.

The following discussions will draw both from traditional models of biomechanics within osteopathy and some current neuroanatomical models from within orthodox science. The aim of the neurological section is to show how science may underpin long-standing approaches within osteopathy.

As the title of this chapter suggests, then, the information presented here is more a catalogue of ideas than scientific analysis.

The osteopathic ideas on spinal motion discussed within this chapter have not been subjected to scientific analysis and therefore cannot be referenced. This is something that clearly needs rectifying, but the hope is that, if these ideas are expressed, people will be encouraged to establish a basis for such approaches within osteopathic practice.

Models emerge in an attempt to analyse practice, and eventually models must in themselves be analysed, to establish their validity. Because of the way that the profession has developed, there are many different styles and models used within daily practice by different practitioners from different schools, and from those practitioners developing their own flavour of osteopathy based on what they have learned and their ongoing experiences.

It may interest the reader to know that not all parts of the profession view spinal biomechanics in the same way. Some practitioners have no idea of the models of Littlejohn and Fryette and some feel there is no other way of looking at the spine. Some feel that these models are outdated and some that to practise without them is to throw away much that is unique and valuable within osteopathy. Some feel that we have abandoned much of what Still said, in an attempt to move towards a more medical model of practice, and some consider that most of what was said by early osteopaths needs to be reviewed in the light of current medical and orthopaedic analysis.

We are all osteopaths, though, and we must have some principles in common. This can be safely said, as models do not define osteopathic practice, only influence the style of its outcome. One of the aims of this chapter (and following ones) is to try to re-establish links and relationships between the different models and approaches and bring a more unified dialogue of motion analysis to osteopathic practice.

Integration and not competition between parts and parties is the key.

At this stage of the book, then, readers have to be introduced to the complexity of interactions between body parts before one can discuss how a variety of movement problems may accumulate and eventually contribute to a variety of clinical situations and conditions. Also, however a problem/injury or dysfunction may have arisen, the accumulated tensions and restrictions throughout the body have the effect of stopping/ interfering with the way the healing mechanisms of the body resolve these disorders themselves; and therefore it is only when one sees how all the parts of the body work together that one can see how management strategies might be devised for the individual presenting with some clinical complaint.

This, then, allows the osteopathic perspective on management to be introduced.

Some clinical references will be made in these chapters, and some more in Chapter 9 (where, readers should note, the consequences of intervertebral articular mechanical restriction of peripheral nerve function are discussed). But it is not until Chapter 10 that all these points can be drawn together, when clinical reasoning and case analysis are discussed. Readers should also note that this chapter does not give all the ideas about spinal movement that are used by osteopaths (more information is included in following chapters).

The spine does not work in isolation. Chapter 5 set the scene for a whole-body model of movement concepts based on tensegrity principles. The spine cannot move independently of the rest of the body, and many other body parts – the arms, legs, pelvis and head – have many influences on the spine, which will affect spinal mechanics and interfere with the dynamics of its movement. It is also important to consider the body cavities and their organs (visceral and neurological), as well as some of the fascial/connective tissue planes that help bind and support the human framework.

One cannot put all this information into one chapter, and so it has been split for convenience sake, although this risks implying that the chosen sections can be viewed as independent biomechanical units. This would be completely erroneous, and over the next few chapters the reader must allow a picture of integrated function to gradually emerge, which we will then consolidate in Chapter 10.

That said, we are ready to travel through a landscape of ideas within osteopathy about the spine – which is more like a story than a justification of information.

MODELS AND THEIR MAKERS

There are several 'models' used within osteopathy regarding the way the body normally moves and where dysfunction may become manifest if various parts of the body start to have adapted movement for whatever reason. Some of these models are of very long standing, such as the classical osteopathy model introduced by Littlejohn and continued by Wernham. Others have evolved over time, such as the reductionist models commonly used in the 1950s and 1960s (when much of the classic model was 'simplified'). Others, such as Dummer, Lever and Lamb, have built upon the classic model, adapting it slightly to their own interpretation. Others, such as Hartman (1997) have, from within a re-evolving 'reductionist' model, developed an increasingly sophisticated method of manipulative technique to the articular structures. Others again have come from a different perspective within osteopathy, not through abandoning various models but by adding to them; these include Sutherland, Korth and Turner, Baral and Latey (1982).

All these practitioners have made an unique and special contribution to perspectives upon body movement and the therapeutic considerations therein, leading to a modern perspective of patterns and inter-relations. Thus has evolved a more all-encompassing, three-dimensional, rational and visionary model of human movement and its relations, which is modern osteopathy.

A. T. Still, founder of osteopathy

Not much mention has so far been made of the American founder of osteopathy, Andrew Taylor Still. This might seem unusual in a book devoted to osteopathic philosophy. However, in the 100 years (and more) of osteopathic practice worldwide since its foundation, there have been many developments and extensions, additions and variations upon a theme within osteopathy. Because of this, it is perhaps no longer possible to say that what is practised now is precisely what was practised by Still. This is not to say that modern osteopathic practice is not related to his work – far from it. Current trends and opinions within osteopathy should be regarded as a direct development and expansion of the original concepts of osteopathy as laid down by A. T. Still.

Osteopathy was founded in the days before antibiotics and modern pharmacology, and many doctors had little that was truly useful in their medical armoury. Still discovered that, if the body was diseased, then manipulating it would be beneficial, and so he developed a whole range of ideas and practices based upon manipulative approaches to the body and advocated their use in an enormous number of conditions ranging from scarlet fever to gall stones, cases of tremor, infections, and respiratory, gastrointestinal and pelvic organ conditions. In other words, regardless of what you presented with, there was a manipulative therapeutic intervention that could help.

Vitalism
Also, Still was very interested in energy within the human force (perhaps arising from his previous work as a magnetic healer – magnetism as a science rather than an emotion). However, within his osteopathic practice he was also thought to be a healer in the broader, spiritual sense of the word. Down the years the 'vitalistic and energetic' components within his work have been played down by some and truly developed by others within the profession. Here already is one path of 'difference'.

Scope of practice

Another difference is that nowhere in the osteo-pathic literature of the time is there the confinement of osteopathic approaches to 'orthopaedic/traumatic conditions' as seems to be the current perception of the scope of osteopathic practice.

Scope of practice has been a deeply contentious issue and, while it is important to recognize the unique benefits that the osteopathic approach has given to the management of conditions that cause back pain, neck pain, headaches and so on, and the management of sports injuries, the original practice of osteopathy was more than this. Indeed, as different osteopaths come into closer contact with other professions it seems that the latter are interested in, if initially wary of, its opinions and approaches to a wide variety of conditions that are proving resistant to orthodox management. Now is a unique time, as the profession gains statutory recognition after much effort, to move the practice of osteopathy forwards to achieve its full potential in healthcare issues.

Still's approach

Still coined many phrases, but some of the most widely quoted by osteopaths are:

- Structure governs function.
- The rule of the artery is supreme.
- Find it, fix it and leave it alone.

As with any such phrases, these maxims require explanation; it is hoped that some idea of their meaning will already be apparent and that, after the following few chapters, they will have been further clarified.

Still's model was one of interpreting physiology in relation to body motion. He had various principles governing his practice, but no 'models' of movement, as such.

Structure governs function

Still felt that structure governed function, which is a reciprocal relationship, as function can also govern structure. We have discussed the role of connective tissues, at a cellular and a general level, including bone formation and remodelling.

These discussions have indicated how the structure (of the extracellular matrix for example) can affect function (by relating ECM dynamics to fluid movement, immunity and cellular communication and activity).

We have also discussed how function can affect structure, in the discussions of the effects of movement on fibroblasts and connective tissue formation and structure, and also how physical force can affect bone remodelling, especially in developing bones. The relationship is reciprocal as, each time the structure is changed, an alteration of its physiological relations will follow.

The phrase 'structure governs function', then, could also be written as 'anatomy governs physiology'. If one is to understand Still's approach, one must appreciate how soft tissue biomechanics within the body relates to physiological efficiency and therefore how problems within soft tissue movement and dynamics relate to pathophysiology.

Anatomy

One thing that should not be in doubt, though, is Still's interest in anatomy, as the above statements indicate. He was vehement that one could not practise as an osteopath without a sound understanding and appreciation of anatomy. Osteopaths today have treasured this interest in anatomy, and consider that there are many interesting physiological relations based on the placement and arrangement of parts within the body. They feel that there is still much to appreciate through the study of form and function. Often, modern anatomical texts seem to show 'standardized' and 'uniform' versions of anatomy and do not demonstrate the exactness of some earlier anatomical descriptions and illustrations (A National Touring Exhibition, 1997). Anatomy is still a growth area, so to speak!

The study of anatomy applied to principles remains to this day the most fundamental aspect of osteopathy practice.

The rule of the artery is supreme

This precept also has already been alluded to – in that fluid dynamics within the body are of prime importance to health, good function and adaptability. This relates not only to blood circulation (whether this is within the general circulation or at a cellular level, controlled by neural signals or aided by passive movements) but also to the lymphatic circulation (from the initial lymphatics to the entry into the venous circulation) and the circulation of cerebrospinal and other serous fluids.

Maintaining an effective circulation will aid tissue health, immunity and the functioning of the nervous system, from the brain to the smallest nerve ending. This then allows effective communication and allows the body to function as a self-regulating, self-healing mechanism.

Find it, fix it and leave it alone

This has caused much head-scratching among osteopaths, but is quite wonderful in its simplicity! The idea is that one should not do unnecessary work to the body as this only 'irritates' or 'fatigues' it, and that one should look closely through all of the body to find what is interfering with its self-regulating and self-healing mechanisms. This includes examining the spine, the extremities, the body cavities and the viscera, to appreciate how the physical restrictions in any of these parts or tissues are interfering with circulation or neural communication, support of the body and its organs, and the emotional well being of the person.

If you can find the main constricting influences, then these should be worked on, and the rest will resolve themselves. Once you have found the problem areas, you should work on them in an effective way so that when you 'walk away' they remain corrected, as far as is possible. You should not need to return time and time again to the same place if you work efficiently, and in the primary areas of dysfunction, and, once corrected, the body should be left alone to make use of this intervention and adapt its physiology and internal health as a result.

Until you have a broad and encompassing view of the human body and its functions, you may not look widely enough and so may not find what it is necessary to treat!

To sum up these tenets, among the many and varied 'definitions' of osteopathy that can be found (Education Department, 1993), the following one, from A. T. Still, is the author's favourite: 'Osteopathy is the knowledge of the structure, relations and functions of each and every part of the human body applied to the adjustment and correction of whatever may be interfering with their harmonious operation' (Webster, 1935).

Still as a teacher

In passing his knowledge on to his pupils Still faced certain challenges, caused by his own strength of opinion. Still did not demonstrate technique, he demonstrated treatments. This fact alone has perhaps led to a range of opinions on what he was actually doing, and many ideas were formulated to help students appreciate what he was doing, how he was doing it, and why.

Still felt that studying technique for its own sake was worthless (although all modern schools do now teach technique as an individual subject). Even if he didn't explain them, Still apparently used a variety of techniques, ranging from articulation and gentle mobilizations to quite strong 'adjustments' or manipulations. There is currently quite a division of opinion within the profession as to the main nature of Still's manipulations: were they akin to articulation and thrust techniques as we would recognize them today, or were they much more gentle – although no less powerful because of it?

The nature of Still's manipulations

Many practitioners with direct experience of the Kirksville school of osteopathy, which Still founded in the USA, and of the Still family (several family members trained as osteopaths over the years) feel that the techniques were articulatory and directly manipulative. Some other practitioners feel that the approach was much more gentle and akin to those techniques coming under the umbrella term of 'balanced ligamentous tension techniques'. These have been passed down through another set of practitioners, who had very close links with those trained directly under Still, such as Sutherland and Wales. Sutherland in particular, as we shall see later, provided a very unique extension of the osteopathic concept through recognizing a type of 'involuntary' motion through the body, and appreciating the value of motion within the membranes surrounding the brain and spinal cord, as well as through the rest of the connective tissues/fascia throughout the body.

This debate continues to this day and cannot be resolved here (although we will return to it briefly later in the text). But one thing is certain: Still did lots of things to the spine, and one way to start would be by looking at a model that emerged from the early history of osteopathy: that formulated by Littlejohn, a pupil of Still's.

J. M. Littlejohn

Osteopathy in Britain has perhaps taken a slightly different format over the years from American osteopathy (not least because of the fact that in the USA osteopaths are trained as doctors as well, whereas in the UK they are not). Osteopathy in the UK was founded by John Martin Littlejohn, who established the British School of Osteopathy in 1917. Littlejohn had trained under Still, and had also been one of his patients. He went on to establish the Chicago School of Osteopathy and was renowned for his interest in physiology. There appeared to be some professional differences between Still and himself and, for whatever reason, Littlejohn came to the UK to continue his work (he was a native of Glasgow).

He developed a whole philosophy of biomechanics, with an attendant physiological analysis that related movement and postural disturbance to function and dysfunction within the body. It has been said that one of the main reasons Littlejohn developed his models was that Still could not easily pass on his own approaches to his students and there was therefore a strong need for something to act as a structure through which to understand the osteopathic approach to treatment. However, another motivation seems to be to give some sort of physiological analysis of the early empirical benefits of osteopathy, to help the validity of the profession.

The widespread influence of Littlejohn

Littlejohn's methods have been a cornerstone of osteopathic practice for many years for many parts of the profession in the UK. It is interesting to note, though, that the school he founded does not now teach his original concepts. There are many possible reasons for that, as we shall see. (Other colleges have continued his work, although only one of these can be said to have remained absolutely committed to his work to the exclusion of all else – the Maidstone College of Osteopathy. Had this not been the case, much of Littlejohn's contribution would have been tragically lost.)

Additionally, because he left the USA, virtually no one in the modern American profession knows about Littlejohn, let alone what his approaches were! This may come as a surprise to some British osteopaths for whom no other approach is as valid, and also to many European osteopaths, for the reason that most of these were trained by ex-pupils of British schools that remained faithful to Littlejohn's approach.

Since Littlejohn was a founder of British osteopathy, his approach will be discussed first, as an introduction to models within osteopathy. Littlejohn wrote much on physiology and medicine but the mechanical analyses discussed here were passed on more by practice than through literature, and the profession must be grateful to John Wernham (among others, including Dummer, Lever and Lamb) for preserving this information.

Littlejohn mechanics

The study of spinal biomechanics has been going on for centuries (Sanan and Rengachary, 1996) and osteopaths have made their own contributions to this debate.

In the previous chapter, we were introduced in an abstract way to the idea that the body moves in a springy, balanced and coordinated manner; and saw briefly that soft tissue activity and tension can influence the pattern of movement in the various articulations of the body. We need to explore this idea of integrated, elastic function in relation to spinal mechanics, and Littlejohn's ideas fit well into this perspective.

Littlejohn mechanics (Maidstone College of Osteopathy, 1960, 1985; Anonymous, 1956) relate to the way the spinal column acts as a flexible unit of interlinked curved sections, within a body where the centre of gravity is considered to lie just anterior to the third lumbar vertebra. The way that gravity acts longitudinally through the spinal column creates an interplay of forces that react with the bony architecture of the spinal curves, leading to a complex set of interactions that were thought to be fairly universal in all humans. It is a model that, among other things, allows for a prediction of where dysfunction will arise and a hierarchical method for releasing areas of the spine in a physiologically appropriate order.

We will concentrate on the spinal biomechanics within his model. Littlejohn contributed much more than this, but it is where we will start.

As stated earlier, this is a review of ideas and is not referenced. Osteopaths need to share what they think before it can be analysed by those with the necessary skills and resources to research it.

The spine as a series of curves

Littlejohn's idea of where various curved sections of the spine started and stopped is different from that within orthodox anatomical texts, as we shall see in a moment. He observed that vertebral shape gradually changes through the curves, thus shifting the traditional 'junctional' areas a little.

Vertebral shape and facet angle governs movement

Generally, the vertebrae are grouped together because of their location: seven cervical vertebrae are in the neck, 12 thoracic vertebrae are in the thorax, and five lumbar vertebrae are in the low back. However, this grouping does not relate so much to the actual shape of the individual vertebrae as to anatomical position. Although orthodox texts describe what a typical cervical, thoracic or lumbar vertebra looks like, Littlejohn was more concerned with transition in shape from one to another, which he thought was more revealing for whole-spine mechanics (because the

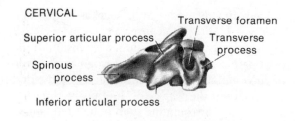

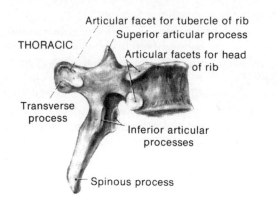

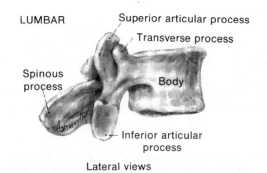

Figure 6.1

Lateral views of the three different levels of vertebra. (Reproduced with the permission of WB Saunders, from Structure and Function in Man, Jacob et al., 1982.)

structure–function relationship was thought to be more revealing than position). The classical shapes of the lumbar, thoracic and cervical vertebrae are shown in Figure 6.1.

Looked at this way, by reflecting on the gradual change of shapes from one type to another, the curves of the spine can be re-described, in accordance with the structure-governs-function principle coined by Still.

Curves and arches

The cervical section of the spine does not really end until the following vertebrae are truly 'thoracic' in shape. This means that the cervical column could be thought of as passing from C2 to the T4 area, and the thoracic spine could go from here to the T9 area (as all these vertebrae are typically thoracic). From T9 onwards the vertebrae start to change shape again, becoming slightly 'lumbar' in design. Therefore the 'lumbar' spine goes from the T10 area to the sacrum (with T10 and T11 considered 'transitional', being neither fully thoracic nor fully lumbar). The upper cervical vertebrae, as they are typically 'atypical in shape', tend to follow rules of their own, and Littlejohn felt that the atlas should be considered more a junction to the occiput than part of the cervical spine proper. The upper cervical area is discussed towards the end of the chapter.

Within these curves, further analyses can be made.

Looking at the facet angles, there are differences in the cervical vertebrae, with a 'change over' at C5, leaving it liable to slightly different movement from the other parts of the cervical spine. This means that above C5 the vertebrae are inclined to move in one way and below it they are inclined into the other direction, with C5 subsequently a little more unstable in its articulations than the other cervical vertebrae, because of the differing movement potentials above and below it. A schematized view of the facet angles is shown in Figure 6.2.

In the thoracic spine the facet angles change at T9/10. The T11 and T12 facets favour extension, whereas the other lower thoracic vertebral facets above this level favour flexion and sidebending more. This means there is a bit of a hinge around the T9/10 area, which is also emphasized by the fact that the T11 and T12 vertebrae have floating ribs (attaching to just one vertebra each) and the other thoracic vertebrae have ribs that are more 'constraining' to thoracic vertebral movement (as one rib attaches to two vertebrae at these levels). The articulations of the ribs with the thoracic vertebrae are shown in Figure 6.3.

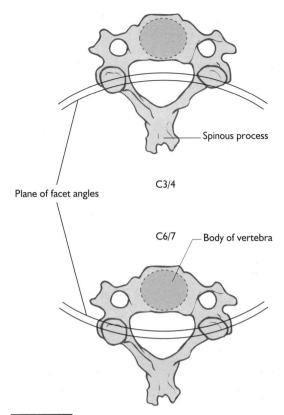

Figure 6.2

A superior view of the cervical vertebrae showing the orientation of the facet planes at C3/4 and C6/7. This different orientation gives different axes of movement in the cervical spine and below C5.

In the lumbar region, the changes that started at T10/11 pass through to L4, with L5 being considered as a separate component to the lumbar spine, forming a junction with the sacrum (much as the atlas was in relation to the occiput).

Put together, these arches were described as **functional arches** (arches in relation to function dictated by structure). These are illustrated in Figure 6.4.

The changeover points between the arches (C5, T9, L5), called interarch pivots, are thought to be more prone to biomechanical dysfunction than other areas because of the changing forces.

The influence of muscle interaction

Muscular anatomy and attachments were considered on top of this pattern, giving leverage to

Figure 6.3

Right lateral view of articulated thoracic vertebrae. (Reproduced from Principles of Human Anatomy and Physiology, 7th Edn, by Tortora & Grabowski; Copyright © 1993, by Harper Collins Publishers Inc.

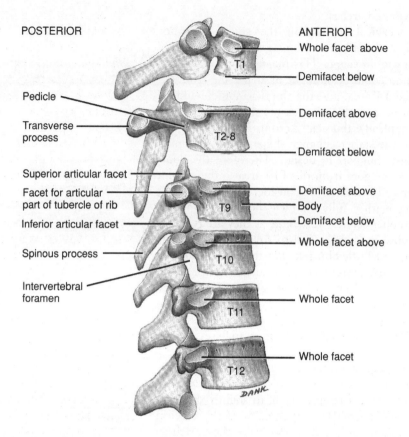

sections of the spine. This added another level of relations within these curves, to give further impetus for certain sites to become more readily dysfunctional than others (in particular C5 and T9).

(Note: These are the leverages that are traditionally described in the Littlejohn model, and some might feel they are a bit too simplistically 'chosen' to 'fit the model'. Nevertheless, they are an interesting introduction into the relationship between parts based on anatomy that should be of interest.)

Muscular leverages on the cervical spine

There is a posterior focus of tension acting between the head and neck, which centres on C2. This is shown in Figure 6.5.

There is an anterior focus around C5. Here the scalenes can be thought of as controlling the neck from C3 down as a group, against the longus capitis muscles acting from the cranium down to C6, against the longus colli running between C2 and T3. All this means that there are pulls that act roughly around the C5 articulation (Figure 6.6).

Muscle leverages acting on the thoracic spine

Posterior and anterior muscular attachments take 'cervical influence' down to approximately T4. The anterior muscle, longus colli, goes down to T3 and the posterior muscles, longissimus cervicis (to T4/5), semispinalis capitis (to T6) and longissimus capitis (to T4/5), all tend to focus neck movement forces/leverages around the T4/5 area.

A 'blocking' influence is exerted by the shoulder girdle/upper limb muscles, which attach broadly along the thoracic spine, through the ribs and scapulae attachments to the axial skeleton between the lower cervical spine and upper two thirds of the thoracic spine – the

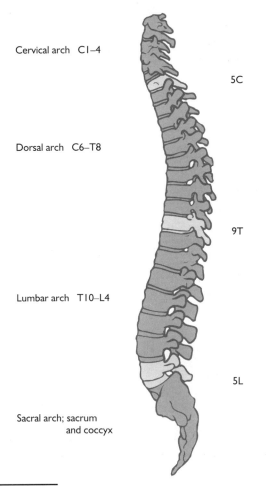

Cervical arch C1–4

5C

Dorsal arch C6–T8

9T

Lumbar arch T10–L4

5L

Sacral arch; sacrum
and coccyx

Figure 6.4

The spine can be divided into functional arches (C1–4, C6–T8, T10–L4, sacrum), as defined by shape.

trapezius and latissimus dorsi muscles being exceptions to this.

Muscular leverages acting on the thoracolumbar area

This is quite an interesting area. The erector spinae muscles take their insertion, as a block, from the sacrum, lumbar and two lowest thoracic vertebrae. This whole block of insertion is supported by the thoracolumbar fascia. Therefore the lumbar spine tends to be braced as a unit when the erector spinae muscles are acting. Any torso movement then has to come from either

side of this block (the L/S area or the T/L area). The 'block' action of the lumbar spine is aided by the combined action of the crurae of the diaphragm and the psoas muscles, which can stabilize the anterior aspect of the spine when working in concert, aided by the function of the abdomen and abdominal turgor (the Valsalva manoeuvre). Torso movement is also principally guided by the action of the abdominal muscles acting between the rib cage and the pelvis. Their action tends to orientate the thorax against the 'block' of the lumbar spine, creating a focus of tension just above the T/L region. This is also exaggerated by the influence of serratus posterior inferior, which runs from the upper lumbars to the lower ribs, creating another block from the lumbars to the lower thoracics (via the ribs); another example is the quadratus lumborum.

Muscular leverages acting on the mid-lumbar region

The psoas muscles and the crurae of the diaphragm (as they 'pull' in opposite directions) create a focus acting around the L3 area, because their actions and attachments overlap at this point. Movement is also focused at L3 because any pelvic action is transmitted here through the fact that L4 and L5 are 'tied' to the pelvis via the iliolumbar ligaments and so move with it.

Muscular leverages acting at the lumbosacral area

The piriformis, coccygeus and levator ani muscles counterbalance the effects of sacral nutation between the ilia induced by weight-bearing forces. The sacrum thus swings between the ilia, with the lumbar spine hinging at the L/S region consequent to this. As L4 and L5 are attached to the ilia, there is the possibility that sacral torsion, which is not fully reflected in the ilia, may create an even greater focus of movement between L5 and the sacrum.

Combining muscular influences with the functional arches

Thus, in this group of concepts, we now have changes in motion, or direction of forces acting

Figure 6.5

Muscular forces
acting around the
axis; posterior view.

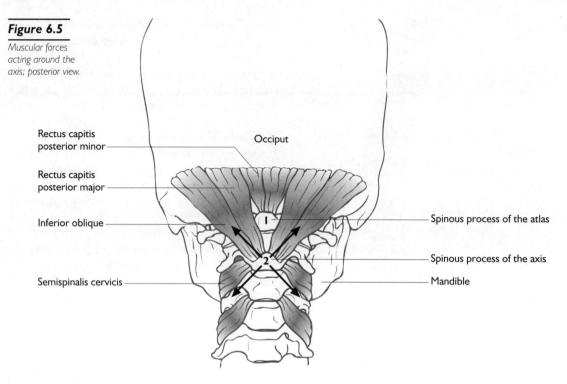

Rectus capitis posterior minor

Rectus capitis posterior major

Inferior oblique

Semispinalis cervicis

Occiput

Spinous process of the atlas

Spinous process of the axis

Mandible

at T4/5, T9/10 and L/S because of hinging between curves, and strain at C4/5, T11/12 and the L3 region because of relative instability in these areas consequent to facet angle, vertebral body shape or muscular attachment.

This view of the spine as a series of interlinked curves was then coupled with a picture of how longitudinal weight-bearing forces acted through the spine. This was an important consideration, as gravity is a powerful force, capable of adapting the spines of differing species depending on whether they are quadrupeds or bipeds and at what relative angles they hold their heads to a vertical axis (Graf *et al.*, 1995). The way the weight of the head is transmitted through the spine to the pelvis could be illustrated by drawing two lines – the anterior and posterior gravity lines, illustrated in Figure 6.7A and B.

These, when combined, created a polygon of forces along the spine and effectively divided the body into two triangular (cone-like) areas, which came together/pivoted around each other just in front of T3/4. These can be seen in Figure 6.7C. These were called the upper and lower triangles,

and the centre of gravity of the whole body was thought to reside in the lower triangle, just in front of L3.

Now, not only is there a picture of a spinal column of interlinked curves that naturally created areas of potential dysfunction through their anatomical arrangement, but also a picture of areas of the body where forces would either accumulate or dissipate through the action of weight-bearing forces and gravity.

The weight of the head and upper triangle accumulates around T4 and, through the placing of the centre of gravity, the body weight acts between the apex of the upper triangle and the base of the lower (leaving L3 and the centre of gravity in the middle of this). Certainly compression could accumulate at L3, but also a sense of instability, as the L3 area would be the first to buckle if the overall relation between the orientation of the upper and lower triangles were to be affected.

This also led to the idea of the spine being separable into three main sections, in relation to these two areas of collected force: i.e. above T4,

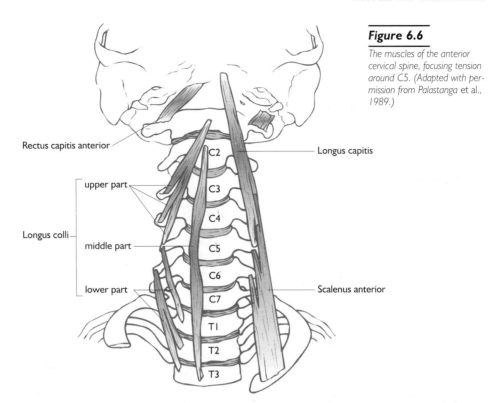

Figure 6.6

The muscles of the anterior cervical spine, focusing tension around C5. (Adapted with permission from Palastanga et al., 1989.)

between T4 and L3, and below L3. These were called the upper, middle and lower arches, respectively. The middle arch was thought to need to be strong to resist the forces acting between the two main weight-bearing points of the body, T4 and L3. Hence T4 and L3 can be thought of as interarch pivots, like C5, T9 and L5. This is shown in Figure 6.8.

Within such a longitudinally compressed curved structure, there is usually one point along that curve that acts rather like a keystone in an architectural arch (i.e. its stability is fundamental to the structural integrity of the rest of the arch). Littlejohn felt that this concept could be applied to the spine, and considered T9 to be the keystone of this strong, central (middle) arch. (The upper and lower arches were thought to be more flexible and fluidic, rather than compressive, and there are many physiological correlations within this relationship that space does not permit discussion of.)

Interestingly, Littlejohn viewed the central arch as the primary arch of the body, because of the above analysis and also because of embryology. During fetal development the whole spine is flexed forwards, and it is only after we are born that the cervical and lumbar (extension) arches develop. Littlejohn felt that the development of movement possibilities within these 'secondary' curves, as he called them, depended on the integrity of the 'primary' (central arch). This 'embryological' relationship was thought to persist through life: if there are problems in the cervical (upper arch) and lumbar (lower arch) curves, look first to the thoracic (middle arch).

Continuing his ideas about the relevance of the developmental changes within the spine, Littlejohn said the following:

> *In the normal individual, the vertebrae are arranged in groups to form a definite series of curves, of which the dorsal and sacral curves are posterior [their convexity is posterior].... The cervical and lumbar curves [although they started out as posterior] are anterior, and represent accessory physio-*

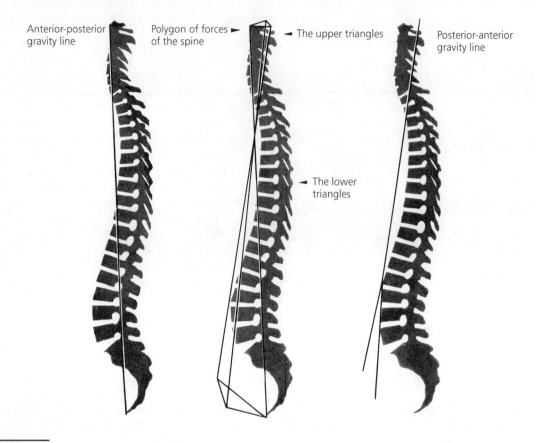

Anterior-posterior gravity line

Polygon of forces of the spine ►

◄ The upper triangles

Posterior-anterior gravity line

◄ The lower triangles

Figure 6.7

Lines indicating the direction of the force exerted by the weight of the head on the spine. **A.** *Anterior–posterior gravity line.* **B.** *Posterior–anterior gravity line.* **C.** *Polygon of forces in the spine created by combining* **A** *and* **B**. *Reproduced with the permission of Maidstone College of Osteopathy from* Institute of Applied Osteopathy, Year Book, *1985.*

logical development. In these two [anterior curve] areas, the development is determined by the shape and size of the discs, while in the posterior curves, the bodies of the vertebrae determine development.

Anonymous, 1956

(This was illustrated by the cervical and lumbar spines – discs are wedge-shaped and vertebrae are square. In the thoracic spine, vertebrae are wedge-shaped and discs are square.)

Littlejohn went on to say:

These [anterior] curves are not embryonic, and appear only when the child begins to assume the erect posture, and form the basis of the locomotor activity of the body.... The posterior curves develop the form, structure and mobility of the column, while the anterior curves are secondary modifications of the posterior curves.

By this he meant that, even in adult life, movement within the thoracic spine can influence the mechanics of the cervical and lumbar spines – which we saw above. He also inferred from this that the embryological foundation of the spinal curves should be considered quite fundamental to later development of integrated spinal function. Working from 'first principles', i.e. from

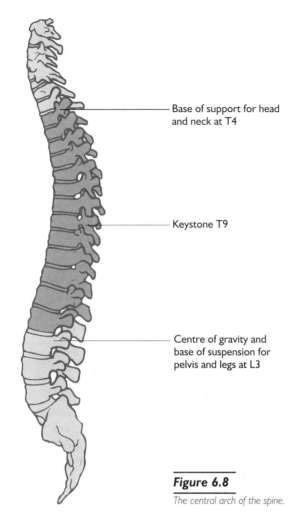

Base of support for head
and neck at T4

Keystone T9

Centre of gravity and
base of suspension for
pelvis and legs at L3

Figure 6.8

The central arch of the spine.

embryology, onwards into biomechanics, if the first area to develop does so unevenly, then any subsequent development will be affected. As stated, this means that one might wish to treat the thoracic area first, because of its influence upon the other curves, even 'after' they have developed.

Littlejohn indicated that although the cervical and lumbar curves naturally rest into extension, when one moves one often does so into flexion, and so an abnormal position for the cervical and lumbar curves is to become restricted into flexion (i.e. loss of lordosis). Following on from this an abnormal position for the thoracic spine is in extension (i.e. loss of kyphosis).

This localizes flexion and extension in different curves, and it is the antagonistic balance and coordination in these separate curves that is the basis of the integrity of the spinal column.

Clinical correlation

This implies that, when one is working with spinal mechanics, for whatever reason, one should encourage the cervical and lumbar spines to become evenly 'extensible' (i.e. the head can tip backwards or the person can bend backwards at the waist) and encourage the thoracic spine to become smoothly 'flexible' (i.e. it can articulate into flexion – as if the person is bending forwards). The key word here is **evenly**.

Many biomechanical problems within the spine tend to appear related to too much extension in the cervical and lumbar areas, and too much flexion in the thoracic area. This is shown in Figure 6.9.

The acutely extended areas are often the ones that express symptoms, but Littlejohn is implying that the 'wrong' bits of the spine are being labelled as dysfunctional, as the symptomatic areas are not the 'primary' areas of dysfunction. In effect, the dysfunctioning curve (Figure 6.9B) could be reinterpreted. This is shown in Figure 6.10.

Littlejohn stated that the acutely curved areas (which were labelled in the first diagram) were reactions due to the restrictions labelled in the second diagram and that it is these latter areas that one should treat to improve spinal motion and so reduce strain at the points indicated. In other words, one should improve the extension within the flexed parts of the cervical and lumbar curves and the flexion in the extended areas of the thoracic curve.

The revised models that we will discuss later led some practitioners to have different approaches, however: the revised models indicate that the painful areas should be explored first, and thereafter any restriction in other areas of the spine; whereas the Littlejohn model suggested that the first place to start would be in the areas of curve that were 'insufficiently curved', i.e. the bits that did not hurt!

Figure 6.9

*Problems caused by unbalanced spinal curves. **A.** Normal, balanced spinal curves (even spread of flexed and extended areas). **B.** Unbalanced curves.*

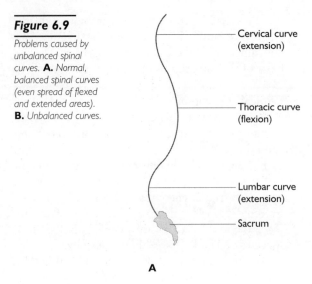

Cervical curve (extension)

Thoracic curve (flexion)

Lumbar curve (extension)

Sacrum

A

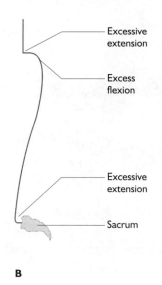

Excessive extension

Excess flexion

Excessive extension

Sacrum

B

Figure 6.10

Unbalanced curves – a different interpretation.

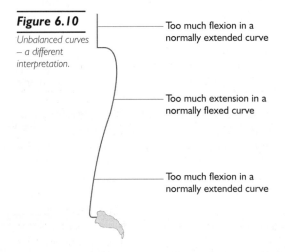

Too much flexion in a normally extended curve

Too much extension in a normally flexed curve

Too much flexion in a normally extended curve

Although these statements are a bit harshly 'cut and dried' and many practitioners would argue nowadays that they would do 'a bit of both', the discussion shows that there are several ways to interpret the same group of findings.

Now, there is an overall picture of a series of interlinking curves, each working in concert as dynamic flexible units under compressive influences; leading to a situation where the spine would naturally be more stable in some areas than others. The spine could now be represented as a series of vertebral arch (curve) groups, with interarch pivots and keystones. (This analysis shows an interesting function for T9: it is supposed to be both a strong keystone and a weak interarch pivot.)

As compressive forces (through gravity) accumulate every day, and these act at certain points of the spine, it was these areas that were thought to accumulate tension first. These areas would tighten as a result and this would have consequences for the function of the interlinking arches, their pivots and the way movement passes through the body as a whole. (This point will be returned to when we discuss Fryette, below.)

Oscillatory movements

Movement was also thought to pass through the body in a series of oscillatory patterns, which would reverberate through the structure in a rhythmic way. As these passed through the spine, the spine would take up this pattern, as the shape of the facets would dictate the way each vertebra would rotate and oscillate. Figure 6.11 shows the axes of rotation for some of the vertebrae.

Because different parts of the spine would naturally rotate about a different axis, there would be a couple of sections within it where oscillatory forces changed abruptly, creating an additional source of potential biomechanical dysfunction.

Therefore because of the differences in axes of rotation caused by the different facet orientations,

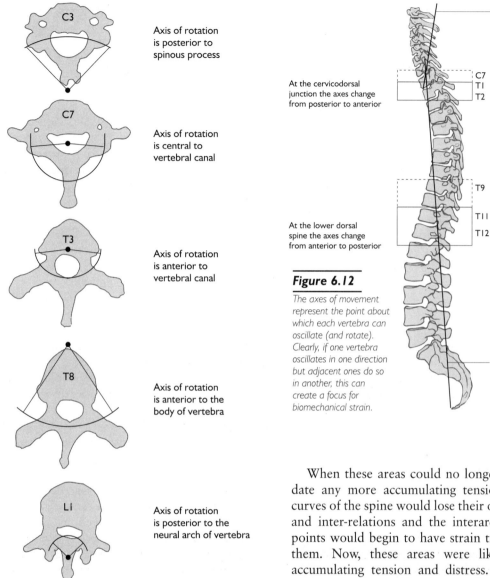

Axis of rotation is posterior to spinous process

Axis of rotation is central to vertebral canal

Axis of rotation is anterior to vertebral canal

Axis of rotation is anterior to the body of vertebra

Axis of rotation is posterior to the neural arch of vertebra

Line joining the axes of movement of the cervical vertebrae

At the cervicodorsal junction the axes change from posterior to anterior

C7
T1
T2

T9

T11
T12

At the lower dorsal spine the axes change from anterior to posterior

Figure 6.12

The axes of movement represent the point about which each vertebra can oscillate (and rotate). Clearly, if one vertebra oscillates in one direction but adjacent ones do so in another, this can create a focus for biomechanical strain.

Line joining the axes of movement of the thoracic and lumbar vertebrae

Figure 6.11

Axes of rotation for some vertebrae.

acting in concert with longitudinally acting gravity forces, oscillatory movements would be in potential conflict in two areas of the spine: C7–T2 and T11/12–L1. This is illustrated in Figure 6.12.

When these areas could no longer accommodate any more accumulating tension, then the curves of the spine would lose their overall spring and inter-relations and the interarch/intercurve points would begin to have strain transferred to them. Now, these areas were likely to start accumulating tension and distress. One of the symptoms that would subsequently be expressed within the body from this was pain at these interarch points.

Clinical correlations
(Note: This adds to the comments on which areas one should treat first that were included above, in the discussion of developmental considerations for spinal movement.)

Clinically, if the person wanted treatment for their symptoms, then the secondary strain areas

137

(the painful interarch pivots) would not be the place to direct treatment, as they were only the effect of stiffness and tension elsewhere, namely the C/T area, T4 area and T/L area. Thus the joints within the arches/curves themselves would need to be freed off in order to make them springy again, adaptable both to oscillatory forces and compressive forces, and so reduce strain at the interarch points.

If the tensions within the curves, i.e. acting at the C/T (upper thoracic), T4 and T/L (lower thoracic) areas, had not been in place too long, their associated soft tissues would not be too chronically contracted and so would respond to treatment in a short period of time. In this situation, any resulting strain at the interarch pivots, e.g. L5/S1, C4/5, could be very quickly relieved by working on the arches (not the pivots). However, if the arches had been chronically restricted for too long, the level of subsequent tension at the interarch points would be similarly tight, and these areas would then start to re-refer back stress to the already compromised areas of primary tension (within the arches, around C/T, T4 and T/L). Thus, depending on levels of tightness, one might need to treat the arches first or the interarch pivots.

The point of releasing strain within the spine
Strange as it may seem, the point of releasing strain within the spine, by whatever model, was not at first simply to reduce pain in these areas, although it was a very effective way of so doing. The real aim of making sure that the spinal articulations improved their mobility, in fact, was that they would then not interfere with structures/tissues related segmentally to them via the nervous system. As mapped out in Chapter 4, articular problems in various points/segments along the spine were considered to have a disturbing influence, through the nervous system, on organs, glands, blood vessels, lymphatic vessels and so on. The purpose was to release the joints so that the nervous system would no longer mediate irritating signals to structures supplied by the same neural segment, and so to bring about an improvement in circulation and nor-

malization of visceral activity, secretion and motion, and, through these effects, a resolution of disease within the body.

Because of the internal structures to which they were segmentally related, sections of the spine when grouped together thus had an influence on various aspects of body function, and these were called **osteopathic centres**. They are illustrated in Figure 6.13.

When a person presented for treatment with some illness or other, this would be analysed with respect to which components of body physiology needed helping (circulation, kidney function – for elimination of waste products, respiration or whatever) and then the spine would be examined to see how movement was able to pass through the relevant osteopathic centre. If restriction was found, the osteopath would work out which other sections of the spine also required work, in order to culminate in an improvement of movement at the spinal area of the relevant 'osteopathic centre'. This would then lead to a normalization of neural processing within the osteopathic centre and a more physiological and healthy functioning of the organs/processes concerned (see Chapter 4).

As stated earlier, Littlejohn's contribution was of ideas and ways of interpreting functional–physiological relations between the spinal mechanics and the osteopathic centres. This related to the way the spine was divided into functional sections, in a structural sense, that could then be correlated as functional areas, in a physiological sense.

The whole concept was (and still is) much more involved and fascinating than is expressed here, but there is unfortunately not time to explain it all in this book, especially as other models need to be explored as well.

Littlejohn's waning influence on some areas of the profession
Littlejohn's influence did wane – which is somewhat surprising if the whole model was so 'complete' and relevant as it is sometimes supposed to be. However, this brief introduction may have left the reader with the idea that such a complex

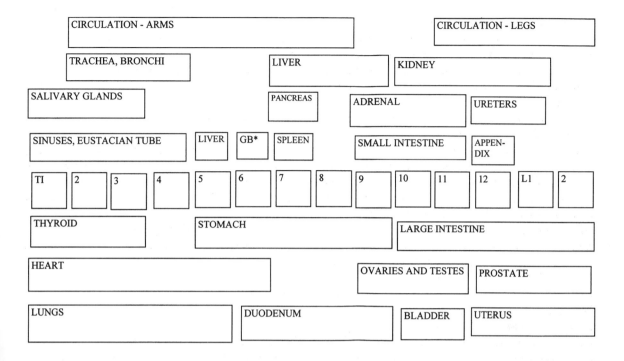

Figure 6.13

*Osteopathic centres – examples of the levels of the spinal column that are segmentally related to the sympathetic supply to various organs/body areas. (Note: some authors may quote slightly different levels – due to the variability in the anatomy of the sympathetic nervous system. Also, the above list is not exhaustive). * Gall bladder.*

set of inter-relations was perhaps a little too confusing, and open to question. This may well have been one of the reasons why in some areas of the profession it fell out of favour to some degree.

There was another, probably much more important reason, though – the discovery of penicillin and the development of modern pharmacology. These developments revolutionized the management of many conditions that osteopaths had up until that time been trying to help through manipulation. Subsequently, the benefits of manipulation were compared unfavourably to those of this new intervention. This gave some impetus to the abandonment of some areas of previous practice when using osteopathic methods in isolation.

Another factor was also relevant – the attempt to gain statutory recognition for UK osteopaths,

who had until that time been practising under common law. There was unease within the orthodox profession about the claims of osteopaths and, when called to discuss his work with parliamentary officials, Littlejohn (for his own reasons) refused to (or could not) justify his ideas and methods to the satisfaction of the committee, which did not help interprofessional relations at the time. The profession was directed to consider its philosophies and practice, and coordinate itself into a more self-regulated and responsible profession, to enable statutory recognition to be awarded (General Council and Register of Osteopaths, 1958).

This in fact took 50 years to achieve, which, along with the other factors mentioned above, led to a drive to simplify and rationalize information given to osteopathic students, to give more time in the curriculum for the orthodox medical model (required for differential diagnostic skills), and to concentrate on certain areas of philosophy that could be more reasonably discussed given neurophysiological understanding at that time. Not all the profession was happy with this direction then, nor are they now, and a great many splits arose on an internal political level as a result, which are only now beginning to be healed.

However, it was indeed these splits that led to new models emerging in some schools, while others attempted to continue as before. But, before discussing these revised models, it is necessary to discuss one other 'traditional' or 'long-held' model, which was also adapted over time.

Fryette

The Littlejohn model of spinal mechanics was allied to another aspect – that of diagnosing local vertebral mechanical function on the basis of vertebral position and alignment. This analysis of local movement has been extensively described by Fryette, and we will review it in a moment. When this section is read, though, it will be clear that this method of analysing joint mobility is also quite complex, and this may have been another reason for the development of other models, based on different assessment categories (movement quality more than position).

Within the broad Littlejohn model of spinal mechanics mentioned before, there was of course a need to work on individual intervertebral relations, to help the overall functions of the curves.

Within this osteopathic practice, then, there developed a complex theory to explain how the local mechanics of the spine functioned and dictate how the restrictions should be released, but also to explain how the positional intervertebral relations/spinal restrictions again related to neurophysiological reflexes that were thought to influence visceral and internal function (as in the osteopathic centres).

Many osteopaths, such as Louisa Burns, had done much work to try to analyse the neurophysiological relations that could possibly link spinal function with visceral dysfunction. There emerged an opinion that not all spinal restrictions could be capable of causing visceral distress; indeed, if they did, then the body would never work at all! Therefore, there had to be some way of recognizing which restrictions were the ones capable of causing such distress through the internal environment.

There was a hierarchy of spinal dysfunction, such that one could distinguish when a restriction was simply a biomechanical event and when it had progressed to one with physiological consequences.

All of this in the early models centred on the way that spinal intervertebral segments moved and the patterns they formed (in their movement) subsequent to biomechanical dysfunction arising. These patterns could be recognized and, as some were considered more perverted in their arrangement than others, these would have more profound and diverse effects (upon the internal environment).

This is the analysis that Fryette made, coupling physiology to intervertebral position analysis.

Intervertebral position analysis

Fryette's analysis starts, though, by relating forces within the curved flexible spinal model that Littlejohn used within his mechanics. Let me repeat an earlier passage, to bring us back to Littlejohn:

> As compressive forces (through gravity) accumulate every day, and these act at certain points of the spine, it was these areas that were thought to accumulate tension first. These areas would tighten as a result and this would have consequences for the function of the interlinking arches, their pivots and the way movement passed through the body as a whole.

Each individual section of the spine (each vertebra) was acting under longitudinal pressure. Because the sections of the spine are curved, forces cannot act in a simple manner. Placing vertical compressive forces (such as gravity) on a curved rod (the spine) makes that curved rod twist to escape the load/pressures induced. To understand how the individual vertebrae of the spine might move in such circumstances, one needs to look at what happens within a straight rod when one bends it.

When one bends a curved rod (which induces compressive forces in some parts of the rod and not others), the rod will twist as it bends. This twisting (torsion) within the rod will be established during small unidirectional bends, but increasingly so if you then try to combine two different directions of bend (such as flexion and sidebending). The direction of the induced twist/torsion pattern depends on how much one bends the rod in one direction before adding the other component.

Sections of the rod would in effect be trying to escape load by twisting out of the path of the induced force. If the combined forces were mild, the rod only needed to torque (twist/torsion) a little to escape serious compression at any particular point. If the combined forces were strong though, the rod would need to torque quite acutely at a particular point, and even so might not be able to dissipate all the compressive forces in so doing. In such a situation, the rod might then become damaged.

Fryette put this analogy into a spinal context: compressive forces acting along the length of the curved spine will induce a tendency to cause the vertebrae of the spine to rotate, to escape the load. The greater the bending (flexion or extension of the spine) the greater the inducement to rotate.

This is interesting in itself, but Fryette considered that, depending on the combination and amount of bends (either flexion and sidebending or extension and sidebending) in the spine, the rotation induced would not always be in the same direction.

Laws of spinal motion according to Fryette
First law: in easy flexion and extension (neutral range), most of the spine will sidebend and rotate to opposite sides. (If the spine is side bent to the left, the anterior portion of the vertebra – the

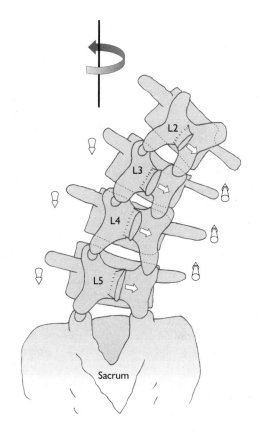

Figure 6.14

The lumbar spine: flexion, rotation and sidebending movement. The person is standing upright and sidebending right at the same time. 'Standing upright' means that the lumbar curve is slightly concave posteriorly – it is held in relative 'flexion'. The vertebrae are rotating about a vertical axis (the bodies are moving to the left and the spinous processes to the right). The bodies thus move into the convexity and the discs can 'escape' pressure and strain.

body – will follow by rotating to the right.) In this situation, the vertebral bodies twist away from compressive forces and the soft tissue structures escape from damaging stresses.

Second law: in extremes of movement, either flexion or extension, the spine will sidebend and rotate to the same side. (If the spine is side bent to the left, the body of the vertebra will now follow by rotating to the left.) In this situation, the vertebral bodies twist in towards the compressive

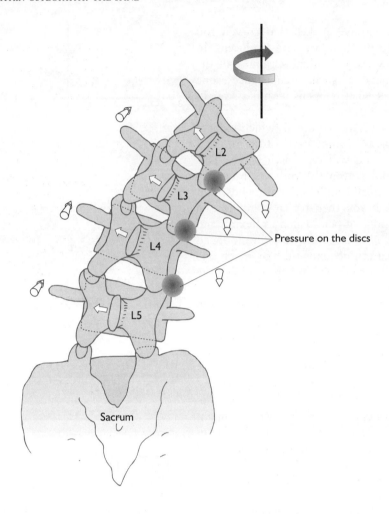

Pressure on the discs

Sacrum

Figure 6.15

The lumbar spine: extension, rotation and sidebending movement. The person is bending forwards and sidebending right at the same time. This flattens the lumbar curve and creates 'extension' in it. (This is a functional/relative description rather than an anatomical one.) With no articular restrictions, all vertebrae follow the pattern of sidebending right, rotation right when the spine is 'extended' (bent forward). However, this pattern of movement compresses the discs on the side of the concavity. The vertebrae are rotating about a vertical axis (the bodies are moving to the right and the spinous processes to the left). The bodies thus move into the concavity, causing pressure on the discs.

forces, as the combination of extreme flexion or extension coupled with the side bending dictates a different behaviour from the curved 'rod' of the spine. Hence, in this case, the soft tissue structures are much less likely to escape damaging stresses.

Spinal movement under combined forces

Lumbar spine motion can follow both of Fryette's laws of motion. If you sidebend the lumbar spine from a relatively neutral position (which is a slight lordosis), then the vertebral bodies will rotate into the convexity. This is shown in Figure 6.14. But, if you start from a relatively straight position (as in body flexion; Figure 6.15), or a relatively bent position (as in marked lordosis) and sidebend it, then the bodies will rotate the other way, i.e. into the concavity.

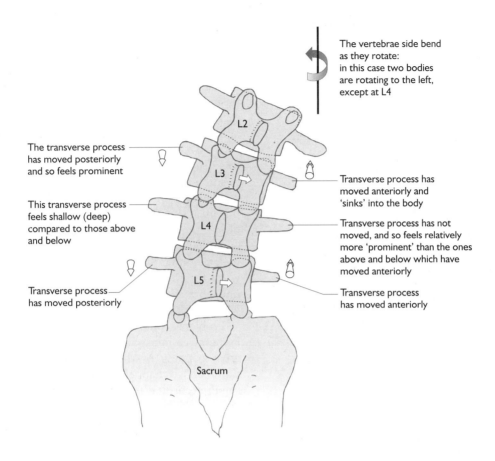

The vertebrae side bend as they rotate: in this case two bodies are rotating to the left, except at L4

The transverse process has moved posteriorly and so feels prominent

This transverse process feels shallow (deep) compared to those above and below

Transverse process has moved posteriorly

Transverse process has moved anteriorly and 'sinks' into the body

Transverse process has not moved, and so feels relatively more 'prominent' than the ones above and below which have moved anteriorly

Transverse process has moved anteriorly

Sacrum

Figure 6.16

The lumbar spine: no movement at L4. The person is standing and attempting to sidebend to the right. The vertebrae are rotating about a vertical axis (the bodies are moving to the left and the spinous processes to the right). Because of articular restriction, the L4 vertebra does not follow the movement of the rest of the spinal column. It will not sidebend to the right and the body will not rotate to the left. Therefore, this L4 restriction is designated a sidebending left and rotated right lesion.

This means that, for sidebending of the lumbar spine in varying positions, you need pliability of the soft tissues acting on the anterior and posterior aspects of the lumbar vertebrae, to allow whichever rotation movement is induced. If the spine becomes restricted in some way, then the normal torsion of the vertebrae will become adapted during general body movement. This is shown in Figure 6.16.

However, the **cervical spine** is different. If the cervical spine is sidebent, the anterior face of the vertebral bodies will always rotate into the concavity, no matter whether the neck was in a flexed or an extended position to start with. Thus the cervical spine operates under Fryette's second law of motion during most movement. This can be seen from Figure 6.17.

It can be seen that the facets on the convex (left-hand) side need to be free to 'open out' in order for the neck to sidebend. Therefore the posterior cervical muscles (erector spinae group) need to be pliable and able to relax to allow this movement.

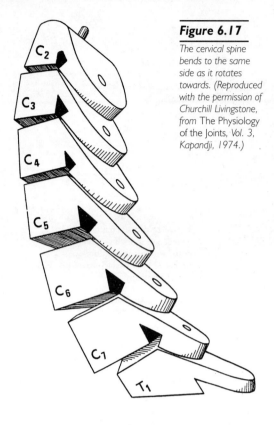

Figure 6.17

The cervical spine bends to the same side as it rotates towards. (Reproduced with the permission of Churchill Livingstone, from The Physiology of the Joints, Vol. 3, Kapandji, 1974.)

Clinical correlation

Interestingly, if the bodies rotate into the concavity (as they do if you sidebend the neck, lean to the side while sitting slumped or lean to the side while standing and stooping down – both these latter acting on the lumbar spine), then the intervertebral discs would come under a lot of pressure (as the movement is following Fryette's second law of motion). So, ergonomically, too much head down at the keyboard and reading pages off to one side is bad for you, and stooping/slouching and leaning over is not healthy either – both scenarios (and many like them) could lead to early disc degeneration and damage!

Normal movement patterns can be distorted

When one moves during the day, the spinal column is naturally coming under a degree of combined bending forces, and so the vertebra should end up rotating first one way and then

another way (in relation to its neighbours), depending on the combination of either flexion or extension and sidebending that that section is exposed to. If the spinal soft tissues are healthy, muscular control is efficient and the relative positions/forces are not maintained for too long, then the spine should remain free from injury and the individual vertebrae should be free to rotate as they need, to escape stress or to return to a neutral position from a potentially damaging position of torsion.

However, it seemed the case to Fryette that this ideal situation did not always occur and that often combined movements/positions were sustained/held for too long, causing stress to accumulate. Now, the locally acting muscles had to work to try to forcibly pull the spinal vertebral units into a less stressful relative position. This is where problems started to occur.

Problems could also arise from stress accumulating at certain points, even without too much gross bending of the spine. This is what was supposed to happen to various points of the spine, according to Littlejohn's model of spinal arches and pivots, if posture was not correctly balanced and maintained.

The theory was that, in the position of stress, the muscles would attempt to retwist the vertebra most under tension, to try to re-establish a better intervertebral relationship. The muscular components would change the relative positions of the vertebrae while the body was still in the combined twisted position but, when the person straightened up, the vertebral alignment pattern would not revert to normal. This was thought to be because the neural control mechanisms had 'locked' that section of the spine into a position where forces were supposedly less. These muscles would then maintain that positional relationship, as the 'least worst option' for the local spinal mechanics given the overall postural picture, and would maintain this even when the person changed their position and so shifted the general force pattern.

If the vertebral malalignment remained in place for some time, then the local muscles would again try to restore normal positioning,

Figure 6.18

A first-degree lesion at L4. The person is standing upright. The L4 vertebra has rotated to the right and sidebent to the right.

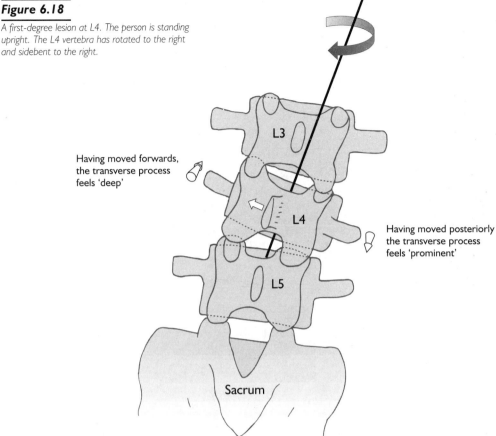

Having moved forwards, the transverse process feels 'deep'

L3

L4

L5

Having moved posteriorly the transverse process feels 'prominent'

Sacrum

but would instead only compound the error, as the spine would now be trying to twist from a position of increased stress. There would now be an even more distorted relationship between the vertebrae than before.

This sort of reasoning led to the idea that there were degrees of lesion that would occur, depending on circumstance or location. The subsequent lesions would each show differing patterns of positional relation.

Degrees of lesion

Lesions that were recent and occurred in not too stressful conditions were called first-degree lesions; those that were longer-lasting or occurred through more serious biomechanical distortion were called second-degree lesions; and those that were very long-lasting were called third-degree lesions.

In **first-degree lesions**, when the articulation was examined it was held in a state of sidebending and rotation to the same side – obeying the first law of motion. These were the most easily reduced category of lesion (Figure 6.18).

Second-degree lesions were when the vertebrae were found to be held in sidebending and rotation to the opposite sides (obeying the first law). In fact, this category of lesion, which was of longer standing than the first-degree lesion, was considered to be an adaptation of the first-degree lesion in which, in an attempt to follow the first law of movement, the spine rotated from the first-degree lesion pattern in the opposite direction, thus giving the second-degree lesion pattern

Figure 6.19

A second-degree lesion at L4. The person is standing upright. The vertebra has derotated out of the position it was in in the first-degree lesion – it has now rotated to the left. It has sidebent to the right.

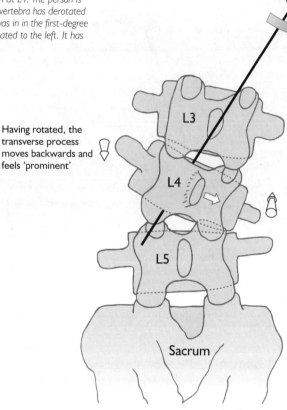

Having rotated, the transverse process moves backwards and feels 'prominent'

L3

L4

L5

Sacrum

Having rotated in the opposite direction to that in the first degree lesion, the transverse process moves forwards and now feels 'deep'

(obeying the first law of motion). This is shown in Figure 6.19.

These lesion patterns are akin to the spine wriggling about under load and getting caught up along the way, with the resulting compromised articular restriction maintained by paravertebral muscle spasm. These lesion patterns were more difficult to resolve and needed more articulation and stretching prior to thrust in order for them to remain corrected afterwards.

Note: In fact, this sort of torsioning has been recognized in the modern 'orthopaedic' descriptions of functional and organic scolioses, and the way in which a functional scoliosis adapts to become organic. Organic scolioses demonstrate several adaptations, including facet joint remodelling in response to the altered forces, a good example of function governing structure.

(Scoliotic forces on the spine are discussed in Chapter 8.)

Third-degree lesions, representing physiology within intervertebral relations, were the most chronic and were, again, a perversion of an unresolved lesion – in this case an unresolved second-degree lesion pattern. In this particularly distorted orientation, the resulting afferent signals to the dorsal horn of the cord were thought to be so disturbed that now they would be capable of disturbing the neural function at that segmental level and lead to the perversion of visceral and vascular function previously discussed with reference to osteopathic centres. Third-degree lesions represented physiological disturbance, whereas the other two lesions were not thought to be capable of inducing this type of reaction.

Reference to Littlejohn

At the risk of confusing matters further at this stage, there is the idea that if one combines Fryette laws with Littlejohn mechanics one can have the situation where certain degrees of lesion are thought to occur either within the curves/arches or at the interarch pivots. So, not only would there be an order of treatment within Littlejohn mechanics (usually mid-arch first, to resolve interarch stain) but the manoeuvres for the mid-curve restrictions (where second-degree lesions were thought to arise) were different from interarch restrictions (where first-degree lesions were thought to operate). Long-standing postural strain would act within the curves and lead to second-degree lesions within them. These, if left in place long enough, would convert to third-degree lesions.

Additionally, the physiological relations of the third-degree lesions could partly be rationalized by looking at which osteopathic centres were located in the segments liable to develop them.

Treatment within the Fryette model

Within Fryette's model, then, one needs to re-establish normal positional relations within the spinal intervertebral segments. To do this, one must 'reverse' the components during a high-velocity thrust manoeuvre to 'overcome' the reflexes that have kept the muscular contraction acting in such a way that it preserved the components of the lesion pattern.

This led to a very 'prescriptive' model of manipulative manoeuvres, which were seemingly more interested in positional relations than in tissue quality and reaction as the prime determinants of treatment methodology (although exponents of this method did 'respect tissue integrity' during the manipulative procedure). It also perhaps led to the very damaging idea that osteopaths 'put bones back into place' – an image that has held back osteopathic progression in the eyes of others external to it.

Confusion from complexity (the opposite of order out of chaos)

As will be appreciated, this is an enormously complex method of analysing what is going on and, as

the treatment involves 'reversing' the components of the lesion, one could not manipulate the vertebral arrangement without having analysed how it was being held in whatever combination of flexion, extension, sidebending and rotation.

It was, and still is a challenging model to learn for osteopathic students and, as many patients were not presenting with 'medical' problems, it seemed the need to be able to recognize when the spinal dysfunction was in a state to cause neural distortion (as per the third-degree lesions) was diminished.

All of this, coupled with an increasing appreciation of the subtleties of spinal motion, led to the idea that such a regulated model was not actually realistic – there were surely many more movement possibilities than simple flexion, rotation or sidebending. Another reason was that, through orthodox analogies such as those relating to scoliosis mentioned above, the same sorts of torsioning force could be recognized without having to really worry about linking the torsions to Littlejohn's curves and so on. Also, the somewhat dictatorial nature of the Littlejohn/Fryette model made one look for and find restrictions in predetermined areas, and this seemed to many to be artificial, too simplistic and not to account for the effects of trauma or surgical injury, nor the effects of disease. There are in fact potentially very many variations in motion patterns within the spine (McGregor *et al.*, 1995), which could come from any number of biomechanical or traumatic insults.

So, when all this was put together, along with a greater appreciation of the anatomical relations of the locally acting muscles and the influence of the differing ligaments of the spine, coupled with the dynamic influence of the intervertebral disc, it became clear to some that a more three-dimensional vision of spinal mechanics was necessary, which could be free from the supposed constraints of a prescriptive/rigid model.

NEW MODELS – THE REDUCTIONIST PHASE AND THE REVISED MODEL

The reductionist phase

There are in essential two 'new models' to consider:

- a simplification of the spinal curve analysis of Littlejohn;
- a simplification of local spinal mechanics from the Fryette model.

As stated before, for a variety of reasons, parts of the profession came to move away from the traditional models within spinal biomechanics. Some of these movements could be described as reductionist in nature, and resulted in a number of different changes of approach (Stoddard, 1983). Some of these have been of enormous value to the profession, such as the refinement of technique carried out by Laurie Hartman (1997), following on from the tradition of superb technicians of that era of change, such as T. Edgar Hall. Some changes were not nearly so beneficial in the long run, such as the loss of real identity with osteopathy as a physiological medical model in its own right, and a subsequent reduction of the common scope of osteopathic practice to such things as the management of orthopaedic conditions, traumatic injuries and sports injuries. It took deep conviction on the part of some other members of the profession for them to remain true to an ideal of osteopathy as a serious medicophysiological model during this period, although, to be fair, it seems that those moving in new directions did not truly wish the demise of a broad scope of practice – it emerged rather by default along the way, subsequently proving difficult to reverse.

The reductionist models – spinal curves
Much of the complex spinal mechanics of Littlejohn's model was put to one side, and what seemed to be retained was the idea of major strain accumulating at T4 (where the upper and lower triangles met) and, in relation to the oscillatory forces, where they came into conflict at C7–L2, and T11/12–L1, although the physiological relations associated with them in the Littlejohn model were somewhat 'lost'.

These areas of potential restriction were 're-described' in a model of junctional areas within spinal mechanics, along the lines laid down by traditional/orthodox anatomical considerations.

The concepts of osteopathic centres were still routinely covered, but students increasingly did not get the chance to explore the management of people for medical conditions (as they did not present), and so even these components seemed to lose relevance as more and more people presented simply for pain-related musculoskeletal problems instead.

If such 'junctional' models are explored for a moment, one can see that Littlejohn's ideas are not required at all in order for certain areas of the spine to be implicated in dysfunction.

The spine is sectioned into four 'curves': sacral, lumbar, thoracic and cervical. The sacral vertebrae are fused and so move as a unit. The lumbar and cervical curves are very much more mobile than the thoracic curve but, if it were not for the ribs, then the thoracic articulations would allow the most movement.

The thoracic facets are very flat, and should allow flexion, extension, rotation and sidebending in large measures. However, in real life (with the ribs in place) the thoracic cage as a whole is quite immobile, permitting mostly a little spinal flexion and extension, with very limited rotation and sidebending. Overall, then, during most gross spinal movements the amplitude is derived from the lumbar and cervical spine articulations. Comparing these two areas, the lumbar spine has a greater range in flexion and extension than sidebending and rotation, and the cervical spine has pretty good movement in all directions.

If we consider all the above, we can see that the most mobile part of the spine (the cervical area) is right next to a very immobile area (the thorax); and that, at the other end, the relatively mobile lumbar spine is between this immobile thorax and the rigid sacrum. This is illustrated in Figure 6.20.

There are therefore 'junctions' or 'hinges' between the different sections of the spine: the lumbosacral, thoracolumbar and cervicothoracic. There is also a 'junction' between the top of the cervical spine and the cranium. Movement through the spinal column as a whole should be as smooth as possible and, if there are areas where the architecture creates 'naturally' abrupt

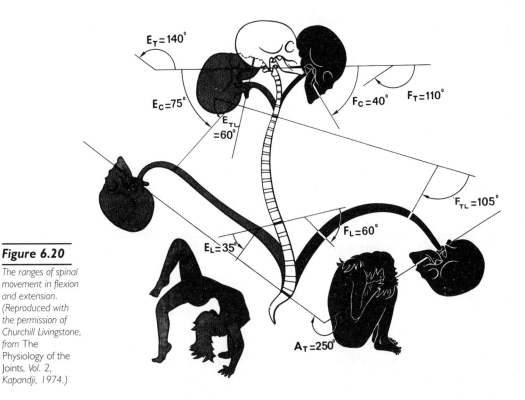

Figure 6.20

The ranges of spinal movement in flexion and extension. (Reproduced with the permission of Churchill Livingstone, from The Physiology of the Joints, *Vol. 2, Kapandji, 1974.)*

changes in movement, then physical forces will tend to concentrate on these junctions. Therefore they are quite likely to suffer stress and strain, particularly if the spine is loaded or the attempted movements are extreme.

Normally, when one attempts to move the spine (in general everyday activities), the movement passes through the cervical and lumbar curves without placing much strain at the individual joints within, until the junctional area is reached, where the movement forces one vertebra to twist against its neighbour. Therefore mid-curve strain (meaning mid-cervical/lumbar spine – or 'within' the cervical/lumbar columns, not at their ends) is not as likely as strain within junctional areas of the spine (except in extreme cases such as whiplash trauma to the cervical spine, where the naturally less stable areas – the mid-cervicals – become damaged even though they are not immediately next to a rigid area). Practically, if the junctional areas then become restricted, transition of movement will be more

compromised and other joints will have strain placed upon them. (If the cervicothoracic area is restricted, then the C6/7 articulation will act as the junctional area and take all the strain, and so on.)

This sort of analysis supposes therefore that mid-curve strain comes as a consequence of that curve having to work differently because the natural junctional area has become restricted over time (for example, subsequent to repeated minor stresses accumulating at this level and encouraging a tightening of the soft tissues in response). In order to get the mid-curve working asymptomatically again, one needs to resolve the junctional areas first.

Under this model, osteopaths would routinely work on the C/T areas, the T4 area, the T/L and often the L/S areas in most cases of spinal dysfunction, wherever there was pain. This is similar to some aspects of the Littlejohn model (oscillatory strain points). However, they would not go into the more detailed analysis of inter-relations between more distant areas of the spine described by Littlejohn's model.

The new models were also 'reductionist' in the sense that the relations within the individual intervertebral segment became much more important than those between diverse vertebrae throughout the spine.

The reductionist models: local spinal mechanics
As stated in the section on Fryette, because of the complexity of that model, a simpler but anatomically accurate model was required and developed that was concerned with local spinal mechanics (between adjacent segments) as well as with the spine in general, which we have just been discussing.

There was first a 'reductionist' model, which had a much narrower outlook, and then a 'revised' model, which began to re-expand in various ways. These will be explored in a moment but, by the time the model was being revised in a dynamic way, the orientation of management and assessment of the spine had changed dramatically from the Fryette/Littlejohn model.

This change had developed in several different directions:

- A recognition had come about of the integrated relationship between all factors influencing spinal motion, such as ligamentous arrangement, intervertebral disc mechanics and consistency, muscular action, fluid columns (maintained in fascial compartments) and the bony architecture of the vertebral bodies and facets.
- This enabled osteopaths to appreciate the spinal column in a very detailed way, with respect to local tissue function, interaction and health, and allowed them to see how changing soft tissue tensions could lead to a whole variety of movement permutations and strain patterns, which could (because of the complex and overlapping innervation patterns within the spinal ligaments and soft tissues) lead to all sorts of pain patterns and presentations.

- This enabled osteopaths to relate soft tissue injury (and the palpatory changes that this induced within and around the joint complex) to the symptom picture of the patient with much greater accuracy than before.
- It also led to a methodology of examination and subsequent 'orthopaedic' analysis of the spinal column (based on tissue quality, soft tissue response to movement and joint range – either single-plane motion or combined-plane motion).
- This in turn led to the practice of describing the 'lesion' in terms of soft tissue distress or injury rather than mere position.
- In this sense, osteopaths could analyse the origin of the symptoms the patient was suffering from, which was correlated to a particular tissue or group of tissues rather than an area of a curve, or a pivot point.

Summing up the major differences between Fryette and the new model, identifying tissues that were causing symptoms became a prime objective of evaluation within this new model, and the method of correction was a more dynamic, individualized release of a 'three-dimensional' restriction than the previous 'artificial' description of planar movement.

'Extra benefit'
This last point meant that now one could determine how to release the joint simply by feeling how it was restricted. This freed osteopaths from much mental anguish, and allowed their palpatory skills to take over – always an aim within any osteopathic technique. The 'release' that is being talked about is the high-velocity thrust, which had previously been performed according to Fryette's principle of position analysis but was now being performed by tissue feel instead. The high-velocity thrust was the mainstay of the reductionist model, which is discussed below.

The reductionist phase – other considerations
This should be seen as part of a development from the Fryette/Littlejohn era to the revised

model within the modern practice of osteopathy in some sections of the profession. As such it need not be fully described as it has been 'submerged' by the revised model that evolved from it. (Note: As stated before, the Littlejohn/Fryette model is still actively being used in some areas of the profession and has not been submerged at all.)

The reductionist 'phase' is worth mentioning briefly, however, as it saw the emergence of one particular technique viewed as being of the greatest value in the eyes of many practitioners – the high-velocity thrust technique (HVT). Up until that point (i.e. within the Littlejohn/Fryette era), during evaluation and treatment there was a 'whole-body routine' called the general osteopathic treatment (GOT). This was a technique where one performed rhythmic, oscillatory and circular movements around the body. One started at a certain point and proceeded to articulate joints around the body in a prescribed manner. At the level of the spine, this movement was continued, but one might consider that the restrictions also needed another type of input and so perform a high-velocity thrust technique to mobilize the joint more directly (in accordance with the principles of Fryette). This mobilization was done as an integral part of the GOT, to help improve the spinal mechanics (with a Littlejohn model in mind). The GOT was thought to be more than a simple whole-body articulation, though, and there were several different physiological effects that could be achieved if the procedure was performed in a variety of ways.

The reductionist model was much less 'physiological' than previous ones – a point that has already been made. The key to improving the patient's spinal mechanics seemed to be local work directly to the joint that had compromised movement, and it was not thought to be so necessary to work through the whole body in such a detailed way. Therefore the full GOT was reduced and there was a concentration on the high-velocity thrust technique.

Also, the concentration on the use of HVTs seemed to be considered a refinement of technique, whereas the general articulatory tech-

niques (within the GOT) came to be seen as a 'preparation' of the joint – something one did just to ease out the area before the thrust, so 'putting aside' the important and dynamic effects that could be achieved through well-performed articulation.

Most treatments consisted of manipulating the joints to relieve local strain, without the same reference to spinal integration as before. Some general articulation and soft tissue massage was performed, but to aid the local manipulation and not in consideration of how these soft tissue tensions could play a significant role on whole-body posture and therefore on local spinal and other articular mechanics (a factor that was always implicit in the Littlejohn model).

Within the orthodox field, Cyriax, an orthopaedic consultant, wrote a book on manipulation that has become a bible for the orthodox approach to manipulation. The Cyriax methods were akin to the reductionist method of joint manipulation and, in the same way that the reductionist osteopathic model did not reflect whole-body physiology, nether did the Cyriax model. However, it did give the impression within the medical world that this orthodox model had 'got all the useful bits' of the osteopathic model, so negating the need for all the confusing, contradictory and questionable aspects of the osteopathic theory.

The osteopathic profession has been trying to reverse this impression ever since, and still has not universally got the message over that osteopathy is more than spinal manipulation!

The whole scope of osteopathic practice was shifting around the time of the reductionist model – and much of the 'medical' work that osteopaths had up until that time been involved with was being superseded by a concentration of interest in orthopaedics and rheumatology. The reductionist model came to the fore for a number of reasons, which have been discussed, but one of the strongest motives must have been 'political correctness' with respect to relations with the orthodox medical profession. Mention has been made of the desire of osteopaths for statutory recognition and a failed attempt at achieving regulation. The orthodox medical profession was at the time very sceptical and suspicious of the claims of osteopaths such as Littlejohn to help liver disease by manipulating the ninth rib on the right, for example, whatever the rationale behind the idea.

The profession was directed to 'put itself in order', which it did, although in the process the scope of osteopathic practice shrank, leaving the profession with the image of specialist practitioners interested in orthopaedics, rheumatology and traumatology.

The revised model was ultimately developed within this scope of practice, and as such has much to recommend it. Osteopaths do have special skills within the above fields of practice, which need to be communicated.

In this context the revised model considered the intricacies of local spinal architecture and soft tissue dynamics, which had relevance both for the development of tissue injuries and their accompanying symptom presentations and in the methodology of technical correction of these articular 'problems'.

Referring back to the major differences between Fryette and this revised model, identifying tissues causing symptoms became a prime objective of evaluation within this model and the method of correction was a more dynamic, individualized release of a 'three-dimensional' restriction than the previous 'artificial' description of planar movement. This model led to some very important developments for clinical practice, which will be summarized shortly.

First, though, it should be pointed out that the high-velocity thrust was not the mainstay of technique for all parts of the profession – another style was emerging.

Manipulation as the mainstay of osteopathic work

There were other conundrums about the nature of technique and how it should be applied that the reductionist model had to contend with. Manipulation is the mainstay of osteopathic work, but the nature of that manipulation could be quite diverse.

The reliance of some sections of the profession upon spinal manipulation by HVT was viewed with despair by other sections. At the same time that this reductionist phase was occurring, another trend within osteopathy (which has eventually come to be considered of profound importance) was developing. Sutherland, an American osteopath, had developed a system of treatment that was gentle, subtle to the point of using minute movement and profound in the effects that could be achieved from such small interventions.

He developed a system of releasing joint problems, whether within the cranium, pelvis or any other part of the body, that revolved around balancing tensions between shifting soft tissue dynamics, within which any joint mobility problems were viewed as consequences of these shifting soft tissue tensions rather than the cause of them (which was the idea within the reductionism model). This model was also much concerned with the physiological effects of releasing soft tissue tensions – another contrast with the 'reductionist camp'.

Thus there was a strong divergence of opinion within the profession as a whole about what 'technique' within treatment was all about.

Interestingly, those followers of Sutherland felt that they had a much better link back to the original methods of Still (as discussed earlier), a claim that was disputed. Using Still's original techniques upon the peripheral joints of the limbs and within the spine, one could sometimes hear the joint 'release' – an audible 'crack' was heard. Remember that Still never discussed his techniques, he only ever demonstrated them within the context of a treatment. Therefore the 'click' was taken as a sign of treatment efficacy, and something to emulate.

This reliance upon the 'click' found its home within the reductionist model. These practitioners had found a reliable way of reproducing this effect within the joint easily and quickly, and the technique became known as the high-velocity thrust. The HVT was considered to be a direct continuation of Still's techniques.

However, the followers of Sutherland's methods also thought that they had the 'true' picture of what Still had been doing. With the methods of Sutherland, when used on the spine and peripheral joints, the gentle positioning of joints and the maintenance of joints in certain positions in relation to a balance in surrounding tissue tension also sometimes produced a 'click'. Sutherland's adherents felt that the idea of gentle movements and re-alignment of joints through subtle tension balancing was the real aim of Still's techniques, and that the 'click' was a secondary outcome, which did not necessarily relate to treatment efficacy. Thus they felt that the 'click' had become some sort of false god to follow!

This caused a bit of a conundrum, as the methods used within the two styles were very different. As stated, in Sutherland's techniques the movements were very small and the 'click' was an occasional 'secondary' occurrence. The other techniques used much faster movements, and larger amplitudes, the 'click' was a major objective, and exponents of this model could not see how the Sutherland techniques could be effective.

The contrast between the styles (and their underlying philosophies) could not have been greater and consequently these two groups within the profession were at odds with each other. Politically these two groups were polarized, which is a shame, as each party could have learned a great deal from the other. Much of their problem lay in the claim put forward by both that their techniques were what Still had used. However, nowadays this division is not antagonistic but much more balanced and respectful than before, with each party recognizing the contribution and value of the other, even if the argument can never be resolved!

So, having noted that not all elements within the profession relied upon the high-velocity thrust, we do need to discuss the ongoing development of the reductionist phase into its revised format, if only because the largest section of the profession has subsequently been taught this way, and it represents the average way that osteopaths practise.

The revised model

Some introductory points:

- When a person presented with some sort of biomechanical dysfunction (back pain and so on), the spinal area that was symptomatic was analysed to appreciate the degree and nature of the soft tissue damage that might or might not be present.
- Determining the type of injury gave insight into potential recovery rates, with mild injuries more quickly healed than disc prolapse, for example. It also gave insights into how much 'manipulating' the area could take – more damaged tissues being considered 'weaker' and therefore dictating the use of less 'invasive' techniques.
- Restrictions in other areas were thought to be quite relevant, along the lines of the 'junctional model' (of common restriction in the C/T, T4 and T/L areas). In these cases, some mobilizing work would be performed on these other areas to give some sort of longitudinal pliability and integration to the spinal column, but the work on the symptomatic segment (or those in close proximity) was thought to be of paramount importance.
- In the Littlejohn/Fryette model the symptomatic area was often actively passed over for treatment until other – often quite distant – areas of the spine had been released; indeed this other work might mean that the symptomatic area could release without being directly worked on. The new model gave the impression to some of its devotees that one had to work directly on the symptomatic area for it to change, for which it has been criticized.

Positive changes within the revised model

The first two points above relate to soft tissue dynamics within motion testing and an appreciation of soft tissue quality as a reflection of tissue health/level of damage. These are aspects that were not as prominent in the early models of osteopathy, and this revision is a positive step to more effective clinical practice. The examination concepts and clinical analysis based upon this will be reviewed in Chapter 10. It has been one of the changes that has led to the wide professional respect in which osteopaths are held by others, and one that has contributed to the maturation of the profession and the gaining of statutory self-regulation status.

Less positive changes within the revised model
The second two points above indicate that the vision of spinal integration was now much more limited, with treatment being much more 'standardized' and less individual. As a consequence the subtleties of relations between parts have become blurred and indistinct for parts of the profession, and they do not necessarily have as many options to fall back on if their 'standard' approach does not resolve the patient's problems.

Also, the loss of identity with the physiological aspects of spinal movement patterns has led to many in the profession not practising as wide a scope of manual medicine as before, which is a great loss both to professional identity within osteopathy and to patients in general.

Integrated practice
However, it is hoped that this book, when viewed as a whole, will illustrate that even if one doesn't use Littlejohn and Fryette, one can still look at movement disorders, reflect on their neural, fluidic and physiological consequences (as described in other chapters) and incorporate a wider model of biomechanics and a better appreciation of manual medicine. One can also incorporate and use the positive aspects of revised thinking – giving a better appreciation of local soft tissue assessment with respect to damage and injury – and come out with an integrated model that also allows a special contribution to be made in the fields of sports injuries, ergonomics and traumatology.

Current practice based on the revised model
The aspects of this subject that have not been discussed are palpation, motion testing, soft tissue evaluation and analysis of examination findings.

As indicated above, these will be discussed in Chapter 10, as there is much to say about them. These palpatory elements, though, do not relate to spinal motion testing alone but to all joints and soft tissues within the body, and so it is only right that they should not be included in the 'spinal' chapter.

What is left to discuss, though, is models of movement patterns based on the cervical spine – and the upper cervical spine in particular, and it is to this topic that we now turn.

IDEAS WITHIN OSTEOPATHY: THE CERVICAL SPINE

Summary of cervical spine mechanics already discussed

The architectural arrangement of the cervical vertebrae, coupled with the shape of the intervertebral discs, makes the cervical area the most mobile part of the spine, and one that works quite differently from the lumbar spine (Bland and Boushey, 1990). This very mobile column must support one of the heaviest structures in the body – the head – in a very finely controlled and subtle way, through numerous movement permutations.

The mid-cervical region is often prone to injury, because it is the least stable part of the spine (structurally) and is the area most commonly damaged in whiplash-type injuries. The cervicothoracic area is also prone to strain, as this is where one very mobile area of the spine meets a comparatively immobile area (the upper thorax and thoracic spine). The neck is prone to strain through upper limb action (the trapezius and levator scapulae muscles insert on to the cervical spine, for example). The neck is also involved in physical postural maintenance through two routes – the nuchal ligament posteriorly and the prevertebral fascia anteriorly.

Several models have arisen within osteopathy that each offer their own perspectives on cervical motion characteristics and how to address problems therein.

Early osteopathic models of head and neck mechanics

Early models centred on resolving tensions and torsions acting from below upwards, coupled with a complex consideration of the atlantoaxial articulation and the atlanto-occipital articulation, to ensure effective head motion upon the cervical column. Some comments have been made on the cervical spine as a whole according to the Littlejohn and revised models, but the upper cervicals have not been included so far.

The upper cervical spine

The Littlejohn/Fryette mechanics hark back to the influence of articular shape as one of the major determinants of joint orientation and torsion patterns. Because of the unconventional shape of the upper two cervical vertebrae, the principles of mechanics that were applied to the rest of the spine could not act in the upper cervical region. Littlejohn himself considered that the cervical column started at C2 (the axis) and that C1 (the atlas) should be considered as a transition vertebra whose role was to support the head upon the cervical column. Hence the C1 and C2 vertebrae were viewed as having special relations and functions due to their shape as well as to their anatomical position.

As the motion patterns that Fryette suggested for the other areas of the spine could not be applied to the upper cervicals, different patterns of restriction/torsion were outlined, in accordance with the anatomical design of the structures involved (Figure 6.21).

According to early osteopathic models the following torsion possibilities applied in the upper cervical region:

- posterior or anterior occiput, left or right;
- posterior or anterior atlas, left or right;
- side-shift of the atlas, left or right;
- right or left rotation of the axis.

Treatment of these torsions would involve performing manipulations that would reverse the components of torsion and so re-align the vertebrae. The evaluation of such vertebral positions

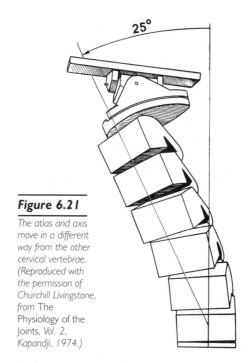

Figure 6.21

The atlas and axis move in a different way from the other cervical vertebrae. (Reproduced with the permission of Churchill Livingstone, from The Physiology of the Joints, Vol. 2, *Kapandji, 1974.)*

depended upon palpating the bony landmarks of the atlas (transverse processes) and axis (the spinous process), as well as through motion testing of the joints involved. As with palpation of the posterior sacrum, there is much soft tissue thickness (both muscular and fascial) to 'feel through' in the suboccipital region of the spine, and this creates problems of interpractitioner agreement on findings of vertebral torsion patterns (especially when coupled with natural anatomical variation in bony shape). Categorizing the vertebral restrictions as changes in relative position has led to some misunderstanding of what the techniques applied in accordance with this model were trying to achieve – namely improved intervertebral motion and improved motion between the cervical spine and the head. Later revisionist models, which concentrated more on a 'three dimensional' picture of articular motion and the soft tissue response to motion, helped to redress this confusion.

(The influence of upper cervical restrictions on the function of the rest of the body was recognized long before the neurological links underpinning them were revealed.)

Osteopathic models – development

Fundamentally, however one worked on the spine, there was a strong opinion that, unless the upper cervical restrictions were eventually resolved, the impetus for adapted posture would remain.

One reason for the great interest in the upper cervical and atlanto-occipital areas was the number of important neural structures in this area, such as the vagal nerves and the superior cervical ganglia, which were thought to be irritated by mechanical restriction in this area and through the dural attachments that concentrated around the upper cervical area. The mechanical behaviour of the dura was thought to be influenced by restrictions and torsions of the upper cervical area, and the effects these were thought to have on the function of neural structures local to the torsion were considered clinically significant. (Note: Dural movement patterns and the concept of biomechanics of neural structures will be discussed in Chapter 9.)

From this type of analysis, there arose a school of thought that advocated treating restriction in any part of the body simply (or rather, solely) by treating the upper cervical region. This is a train of thought that is very prominent in other manipulative professions – chiropractic, for example). Such a concentration on one or two areas of the body was typical of the reductionist models of treatment that arose during the mid part of this century, which have already been referred to in the sections on spinal mechanics.

However, there is a particular model of osteopathy that still orients itself around a positional relationship between the upper cervicals, and between them and the occiput, which has specific relevance in traumatic injuries of the spine such as whiplash.

The influence of trauma on the positional relations of the upper cervical spine

The specific adjusting technique (or SAT model) was introduced by Parnell Bradbury, a chiropractor, and Thomas Dummer, an osteopath (the latter developing it into its current form), in order to resolve the special movement problems of the upper cervical region that were thought to arise from whiplash-type trauma, whether from road traffic accidents or some other incident such as falling and hitting the head. Higher-speed impacts were/are considered to cause a very particular reaction in the soft tissues around the upper cervical articulations that could not simply be reduced by correcting, for example, either a posterior occiput or an anterior atlas (as would have been the case in the Fryette approach).

This SAT model remains strongly convinced of the need to evaluate the upper cervical region according to positional principles, but in a more three-dimensional perspective than was the rule under the Fryette model.

The suboccipital muscle group is thought to function very much more as a proprioceptive system than a prime mover system, although clearly activity in these muscles will influence joint position. In high-speed trauma and impact situations, the motion that reverberates through this region engages all these muscles so that they contract to combat the particular torsion that the area is being subjected to. The impetus to stabilize the region is so strong that, after the motion has stopped, the muscular group remains highly contracted in a pattern of contraction corresponding to the particular motion that passed through the area.

The more or less planar joint surfaces of the occiput – atlas articulation, the swivel articulations of C1 and C2, and the curved shape of the vertebral body of C3, with its flat antero-posterior-oriented facets – allow a highly variable number of movement combinations, and hence a highly variable arrangement of restriction combinations in this area.

The SAT model posits that one must acknowledge each component of the pattern and ensure that it is resolved. Often, in a less analytical approach to this area, the joints would be mobilized, but not in a specific enough direction to reverse the components associated with the trauma. The joints would thus remain in the torsioned pattern, despite repeated attempts to release it with 'standard' manipulative approaches. Because of the emphasis on anatomical relations, the whole pattern of restriction found in each individual is described as a 'positional lesion', to separate it from other restrictions of the upper cervical region that do not have the same origin or quality. Because these restrictions are not often recognized for what they are patients can suffer symptoms for years despite treatment.

This model certainly has strengths, in that it emphasizes the need for a very careful assessment of the upper cervical area, with respect to post-traumatic consequences. It also describes the quality of the soft tissue tensions as being more restricting of joint motion than is the case in the rest of the spine. These 'positional' restrictions are very much more immobile than other articular restrictions, and recognizing them from this quality of complete immobility, coupled with a history of whiplash or impact trauma, identifies the patient as needing the careful attention of the SAT model.

In treating such cases, special care must be taken to ensure that all components of the torsion pattern are addressed during the manipulation, which requires a careful analysis of the pattern in three dimensions so that all the relevant leverages can be worked out in advance – it is only combining all leverages, and not just some of them, that creates the success of the technique.

Moreover, the SAT model embodies the idea that how the practitioner approaches the technique mentally is as important as the anatomical approach. This stems from quite mechanistic principles in the sense of the physical force of momentum having been suddenly arrested by the action of elastic and contractile tissues (the sub-occipital muscles, ligaments and fascia), leaving behind stored mechanical energy in the tissues equivalent to the original trauma. In order to release this stored mechanical energy, the type of manipulation must be very specifically chosen with respect to the energy that is put into the technique. This does not mean that the manipulation is big and uses long leverages and amplitudes (which could be extremely dangerous), but

that it is directed mentally with a view to providing an extra impetus within a highly controlled and well-contained manipulation. This 'mental direction' of technique is a concept that is not universal among manipulative procedures. It is additional to the careful thought processes that are always engaged during assessment and treatment, and represents an attempt to instil a higher degree of energy within the treatment to trigger the release of the stored mechanical energy and 'shock' within the tissues consequent to the original trauma.

The one major criticism of the technique is that it relies upon X-ray evidence of the relative positions of the vertebrae – which is needed to work out the directions required within the corrective manipulative procedure. The use of X-rays is questionable for a number of reasons, exposure to radiation being a prime consideration and the difficulty of trying to establish a three-dimensional relationship from a two-dimensional record being another. It does seem a shame that, given the palpatory skills of osteopathic practitioners, exponents of this technique cannot find a way around the use of X-rays in this valuable approach to upper cervical problems.

In addition to these considerations of the cervical spine, the SAT model also has applications for the whole spine; in order to prioritise and rationalise which area(s) of the spine are treated, in which order.

Contraindications to manipulation of the cervical area

The other problem with this approach is that one is working in a highly sensitive area: vertebral artery damage and spasms (with subsequent ischaemic injury to brain tissue) can occur after high-velocity thrust work in this area. This is a relative contraindication for all manipulators, whether they are orthopaedic consultants, chiropractors, physiotherapists, osteopaths (regardless of the model they are following) or anyone else who uses spinal manipulation. Careful evaluation prior to treating the patient is necessary before each application of such techniques (Randell, 1998).

The reductionist model for the cervical spine

As we discussed before in the section on spinal mechanics, this model was more concerned with appreciating restriction following a three-dimensional motion evaluation of the area than with working out the more 'two-dimensional' relationships described within the Fryette model. Thus some of the constraints imposed by the Fryette model could be dispensed with by relying more on the soft tissue dynamics around a joint to indicate how the articulation could be manipulated. This led to a more individualized approach to each manipulation than was possible under the Fryette model and allowed the reductionist practitioners some greater individuality in their treatments than before. This perhaps moved them towards the complexity of the SAT model, without having to go through the same 'technical analysis' of joint position as described by X-ray (although it has to be said that the 'energetic' components of the SAT model would still not have been so adequately addressed).

The revised model for the cervical spine

The revised model followed on from the reductionist approach but also harked back to the original principles of A. T. Still: that one should know anatomy thoroughly in order to understand how the body operates. As the detail and relevance of the soft tissue anatomy within the body was increasingly appreciated, it became clear that, to understand the complexities of head and neck mechanics, much more needed to be considered than the articulations of the occiput, C1 and C2.

Other important considerations for head and neck mechanics

Other considerations in head and neck mechanics include the soft structures of the anterior throat, the mandible, hyoid and other oral structures (such as the tongue) – all of which, when coupled with the head and cervical spine, make up the **stomatognathic system.**

The stomatognathic system is discussed in Chapter 8, simply because of its extensive links with the thorax and upper limb. We will need to reflect back on cervical motion when these areas are analysed.

WHOLE SPINAL BIOMECHANICS: SUMMARY AT THIS POINT

One of the main differences between the 'old' and the 'new' models discussed is the different ways in which reciprocal relations are thought to work along the length of the spinal column, and how influential dysfunction in one area is thought really to be to another area. As we have seen, some osteopaths consider that there are many more inter-relations than others, if only because of the historical accident of where they trained.

All other parts of the debate so far to one side, if we want to reflect on how one should view the spine and its mechanics, what better way than to review this through the eyes of neuroanatomy.

If we look at some aspects of the neuronal control of spinal movement, we can see that these indicate that there are potentially many more inter-relations between spinal areas than the new model 'allows' for (although neurophysiological knowledge has not yet established enough pathways to account for all aspects of the 'old' model).

It may be that the following information will give heart to those who are unsure of the wider implications of the older models and do not want to rely upon dogma as a rationale. And, if one's view on the inter-relations between parts is not yet fully developed, then this section may give insight that there is much more to appreciate and learn within the subject of spinal movement dynamics!

THE AXIAL SKELETON: CURRENT NEUROPHYSIOLOGICAL INTER-RELATIONS

This discussion aims at pointing out that, whatever the pattern of motion that emerges, there is a pattern: balancing all the movement possibilities within the axial skeleton and then coordinating this with the appendicular skeleton, there is a need for whole-spine communication on a neurological level, which establishes certain inter-relations and areas of reciprocal influence.

To appreciate these ideas, we need to review the basic arrangement of the motor system (Figure 6.22).

These are the basic inter-relations within the central nervous system that relate to the smooth and integrated control of motion, which we have already discussed in Chapter 3.

Locomotor skills are learned, and become 'automatic'. Patterns of movement control are laid down in the central nervous system, such that, when the desire for a particular motion is acted upon, the higher centres send down the instruction for that motion to the spinal cord, which triggers a preset pattern of activity within the relevant muscles. This motor activity can be slightly adjusted according to feedback mechanisms, and so the patterns can be slightly adjusted and refined through experience.

As we continue through this chapter, and discuss the relations between different body parts, the complexity of such 'patterning' will become apparent. For now, in this section on spinal mechanics, we shall confine the discussion to the axial skeleton – the spinal column.

The topographical arrangement of the spinal motor neurones gives some insight into potential patterns of control.

Spinal motor neurones are topographically organized into medial and lateral groups that innervate proximal and distal muscles. The spatial organization is such that the motor neurones innervating the most proximal muscles are located most medially, while those innervating more distal muscles are located progressively more laterally. The lateral motor system innervates the distal musculature of the limbs. Fine movements of the hands and fingers are mediated through this system. The medial motor system innervates the axial and the proximal limb musculature and is involved in balance and postural movements.

Those motor neurones of the medial motor system particularly associated with the control of

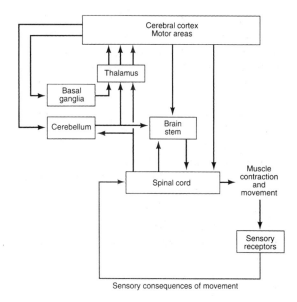

Figure 6.22

The motor system consists of three levels of control. The motor areas of the cerebral cortex influence the spinal cord both directly and via the brain stem. All three levels receive sensory inputs and are also under the influence of the basal ganglia and the cerebellum, which act on the cerebral cortex via the thalamus. (Reproduced with the permission of Appleton & Lange from Principles of Neural Science, *3rd edn, Kandel et al., 1991.)*

the muscles of the spinal column are arranged into particular groups, and the interactions between these groups and the rest of the motor control system hint at some interesting relationships.

A pattern-generating centre within the spinal cord
The propriospinal system is a system consisting of interneurones that originate, travel, terminate and exert all their influence within the spinal cord itself. It is shown in Figures 6.23 and 6.24.

One function of this system is to transmit motor commands from the cerebral cortex: axons of the corticospinal projection terminate on these cells. Another is the transmission of slow nociception up to the higher centres. In addition, the role of the propriospinal system is to connect the parts of the cord that provide segmental innervation of the spine and neck muscles, and allow these to interact with the proximal muscles of the upper and lower limbs.

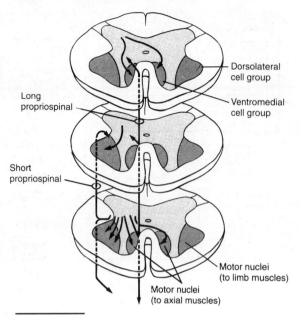

Figure 6.23

Medial motor nuclei are interconnected by long propriospinal neurones whereas lateral motor nuclei are interconnected by short propriospinal neurones. (Reproduced with the permission of Appleton & Lange from Principles of Neural Science, *3rd edn, Kandel et al., 1991.)*

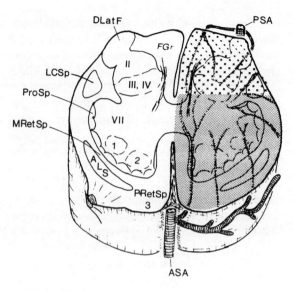

Figure 6.24

The propriospinal system. ALS = anterolateral system; ASA = anterior spinal artery; DLatF = dorsolateral funiculus; FGr = fasciculus gracilis; II–IV = laminae II–IV; LCSp = lateral corticospinal tract; MRetSp = medullary reticulospinal tract; PRetSp = pontine reticulospinal tract; ProSp = propriospinal tract; PSA = posterior spinal artery; VII = lamina VII; 1 = lateral motor nucleus; 2 = medial motor nucleus; 3 = lateral vestibulospinal tract. Reproduced with the permission of Lippincott Williams & Wilkins from Medical Neuroanatomy, *Willard, 1993.*

There are three parts to the propriospinal system, long, medium and short, relating to the length of the fibres – in other words how many segments they span: some span just a few segments and some run practically the whole length of the cord. (The section of the cord they are within is concerned with low-threshold mechanoreceptor input.)

This pattern of organization allows the axial muscles, which are innervated from many spinal segments, to be coordinated during postural adjustment.

Several papers indicate links in singular directions (of effect) between the lumbar and cervical cords (Berezovskii and Kebkalo, 1992; Sandkuhler *et al.*, 1993) and between the lumbar, thoracic and cervical cords (Bolton and Tracey, 1992); and also reciprocal connections (Robbins *et al.*, 1992). Studies confirm that afferents from each muscle activate a specific subset of neurones, and they also suggest that the projections of each subset are divergent, implying that individual neurones project on to diverse motor nuclei, an organization that would favour the coordination of multijoint movements (Mazevet and Pierrot-Deseilligny, 1994).

The propriospinal system represents a broad network of reciprocal inhibitory and excitatory connections running between multiple segments of the spinal cord. The greatest areas of interconnection appear to be between the lumbar and cervical cords (with some sections of the propriospinal system absent in the thoracic cord).

This network of interneurones seems capable of generating rhythmic patterns of activity between different sections and areas of the paravertebral muscles, with activity in one area of the paravertebral musculature triggering responses in other areas, some adjacent and some distant. These patterns of rhythmicity can be ipsilateral or bilateral.

In general, there is evidence that gravity plays a role in the control of posture (Mittelstaedt,

1995, 1996). If we stood still all the time, then gravity could be compensated for relatively easily. Our bodies have therefore a centre of mass, and a degree of inertia that must be overcome during movement (Pearsall *et al.*, 1996). In overcoming this inertia through muscle activity, we end up with a degree of momentum that needs to be controlled to maintain a stable cycle of motion during gait and other actions. Muscle patterning must therefore take into account the permutations of movement in the whole body, and the propriospinal pathway would enable monitoring and intercoordination of such movements. It seems to act as a spinal pattern generator that, although normally somewhat inhibited by higher-centre activity, is not completely subservient to it.

Remember that this is a sensory proprioceptive system, which monitors activity in one section of the spinal column and feeds this information to other areas so that muscle activity in these other areas can be appropriately adjusted as required to maintain posture and stability in motion. It is a sensory-driven system: change the sensation in one part (by altering its motion) and this will trigger a response elsewhere.

How does this compare with the models discussed above?

The Littlejohn model suggested a widespread inter-relation between parts, which implied that manipulating/mobilizing sections of the spine would immediately cause a reaction and difference in distant parts. Practitioners using this model are quite used to releasing restrictions in one area not by treating them directly but by working on distant areas of the spine. The other model, by contrast, does not seem to leave such an impression, and certainly many practitioners working within it do not have the same sense of diverse reactions becoming apparent in such an immediate time-frame.

The complexity within the neural control of movement and the mechanisms of pattern generation through the whole body, not just the spine, should expand the way that some practitioners work – leading to a much more dynamic acknowledgement of the interaction and influence between parts.

Spinal curves and head orientation

The preceding section has involved a discussion of spinal mechanics, in the absence of the pelvis or other parts of the body, which we will partly address now. Within this there are also one or two other points about spinal mechanics and curves that can be made, to help illustrate the differences and similarities between the osteopathic models discussed so far, and to help bring into context the influence of the special centres of balance on the control of posture and locomotion.

Whatever movement patterns are initiated within the spinal column, the positioning and orientation of the head is very influential.

Ultimately, the whole spine is oriented so that the head is level on the top of the spinal column. The special senses (eyes and ears) need to be horizontal, and the balance of the whole body is dependent upon this being maintained.

The spinal mechanisms mentioned in the preceding section (the propriospinal system) are involved in this relationship. Much muscular activity in the spinal muscles, particularly in the cervical area, will be coordinated so that the head is level regardless of what is happening at the pelvis. This mechanism is explained below.

Vestibular and neck afferents converge on vestibular nuclei and propriospinal neurones

Inputs from the otolith organs and proprioceptive inputs from neck afferents are relayed to the vestibular nuclei. Vestibular neurones project to the spinal cord through two vestibulospinal tracts and influence spinal circuits indirectly through connections with the pontine and medullary reticular formation. Reticular neurones in turn project to the spinal cord in two reticulospinal tracts. Both the vestibulospinal and reticulospinal tracts excite interneurones and long propriospinal neurones responsible for distributing the patterns of excitation and inhibition within the axial muscles (Kandel *et al.*, 1991).

The pattern of activity in segmental paravertebral muscles will be initiated in such a way that the head is level. This means that there may be small areas of altered segmental spinal mechanics designed to adapt the overall balance of the spinal curves (arising from differences in sacral inclination), leading to a horizontally oriented head.

These local alterations should be considered as a segmental adjustment to an uneven sacral base plane. These local torsions can present as restrictions in spinal movement, and may be painful, because of the constant muscular activity required to maintain them (leading to relative ischaemia, build up of lactic acid and so on, leading to pain and discomfort). This theme will be returned to in a moment.

Learning to keep the head balanced and horizontally oriented

Spinal movement patterns and coordination of posture through the balance mechanisms are learned events that are dependent upon proprioceptive information at the level of the pelvis. There have been several studies that would seem to back this view: they illustrated the way in which muscle activity involved in stabilizing spinal movement is initiated at the level of the pelvis (Yasukouchi and Isayama, 1995); and, in exploring the development of postural reflexes, again, detect muscle activity first in the pelvic part of the erector spinae musculature (Hirschfeld and Forssberg, 1994).

Development of standing posture in babies and toddlers

Babies are born with flexed spinal columns and only develop extension in the cervical and lumbar regions as they try to move around. The 'practising' of head lifting and then sitting, prior to standing, gives the opportunity for the above-mentioned neural reflexes to establish effective patterns and links, so that, as the baby develops into a toddler and eventually an adult, the neural control of posture is correctly established. This developmental process will be returned to later on.

Reciprocal relationship between the mechanics of the lumbar spine/pelvis and the head/neck mechanics – clinical relevance

- Movement restrictions in the pelvis or low lumbar region alter spinal mechanics, so that

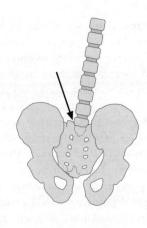

A

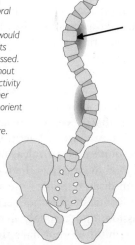

B

Figure 6.25

*Sacral torsion and spinal balance. **A.** Sacral sidebending. An uneven sacral base plane (arrowed), caused by sacroiliac restriction and torsion, means that the vertebral column is unevenly supported. The spine would be at an odd angle if its balance was not redressed. **B.** Adaptation throughout the spine. Muscular activity in the cervical and other areas (arrowed) will reorient the spine to preserve horizontal head posture.*

the upper neck has to move differently to compensate. This is illustrated in Figure 6.25.

If the neck muscles have to work hard over a long period of time to maintain the horizontal

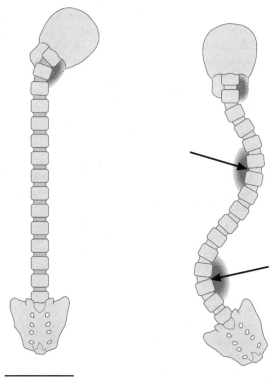

Figure 6.26

Cervical torsion and spinal balance. **A.** *An unacceptable head position can arise due to tension in the cervical muscles (arrowed).* **B.** *If neck tension is not released, then the muscles in the rest of the spine and pelvis will be contracted (arrows) to induce a sacral inclination, so balancing the curves of the spine.*

orientation of the head, then they will become painful. However, releasing tension at the level of the neck will only be temporarily effective if the lumbar/pelvic articulations are not released.

- Movement restrictions in the cervical region (perhaps as a result of working too long in front of a computer, or having some sort of injury to the neck, e.g. whiplash) will lead to the abovementioned neural mechanisms altering the activity in the rest of the spine and pelvis, so that the head will be returned by this indirect route to a horizontal orientation. This is shown in Figure 6.26.

This is the opposite relation to the one above, and means that some cases of low back pain or pelvic pain may be secondary to altered spinal mechanics in the head/neck region.

- In the same vein, movement restrictions within the thoracic section of the spine can affect the way that overall spinal mechanics affect head position, in that it alters the flexibility of the spine as a whole, requiring more reciprocal compensation at either the lumbar or cervical areas for any changes in mechanics at these levels than would otherwise have been necessary.

The role of the reciprocal relationship between the spinal curves again proves to be important to locomotion and posture, with respect to balance.

Referring back to osteopathic models

The revised model

The neural inter-relations just described were easily fitted into the revised osteopathic model because spinal mechanics were important to balance control systems.

We have mentioned that spinal patterning is a learned activity and that head orientation upon the spine develops as the infant first learns to lift its head. When the infant starts to sit, the influence of the pelvis and any rocking motion therein is transferred up the spine, and in this way the infant learns to control overall spinal movement upon a dynamic base, so that head stability can be preserved.

This adds weight to the idea that learned patterns of spinal relations can be distorted by changing the movement possibilities of various spinal areas (through the effects of restrictions). Both the revised models and the Littlejohn models can be correlated to this idea.

The point was made earlier that the revised model did not seem to indicate the range of intricacies within spinal mechanics compared to the Littlejohn model. However, it is through an understanding of the mechanisms of the neural control of balance and posture that the followers of the revised model can gain additional 'freedom' to work on diverse areas of the spine to good clinical effect.

The Littlejohn model

The relation between curves and pivots has been previously introduced and this lends itself very well to the above-described neural mechanism. This will not therefore be rediscussed at this point, but taken as read.

SUMMARY OF SPINAL MECHANICS

Many inter-relations have been discussed, and many different ways of viewing the spinal column as a coordinated whole have been introduced. Some of these may initially seem complex and others too simplistic. However, the ways in which these models developed may illustrate that they need not be divergent visions of spinal motion but different perspectives/sides of the same coin, each with 'different' parts of the whole puzzle.

The spine acts as an intercoordinated whole and should be examined and treated as such.

However, the body is more than just a spine, and it is time to consider the influence of other body parts, starting with the next chapter, on the pelvis and lower limbs.

REFERENCES

Anonymous (1956) *1956 Year Book*, Osteopathic Institute of Applied Technique.

Berezovskii, V. K. and Kebkalo, T. G. (1992) Descending neuronal projections to the lumbar division of the cat spinal cord. *Neuroscience and Behavioral Physiology*, 22, 171–174.

Bland, J. H. and Boushey, D. R. (1990) Anatomy and physiology of the cervical spine. *Seminars in Arthritis and Rheumatology*, 20, 1–20.

Bolton, P. S. and Tracey, D. J. (1992) Spinothalamic and propriospinal neurones in the upper cervical cord of the rat: terminations of primary afferent fibres on soma and primary dendrites. *Experimental Brain Research*, 92, 59–68.

Education Department (1993) *Competences Required for Osteopathic Practice (C. R. O. P.)*, General Council and Register of Osteopaths, Reading, Berks.

General Council and Register of Osteopaths (1958) *The Osteopathic Blue Book*, General Council and Register of Osteopaths, London.

Graf, W., de Waele, C. and Vidal, P.P. (1995) Functional anatomy of the head-neck movement system of quadrupedal and bipedal mammals. *Journal of Anatomy*, 186, 55–74.

Hartman, L. (1997) *Handbook of Osteopathic Technique*, 3rd edn, Chapman & Hall, London.

Hirschfeld, H. and Forssberg, H. (1994) Epigenetic development of postural responses for sitting during infancy. *Experimental Brain Research*, 97, 528–540.

Jacob, S. W., Francone, C. A. and Lossow, W. J. (1982) *Structure and Function in Man*, 5th edn. W. B. Saunders, Philadelphia, PA.

Kandel, E. R., Schwartz, J. H. and Jessel, T. M. (1991) *Principles of Neural Science*, 3rd edn. Prentice Hall, Englewood Cliffs, NJ.

Kapandji, I. A. (1974) *The Physiology of the Joints*, 2nd edn, Churchill Livingstone, New York.

Kuchera, W. A. and Kuchera, M. L. (1992) *Osteopathic Principles in Practice*, 2nd edn, Kirksville College of Osteopathy, Kirksville, MO.

Latey, P. (1982) *The Muscular Manifesto*, 2nd edn, Philip Latey, London.

McGregor, A. H., McCarthy, l. D. and Hughes, S. P. (1995) Motion characteristics of the lumbar spine in the normal population. *Spine*, 20, 2421–2428.

Maidstone College of Osteopathy (1960) *The Mechanics of the Spine and Pelvis*, Maidstone College of Osteopathy, Maidstone, Kent.

Maidstone College of Osteopathy (1985) *Littlejohn*, Maidstone College of Osteopathy, Maidstone, Kent.

Mazevet, D. and Pierrot-Deseilligny, E. (1994) Pattern of descending excitation of presumed propriospinal neurones at the onset of voluntary movement in humans. *Acta Physiologica Scandinavica*, 150, 27–38.

Mittelstaedt, H. (1995) Evidence of somatic graviception from new and classical investigations. *Acta Oto-Laryngologica – Supplement*, 520,186–187.

Mittelstaedt, H. (1996) Somatic graviception. *Biological Psychology*, **42**, 53–74.

National Touring Exhibition (1997) *The Quick and the Dead. Artists and Anatomy*, P. J. Reproductions.

Palastanga, N., Field, D. and Soames, R. (1989) *Anatomy and Human Movement*, Heinemann Medical, Oxford.

Pearsall, D. J., Reid, J. G. and Livingston, L. A. (1996) Segmental inertial parameters of the human trunk as determined from computed tomography. *Annals of Biomedical Engineering*, **24**,198–210.

Randell, P. (1998) Clinical patient screening: a clinical protocol for osteopaths: Part II. *Osteopathy Today*, **4**, 16–17.

Robbins, A., Pfaff, D. W. and Schwartz-Giblin, S. (1992) Reticulospinal and reticuloreticular pathways for activating the lumbar back muscles in the rat. *Experimental Brain Research*, **92**, 46–58.

Sanan, A. and Rengachary, S. S. (1996) The history of spinal biomechanics. *Neurosurgery*, **39**, 657–669.

Sandkuhler, J., Stelzer, B. and Fu, Q. G. (1993) Characteristics of propriospinal modulation of nociceptive lumbar spinal dorsal horn neurons in the cat. *Neuroscience*, **54**, 957–967.

Stoddard, A. (1983) *Manual of Osteopathic Practice*, 2nd edn, Hutchinson, London.

Tortora, G. J. and Grabowski, S. R. (1993) *Principles of Anatomy and Physiology*, 7th edn, Harper Collins College, New York.

Webster, G. V. (1935) *Sage Sayings of Still*, Wetzel Publishing, Los Angeles, CA.

Willard, F. H. (1993) *Medical Neuroanatomy*, Lippincott, Philadelphia.

Yasukouchi, A. and Isayama, T. (1995) The relationships between lumbar curves, pelvic tilt and joint mobilities in different sitting postures in young adult males. *Applied Human Science*, **14**, 15–21.

7

COMPARISONS AND CONTRASTS IN BIOMECHANICAL MODELS: THE PELVIS AND LOWER LIMB

IN THIS CHAPTER:

- The pelvis
- The influence of sacral biomechanics on spinal curves
- The sacroiliac joints
- Pelvic mechanics within osteopathic models – Mackinnon, Fryette, Mitchell
- Gait
- Muscle energy technique and motor learning
- Revised models of pelvic motion
- The influence of the lower limb on the axial skeleton
- The lower limb – the hip, the knee, the foot
- Muscles and connective tissue interactions during lower limb movement
- Ossification within the lower limbs, and its significance to osteopaths

INTRODUCTION

None of the discussion in the preceding chapter of spinal movement patterns has included the influence of the pelvis, which is clearly an artificial situation – and as we shall see the various models within osteopathy did not exclude this area.

As with the previous chapter, the aim of this chapter is to indicate the reciprocal and complex links both within the pelvis and also between the pelvis and the rest of the body. When considering biomechanical relations and pain and dysfunction patterns within the pelvic area, it is necessary to place it in context within the rest of the body.

Very few specific treatment/management strategies will be discussed here, but these will become more apparent as the remaining chapters unfold.

Integration between parts is the key focus.

As with the previous chapter, a lot of the osteopathic models are not referenced, although there is much more supportive orthodox research that relates to the pelvis and lower limb than the traditional osteopathic models of the spine.

THE PELVIS

The pelvis is a complex biomechanical area, which has many conflicting demands upon it. With respect to spinal mechanics, the sacrum needs to be relatively level in order for the spine to be correctly oriented in static posture; and it needs to be symmetrically mobile during locomotion to ensure the transference of a uniform oscillation of motion through the spinal column. Indeed, there is a reciprocal relationship between the spine and the sacrum, as in other areas of the spine: the sacral base certainly does change during activity, and walking/running in particular (Inman *et al.*, 1981). This means that the spine has to be flexible enough to cope with the cyclical/oscillatory motion of the sacrum. (If it does not then this can create strain, and possible confusion in the neural monitoring and control of spinal activity.)

Spinal curves in relation to sacral mechanics

Readers should not forget the final section of the preceding chapter on spinal curves and head orientation. There the influence of pelvic orientation on the control of movement and balance for the spine, head and higher centres was introduced. It is important to keep those points in mind when reflecting on the variety of movement possibilities within the pelvis and lower limbs, and their potential influence on spinal movement patterns.

Figure 7.1 shows how sacral inclination can influence spinal mechanics, in at least two planes.

This need for the spine to act as a curved rod, which needs to be elastic and adaptable to accommodate motion, has already been introduced, but not from the perspective of pelvic (sacral) inclination, where spinal flexibility to accommodate changes in sacral base planes is required. The converse also applies: should there be immobility/changed motion within the spinal column, then this might produce an impetus for altered pelvic motion. (This point will be returned to later.)

There are two main ways that the inclination of the sacrum can be changed:

* by local motion of the sacrum between the ilia;
* by motion of the whole pelvis on the hip joints (either unilaterally or bilaterally).

These aspects will be discussed individually, starting with motion in the sacroiliacs.

The sacroiliac joints

For many years the idea of motion at the sacroiliacs was denied vigorously by the orthodox profession. However, the sacroiliacs are not like other areas of the body that are thought to be somewhat evolutionarily unnecessary: their motion possibilities, although small, are incredibly important for efficient biomechanical function, with many factors influencing their function (Walker, 1992). Indeed, the sacroiliac joints develop significantly during life and alter their structure from the neonate to the adult, implying that they adapt to changing movement demands throughout life (Bowen and Cassidy, 1981). They are very complex structures, which, while they may not move like the hips or spinal articulations, nevertheless allow a degree of subtle movement that is very important for biomechanics of the spine and pelvis (Takayama,

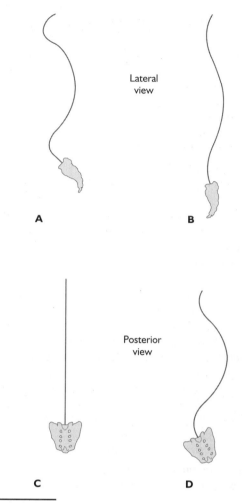

Figure 7.1

Influence of sacral inclination on spinal curvature. **A.** *'Anterior' sacral position gives accentuated curves.* **B.** *'Posterior' sacral position gives diminished curves.* **C.** *Level sacral position (horizontal) gives a straight spine.* **D.** *Lateral inclination of the sacrum gives lateral curves.*

1990; Kissling and Jacob, 1996). There are differences in the structural arrangements of male and female pelvises (the latter having more mobile sacroiliac joints; Brunner *et al.*, 1991) which reflect the different functions of the male and female pelvis. Additionally, the arrangement of soft tissues around the sacroiliacs, the lumbosacral junction and the pelvic outlet is complex and ensures a highly integrated mechanism to orientate sacral motion between the ilia and the spinal column (Vukicevic *et al.*, 1991) and between the trunk, pelvis and lower limb (Snijders *et al.*, 1995a).

Ligaments guiding the sacrum

The sacrum is suspended between the ilia, and the integrity of the articulation is maintained by the ligamentous structures of that joint (Gerlach and Lierse, 1992). It seems that the joint achieves a strong shock-absorbing function through the structure of its ligamentous arrangements (Wilder *et al.*, 1980) and that the pelvis is capable of storing a degree of elastic energy (which helps in locomotion and stability; Dorman, 1995). Any dysfunction of the ligaments will lead to instability/altered movement of the sacrum and hence to lumbar spine dysfunction and strain; and the sacroiliac joints may be responsible for pain in the low back, buttocks, pelvis and proximal lower extremities (Daum, 1995). Forces generated within the pelvis are strong, and if there has been for some reason a fusion of the lumbosacral spine and/or sacroiliac joints, this causes a shift of forces through the bony aspects of the pelvis, hip joints and symphysis pubis. This can result in much pelvic girdle pain, and even in fractures of the pelvic rami or iliac wing (Wood *et al.*, 1996).

The ligaments of the posterior spine and pelvis, coupled with the thoracolumbar fascia, form a sling/sheath in which the sacrum is embedded. The sacroiliac joint is considered a self-locking mechanism, where the complexity of ligamentous and muscular relations tries to overcome the dilemma of stability versus mobility (Dorman and Vleeming, 1995). The sacrotuberous and sacrospinal ligaments transfer forces acting through the thoracolumbar fascia and sacrum to the inferior pelvic outlet, where they join a sort of annular arrangement of fibres that sweeps forwards from the tuberosities, along the inferior pubic rami to the inferior part of the symphysis pubis. Standard texts (Kapandji, 1974) discuss movement of the sacrum between the ilia as nutation or counternutation, and this ligamentous arrangement (including the intraosseous ligaments; Vukicevic *et al.*, 1991) is designed to permit (and guide/limit) this, and other types of motion (such as rotation of the sacrum between the ilia).

Figure 7.2 shows the anterior and posterior ligaments of the pelvis, the iliolumbar ligaments, and the sacrotuberous and sacrospinal ligaments. These ligaments all guide/limit a variety of pelvic torsion patterns.

When weight acts from above, the posterior/inferior ligamentous fibres can absorb and limit sacral excursion into nutation, and provide elastic recoil potential to help return the sacrum to a neutral position. It seems that the long dorsal intraosseous ligament (not shown in Figure 7.2. but passing from the tubercle of S3 to the ilium) acts as a pivot for this aspect of sacral motion (Vleeming *et al.*, 1996) and creates (among other tissues) a pathway where ilial motion can engage the sacrum and hence induce movement through it to the lumbar spine. The fan-like arrangement of the anterior sacroiliac and iliolumbar ligaments reinforces the idea that the sacrum cannot move without influencing the ilia or lumbar spine, and *vice versa*.

Other activities are thought to influence sacral and iliac motion – sitting in a very flexed position, having the low back very extended, kicking a ball harshly or landing heavily on one foot, for example. All of these things could lead to the ligamentous suspensory mechanism that holds the pelvis being injured or stressed/strained in some way, leading to a slight 'giving' in the structural integrity of the pelvis (Vleeming *et al.*, 1995a) and allowing a lesion pattern/torsion to appear. However, some activities such as prolonged sitting are not thought always to be as bad for spinal and pelvic integrity as one might imagine (Snijders *et al.*, 1995b).

The lumbosacral junction

As already stated, it is impossible to consider the mechanics of the pelvis without discussion of their relation to the spinal column. Although this relation has been alluded to it is important to consider the relation between the lumbar spine and the pelvis in more detail, as this is where most stresses and strains arising through poor

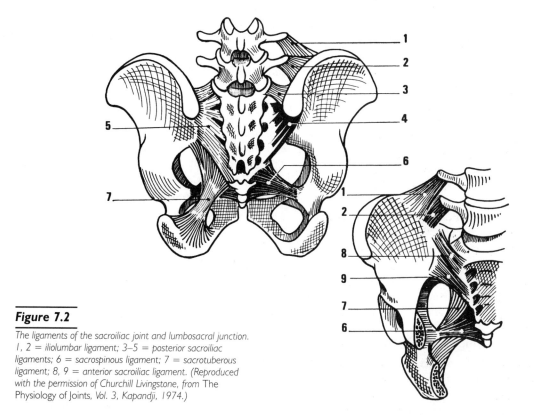

Figure 7.2

The ligaments of the sacroiliac joint and lumbosacral junction.
1, 2 = iliolumbar ligament; 3–5 = posterior sacroiliac
ligaments; 6 = sacrospinous ligament; 7 = sacrotuberous
ligament; 8, 9 = anterior sacroiliac ligament. (Reproduced
with the permission of Churchill Livingstone, from The
Physiology of Joints, Vol. 3, Kapandji, 1974.)

movement coordination between these parts are
manifest.

The fifth lumbar vertebra is 'suspended'
between the two ilia, and floats between the rest
of the lumbar vertebral column and the sacrum.
The anatomy of the lumbosacral connection is
complex, with many muscular, fascial and ligamentous structures acting in concert to guide and
support movement in this dynamic area (Willard,
1995). The stresses and strains acting upon the
fifth lumbar vertebra are quite complex, and the
iliolumbar ligaments are designed to cushion and
guide its position in relation to surrounding
structures (Leong *et al.*, 1987).

Clearly if several movement torsion patterns
within the pelvis combine with any that are present in the spinal column, then the force acting
through the lumbosacral region can more easily
cause distress and injury at the lumbosacral articular disc than if patterns act in isolation. This
interplay of forces may have particular relevance

for the high proportion of discal injuries and
peripheral neuropathies at this (lumbosacral)
level, and may compromise the ability of the local
soft tissues to stabilize a case of spondylolisthesis
(Friberg, 1991). Interestingly, the article referenced above (Leong *et al.*, 1987) states that the
iliolumbar ligament is not present at birth but
develops during the first decade. This may mean
that exploring and resolving movement and
locomotion patterns in young children may be
relevant to try to ensure efficient lumbosacral
mechanics and integrity in later life. (This
delayed development of the iliolumbar ligament
has been disputed by some other authors;
Hanson and Sonesson, 1994.)

*Nutation and counternutation are not the only
directions of sacral (and therefore pelvic) motion*
When the relationship of the ligamentous
support to nutation and counternutation of the
sacrum was mentioned above, it implied that

there was the same movement in both sacroiliac joints at the same time. In fact, each articulation can move independently of the other, as necessary (Dontigny, 1995). This occurs in walking, where movement across the sacroiliacs is quite complex (as will be discussed below). The variation of stresses that can be imposed in this area is illustrated by studies that indicate stress patterns across the sacrum and sacroiliac cartilages (and the symphysis pubis; Putz and Muller-Gerbl, 1992). These indicate that all aspects of the sacroiliac articulations are involved at different stages of the walking motion, and that the strain patterns induced across the sacrum can be strongly variable, indicating perhaps that uneven gait cycles are not unusual. Gait is discussed in more detail later in the chapter, where a three-dimensional picture of sacral/pelvic motion is built up.

Forces accumulating within the pelvis

There is a potential conflict between torsional forces acting on the sacrum from above (via the spine) and those acting from below (via the legs and ilia), which the ligamentous arrangement of the area must accommodate. In osteopathic theories (see below) torsions acting through the spine on to the pelvis twist the sacrum in relation to the ilia and give 'sacroiliac' lesions; whereas those acting upwards through the leg on to the pelvis twist one ilium on to the sacrum and give an 'iliosacral' lesion.

Torsion acting from above

If the weight of the body acts evenly upon the lumbar spine, then the sacrum will remain level and incline towards nutation. If the forces act unevenly upon the lumbar spine, then the sacrum will be moved unevenly between the ilia. For example, if you twist your upper body, then there will be more load on one lumbosacral joint compared to the other. This, coupled with the uneven pulling of the iliolumbar ligament, will start to twist the sacrum – and this torsion will presumably need to be balanced by activity in different sections of the ipsilateral and contralateral sacrotuberous and sacrospinous ligaments of the

sacroiliac articulations (depending upon the actual direction of sacral movement induced). This will mean that there are different stresses acting simultaneously in each sacroiliac joint.

Torsions acting from below

The actions and biomechanics within the lower limb have a strong influence on pelvic mechanics and lumbosacral function (Dananberg, 1995). The strains imposed on the sacrum are more complicated during walking, as the ilia move and are engaged differently at different stages of the gait cycle (Vleeming et al., 1995b). As one ilium moves, it transmits forces across one sacroiliac joint and may twist the sacrum on that side. As the action of walking proceeds, then that ilium will be moved differently and may now twist that side of the sacrum in the opposite direction. In fact, the sacrum comes under quite conflicting demands during walking, as there is activity in both ilia at once: the ilia are often rotating in different directions during different phases of the gait cycle. So, the left side of the sacral base might be required to move anteriorly at the same time as the right side is required to move posteriorly. Couple this with the fact that there is also a sideways tipping of the sacrum during gait (as one leg is raised, put down and raised again) and the three-dimensional oscillation of the sacrum becomes more evident (Dontigny, 1995). (As stated above, the subject of gait will be expanded upon later.)

Viewed in this manner, the movement of the sacrum can be imagined as oscillatory/floating, and is in fact involved in coordinating motion between the arms, legs and spine, the long dorsal sacroiliac ligament having particular relevance for this integrating role, through its attachments to the erector spinae muscles, the posterior layer of the thoracolumbar fascia and the sacrotuberous ligament (Vleeming et al., 1996).

The symphysis pubis

As we shall see, many of the osteopathic models tend to focus on motion patterns between the ilia and the sacrum and to consider the symphysis pubis much less than is reasonable.

The motion within the symphysis pubis is not solely of importance within the obstetric patient, when its function is very relevant within peripartum pain syndromes (Mens *et al.*, 1996). In fact there is no major difference in joint morphology in males and females, nor between different age groups (in people with no history of disease of the joint – Sgambati *et al.*, 1996). This may not be illogical when one considers that it is a necessary feature of force distribution and motion coordination within the male **and** female pelvis. Lack of integrity of this joint can lead to many instability syndromes and pain syndromes within the pelvic, lower back and lower abdominal regions (Maclennan and Maclennan, 1997). It may also be implicated in many sports-related groin pain syndromes (Ekberg *et al.*, 1996).

The pubic joint can experience a high degree of load-bearing, with the pelvic girdle muscles helping to stabilize load transfer across the pubic area (Dalstra and Huiskes, 1995). Normal movement possibilities of the symphysis pubis include vertical shear and slight rotatory motion, as indicated in Figure 7.3.

Pelvic mechanics within osteopathic models

The above description will hopefully hint at the multitude of different possible motion relationships between the lumbar spine, sacrum and ilia (and from there both to the whole spinal column and to the lower limbs). The pelvis remains an area of the body that resists practically all attempts to reduce its movement patterns and diverse functional relations into a few simple rules. It is an enormously complex area, and successful treatment can give enormous benefit throughout the body. However, if some aspect of the pelvic torsion/movement problem is not recognized/addressed, the patient may continue to suffer a variety of symptoms for years, despite continuing treatment.

The methods and analyses that osteopaths have gone through over the years trying to resolve the conundrum of pelvic motion give telling testimony to its complexity.

There have been a wide variety of attempts at 'defining' the motions within the pelvis into pre-

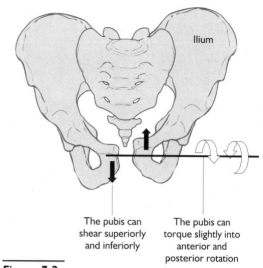

Ilium

The pubis can shear superiorly and inferiorly

The pubis can torque slightly into anterior and posterior rotation

Figure 7.3

Movements of the pubis.

dictable patterns, so that they could be addressed during treatment and the relationships normalized. However, within the early models, it seemed that the three-dimensional nature of the relationships needed to be broken down into a more 'mechanistic' rather than a 'fluid/floating' dynamic analysis in order to be practically addressed.

Two models of pelvic mechanics will be discussed to begin with: one based upon the Fryette model and the other being the Lindlahr–Mackinnon model (known simply as the Mackinnon model). Both of them have their foundations within the overall Littlejohn model (as was discussed in the previous chapter on the spine) but, as will be seen, the Mackinnon technique did not use as many rotatory components as the Fryette analysis. After that we will briefly discuss other models, such as the Mitchell model, and another that incorporates a different motion concept to the preceding ones.

Note: The first three of these – Mackinnon, Fryette and Mitchell – basically revolve around whether the ilium is twisted upon a balanced sacrum or *vice versa*, producing the above-mentioned 'iliosacral' or 'sacroiliac' lesions, which will be discussed.

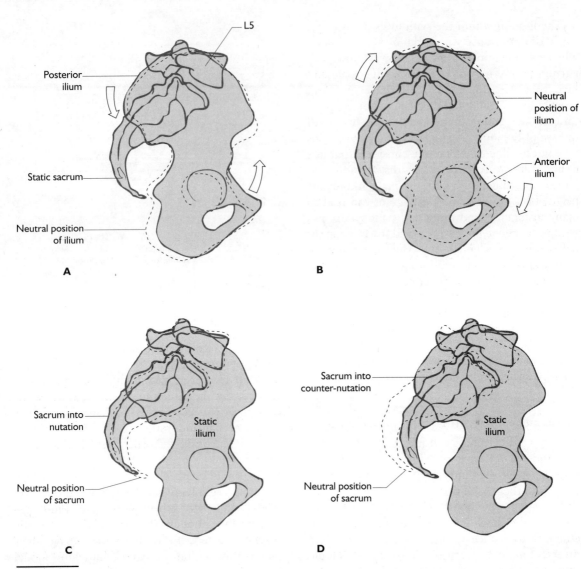

Figure 7.4

Ilial and sacral torsion. **A.** *Posterior rotation of ilium.* **B.** *Anterior rotation of ilium.* **C.** *Anterior rotation (nutation) of sacrum.* **D.** *Posterior rotation (counternutation) of sacrum.*

The Mackinnon model (as recorded by Jocelyn Proby, 1930)

This is the simpler of the two, and is based upon the relation between the ilia and the sacrum. This relationship is a little more 'two-dimensional' than the 'floating and oscillatory' pattern discussed in the earlier part of this chapter. In this model, either the sacrum or the ilia is considered 'static' and the other part is examined to see how it is orientated in relation to the static bone. In total there are 'five' types of distorted pattern that are recognized:

- inferior-lateral innominate (ilium) – giving a short leg on that side;
- superior-medial innominate – giving a long leg on that side;
- anterior ilium (posterior sacrum);

- posterior ilium (anterior sacrum);
- tilted sacrum.

Some of these torsions are shown in Figure 7.4.

Inferior-lateral indicates that the position of the posterior superior iliac spine has moved from its normal position to one that is slightly lower (inferior) and further away from the spinal column (more lateral). This torsion of the ilium gives a short leg as it 'raises' the height of the acetabulum, 'drawing the leg with it' (Figure 7.4A).

Superior-medial indicates that the position of the posterior superior iliac spine has moved from its normal position to one that is slightly higher (superior) and closer to the midline (more medial). Here the acetabulum is 'lowered', thus 'lengthening' the leg (Figure 7.4B).

In **anterior** or **posterior ilium**, the ilium shifts anteriorly or posteriorly without rotating. There is no difference in leg length.

Tilted sacrum relates to sacral nutation or counternutation. It can be associated with pain or tension at the level of the sacrococcygeal articulation. There is also no change in leg length in this case (Figure 7.4C, D).

These 'lesions' could occur unilaterally or bilaterally (in a sort of 'equal and opposite' relationship) and could occur either singly or in combination on either side. They were considered to have individual effects upon the spinal curves (Figure 7.5).

Treatment would be to 'reverse' the components/position of the lesion pattern, using a direct manipulation to the sacrum or ilium, which would then restore the spine to normality. If the lesion was long-standing, then the curves within the spinal column might become 'fixed' and so become a maintaining feature for the pelvic lesion pattern and require treatment in their own right. (This links the management of spinal disorders as discussed under the Littlejohn mechanics of spinal motion, introduced in Chapter 6, with pelvic mechanics.)

Historical perspective. In the parts of the profession that were more inclined to follow the

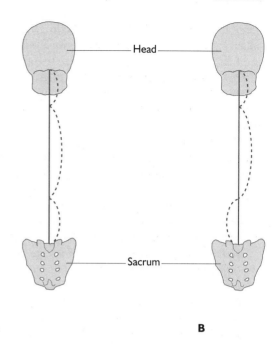

A   **B**

Figure 7.5

A. *The spinal curves associated with an inferior-lateral ilium on the right.* **B.** *The spinal curves associated with a superior-medial ilium on the left. If there are thought to be several superimposed lesions, then the curves are referred to. They are thought to 'dictate' the most 'important' of the sacroiliac lesions.*

reductionist/revised models of spinal mechanics, this model of pelvic mechanics was more frequently used, and most parts of it were retained while the general osteopathic approach was being adapted as previously discussed. Interestingly, although the 'positional' aspects of the spinal mechanics (where a vertebral complex was considered to be held in a relatively flexed, sidebent and rotated position, for example) were gradually put aside for a more dynamic picture, it is perhaps curious to note that many aspects of the 'positional' relationships within the pelvic model were retained.

One other point is worth noting: there were many physiological consequences thought to be associated with iliac lesions (through the influence they could have upon pelvic nerve function, including the pelvic parasympathetic nerves).

The Fryette model did not highlight such specific associations (although the link was implicit). However, the knowledge of the influence upon spinal curves, and the physiological relations mentioned below, were not really carried forward into common osteopathic practice in later years.

The following quote from Jocelyn Proby's account of the Mackinnon technique makes the following observations:

> *The first point to be noted is that right innominate lesions seem to produce a very special effect upon the gastro-intestinal system, while left innominate lesions mainly influence the genito-urinary and circulatory systems, including function of the heart itself. Thus, when a patient is suffering from headache, indigestion, flatulence, gastric ulcer, disturbances of bowel function, haemorrhoids, etc., it is practically certain that a right innominate lesion will be found, though the migraine type headache is very commonly associated with a left innominate lesion. On the other hand, a patient with heart trouble, menstrual trouble, bladder or prostate trouble, night emissions, etc., is almost certain to have a lesion of the left innominate bone.*
>
> Proby, 1930

The mechanisms behind such relations were not explained, other than by some association with the nervous system. However, although these observations were made several decades ago, more modern authors are also noting some similar relations (although not so extensive). Jean-Pierre Barral, for example, has related problems in the right sacroiliac articulation to large-bowel dysfunction, and those within the left sacroiliac articulation to genitourinary problems (Barral and Mercier, 1988).

(Note: The Mackinnon model does not discuss the influence of the hip articulations, or the muscular components of the pelvic girdle, but considers the relationship to be governed principally by the ligaments of the pelvis. The muscular and hip joint relations will be returned to later, when different models/views are discussed.)

'Fryette' model

This model is slightly more three-dimensional. It uses the same torsion pattern of combined sidebending and rotation that is used in the Fryette analysis of spinal mechanics (which is related to the Littlejohn model of spinal mechanics) and looks at the sacrum as a sort of continuation of the spinal column that happens to find itself between two ilia (it is a precursor of the technique/methods of Fred Mitchell). This model is strongly concerned with sacroiliac lesions (meaning that the dysfunctional part is the sacrum, not the ilium).

Fryette considered the sacrum to be fundamentally important to body function and biomechanical integrity, and said of it: 'Little wonder that the ancient phallic worshipers named the base of the spine the Sacred Bone. It is the seat of the transverse centre of gravity, the keystone of the pelvis, the foundation of the spine. It is closely associated with our greatest abilities and disabilities, with our greatest romances and tragedies, our greatest pleasures and pains' (Fryette, 1954) (which sounds a bit as if one should consider sacral 'emotion' as much as sacral motion!).

Sacral motion (Kuchera and Kuchera, 1992)

The types of motion within this model can be surmised by looking at what happens to the sacrum during locomotion. Different parts of the gait cycle show the sacrum in differing degrees of sidebending, rotation and nutation/counternutation. The axes of motion are complex, and are briefly discussed below.

Axes of sacral motion

Within this model the axes of sacral motion are considered to be composite, as though the sacrum is 'floating', and are best understood by the following illustration.

The idea of the sacrum as having a motion within three dimensions is gaining some support

Figure 7.6

'Spherical' motion of the sacrum.

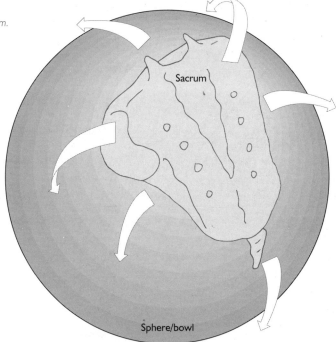

(Levin, 1995). The 'axes of movement' of this 'floating' of the sacrum might best be described by picturing the sacrum as moving on a part of a sphere, as shown in Figure 7.6.

If one assumes that the ilia are stationary and identically orientated, and that the sacrum 'floats' around in between them by using the upper and lower poles of the sacroiliac joints as pivots, two composite axes of sacral motion emerge. One sacral torsion using this axis analogy is shown in Figure 7.7.

Figure 7.8 shows a summary of the palpatory findings associated with the variety of sacral torsion found within this analogy.

If the sacrum becomes twisted between the ilia, as a result of following spinal torsion patterns from above, under the influence of weight and gravity, then the sacrum may become 'fixed' into an awkward relationship, based on its movement around these axes.

As is indicated in these figures, there are also relations with leg length, which are mediated more through the action of the piriformis muscle than as a consequence of acetabular height following ilial rotation (as per the Mackinnon model). Remember that the Fryette model assumes that the ilia remain level in relation to each other, and to a horizontal plane. The sacrum twists between them, irritating the piriformis on one side and causing it to tighten. When piriformis contracts, the femur is taken into external rotation, which causes the leg to appear longer than the other (this 'lengthening' occurring because of the shape of the femur and the way it articulates with the ilium in this rotated position).

Evaluation

These different lesion patterns are diagnosed by palpatory examination. Figure 7.7 illustrates that identifying how the sacrum is twisted depends on palpating bony landmarks, assessing the relative depths of the sulci and looking at the amount of easy spring present on pushing the lumbosacral articulation into extension, all coupled with measuring the leg lengths.

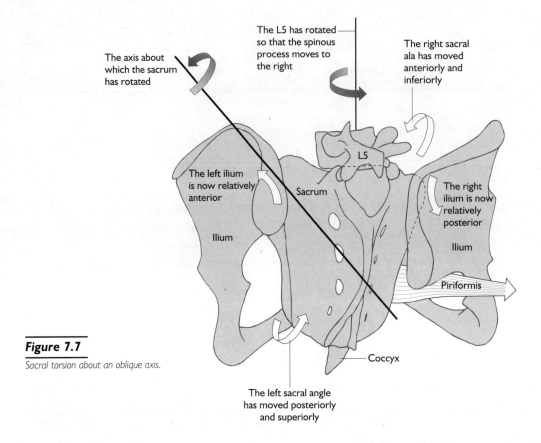

The L5 has rotated so that the spinous process moves to the right

The axis about which the sacrum has rotated

The right sacral ala has moved anteriorly and inferiorly

L5

The left ilium is now relatively anterior

Sacrum

The right ilium is now relatively posterior

Ilium

Ilium

Piriformis

Coccyx

The left sacral angle has moved posteriorly and superiorly

Figure 7.7

Sacral torsion about an oblique axis.

Combining lesion patterns

Additionally, the whole picture could become confused if there is a lesion of the ilium super-imposed upon this sacral torsion! This leads us on to a discussion of iliosacral lesion patterns within the 'Fryette' model.

Lesion patterns within the pelvis that could not be explained through the above methods were often thought to be associated with some lesions of the ilium on the sacrum, where the ilium was considered to be 'shunted'/sheared either superiorly or inferiorly on the sacrum.

Treatment within the 'Fryette' model is based upon a series of precise reversals of all the above components of either sacral torsion or ilial position. These could be done through various manipulations, with a contact on the ilium or the sacrum, or even with two practitioners working together to try to deal with several components of the torsion pattern simultaneously.

The Mitchell model/technique (Mitchell, 1965; Mitchell and Mitchell, 1995)

If the preceding model seems somewhat over-loaded with detail, then the following one may seem even more so.

As hinted at the beginning of this section, over time, osteopathic practitioners were increasingly convinced that the movement patterns and dysfunctions within the pelvic area were far more difficult to resolve than those in other areas of the body, simply because of the complex and diverse functions of the pelvic girdle to which its structure must be subservient.

Therefore, as treating the patient in accordance with the lesion patterns from the preceding models did not lead to a satisfactory outcome in all cases, increasing efforts were made to develop a more all-encompassing method of evaluation and treatment. Fred Mitchell, an American osteopath, came up with proposals that have now

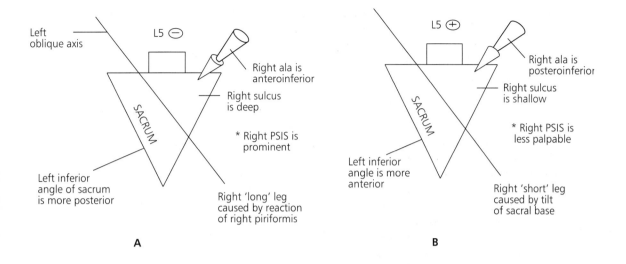

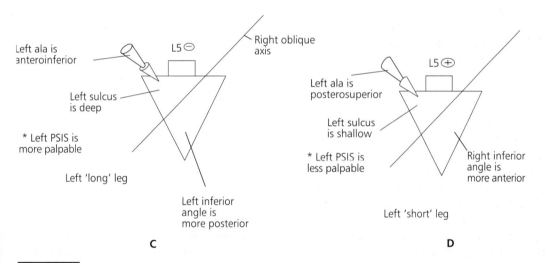

Figure 7.8

*Sacral torsion on the left and right axes (posterior view). **A.** Left–left sacral torsion. The sacrum turns around the left axis and the face of the sacrum looks more to the left. **B.** Left–right sacral torsion. The sacrum turns around the left axis and the face of the sacrum looks more to the right. **C.** Right–right sacral torsion. The sacrum turns around the right axis and the face of the sacrum looks more to the right. **D.** Right–left sacral torsion. The sacrum turns around the right axis and the face of the sacrum looks more to the left. PSIS = posterior superior iliac spine; L5 − = L5 is in extension – no resistance to pushing it into extension; L5 + = L5 is in flexion – there is resistance to pushing it into extension.*

become embedded in very many parts of osteopathic practice throughout Europe and America (although not all current British osteopaths adhere to the following!).

The following quote from one of Mitchell's papers discusses the need for a fulsome method of pelvic management:

> *The pelvic girdle is the cross-roads of the body, the architectural centre of the body,*

*the meeting place of the locomotor appara-
tus, the resting place of the torso, the temple
of the reproductive organs, the abode of the
new life's development, the site of the two
principal departments of elimination, and
last but not least, a place upon which to
sit.*

*When the osteopathic physician appreci-
ates the relationship of the bony structures
of the pelvic girdle to good body mechanics,
circulation to the pelvic organs and lower
extremities, reflex disturbance to remote
parts of the organism through endocrine or
neurogenic perverted physiology, and can
master the diagnosis and manipulative
correction, he has a basic tool from which
all therapy can begin.*

*This knowledge helps take him out of the
symptom-treatment class and sets him apart
as the physician* par excellence. *The sacroiliac and ilio-sacral and symphysis pubis
lesions are technical and complicated. The
technique for the correction is not difficult,
and is worth knowing.*

Mitchell, 1965

Mitchell's approach

One of the main reasons that the two preceding
models were not adequate is that they related
lesions as one mobile bone against a static bone,
whereas in reality this was not the case, as can be
seen if the changes in relations of the pelvic bones
and lumbar spine during gait are examined (see
below). In effect, Mitchell put together the lesion
patterns of both Fryette and Mackinnon, and
then added a few more of his own! He additionally proposed a novel system of muscle
evaluation complementing the biomechanical
'positional' analysis of the pelvis, which will be
discussed in a moment.

Gait

This discussion takes the idea of sacral motion
into a more three-dimension dynamic than
previous models, and is the development of
sacral motion that was referred to at the beginning of the chapter.

During gait, the sacrum floats between the ilia,
orienting itself around these axes, and if one
takes 'snapshots' of the relative positions of the
sacrum, lumbar spine and ilia during movement,
several 'patterns' emerge at different stages of the
gait cycle. Normally the sacrum would return to
a neutral balanced and symmetrical position in
the standing/static/seated positions, but may
become restricted and 'twisted' along these axes,
thus altering pelvic balance. This would clearly
mean that any future pelvic motions would not
be able to follow the same oscillatory patterns as
before, and soft tissue strain and symptoms
would follow as a result.

The gait cycle is as follows.

- During left leg weight-bearing and the
  beginning of the right leg swing phase,
  there is a right lumbar convexity, the wing
  of the left ilium begins an anterior movement and the wing of the right ilium starts
  posteriorly; there is a left-on-left sacral
  torsion.
- During toe-off on the weight-bearing left
  leg and the end of the right leg swing
  phase, there is no sacral torsion, no lumbar
  convexity, the left ilium is as far forward as
  it is going to go and the right ilium is still
  going backwards.
- During right leg weight-bearing, there is a
  left lumbar convexity, the right ilium starts
  to go forwards and the left ilium starts to
  go backwards; there is a right-on-right
  sacral torsion.
- During toe-off on the weight-bearing right
  leg, there is no sacral torsion, no lumbar
  convexity, the right ilium is as far forwards
  as it is going to go, and the left ilium is still
  moving posteriorly. This completes one
  complete gait cycle.

The most commonly recognized lesion patterns
within this osteopathic model were as follows:

- bilateral flexion of the sacrum between the
  ilia;
- unilateral flexion;

- bilateral extension;
- unilateral extension;
- torsion on the left oblique axis to right and left (as per Fryette);
- torsion on the right oblique axis to right and left (as per Fryette);
- symphysis pubis superior on the left;
- symphysis pubis inferior on the left;
- anterior innominate (ilium) on the right;
- posterior innominate (ilium) on the left.

Evaluation
As with the Fryette model, these lesions are all recognized by comparing bony landmarks, such as iliac spine heights, levels of the symphysis pubis, heights of the medial malleoli, and so on, but also by comparing soft tissue/muscle state (which will be referred to in a moment).

Problems with using bony landmarks as a diagnostic criterion
Because of the diverse soft tissue attachments on to the posterior sacrum and the variability of bony anatomy of the sacrum and ilia (where sacral spines are often missing, extra, altered in size or orientation, or the ilial spines are similarly variable in size and shape), comparing relative positions of bony landmarks may give a false impression of the motion relations between these bones.

There are so many situations of different practitioners coming to differing conclusions when examining the same patient that the complete accuracy of this mode of diagnosis must be questioned. This does not necessarily negate the model, which should be commended for its attempts to cover as many variations of pelvic torsion patterns as possible, but indicates the need for caution in being dogmatic with findings.

However, there are ways of reducing error, through an assessment of the muscular system. If the relative lengths, elasticity and strengths of differing groups of muscles or individual muscles are compared during the evaluation of the patient, patterns of muscular dysfunction can be identified and correlated with palpatory findings, and a more accurate assessment of dysfunction achieved.

Muscle evaluation
At the very beginning of this section on the pelvis mention was made of the sacrum being within a fascial sleeve/sheath, which orients the position of the sacrum according to how different muscles influence the fascial structure. The Mitchell model adheres to this concept as it is concerned with trying to re-establish normal relations between diverse soft tissues in the area and to re-coordinate appropriate neural control of the area through the normalization of these differing soft tissue tensions. This would lead to a re-establishment of normal pelvic bony alignment.

Mitchell was very concerned with the balanced function of all the muscular components that influence pelvic motion and contribute to the diverse 'positional' lesion patterns already described.

If, for whatever reason, the muscle lengths acting upon the area were altered from normal (perhaps through injury), then this would begin to alter the tensions acting upon the pelvic bones and begin to twist them. Additionally, through the phenomenon of reciprocal innervation involved in the patterning within neural control of motion, if one muscle is too tight, then a related muscle would be 'relaxed' in order to accommodate the increased tension of the first muscle (as part of the standard agonist and antagonist relationships within muscle groups). This lessening of tension in the second area would further alter the tensional relations throughout the pelvic region, resulting in an uneven 'suspension' of the sacrum and other pelvic bones, leading to torsion, stress and strain within one or more of the articulations between these bones. Testing the relative elasticity and stretch within the various muscles gives some idea of which muscles are too tight and which are too loose, which helps decide how the pelvis is being twisted.

Treatment
Treatment is directed at correcting these soft tissue imbalances, and the technique used is called 'muscle energy technique'. This approach to the treatment of the torsions found makes it the most sophisticated model so far.

It is useful to consider this technique for a moment, as it brings the role of soft tissues within articular mechanics to the fore. As we go through the rest of this chapter, considering different concepts and models, we shall see that increasingly the models incorporate the soft tissue component far more than was previously the case.

Muscle energy technique (Mitchell and Mitchell, 1995)

As stated, then to accompany Mitchell's approach to soft tissue-guided/induced pelvic torsion, a method of treatment that would address the soft tissue imbalances was conceived. One should note that this technique can be applied throughout the body and is not confined to the pelvic area.

Muscle energy technique was thought to influence the neural control of the various muscle groups (after it had become adapted in some way to whatever soft tissue injury/strain had created the torsion pattern in the first place).

We have discussed in part the neural control of muscle activity; to appreciate the therapeutic advantages to the muscle energy approach, it would be helpful to consider some other aspects of the neural control of motion.

Motor learning, and neural control of muscles
Eyal Lederman, in his recently published book *Fundamentals of Manual Therapy* (Lederman, 1997), has done much work to clarify the mechanisms underlying the role of manual therapy in motor learning, and the clinical relevance of various types of manipulations on this system, which we will touch on below.

Mention has been made in preceding chapters of the need for proprioceptive feedback (through mechanoreceptors, for example) to help guide and modify motor activity during a certain action. Also, it is known that the motor system can learn new tasks, and increasing subtleties of motion, through experience based upon the responses it has through these feedback loops.

Lederman states:

Proprioceptors do not control the motor centres but provide information with which the motor system 'decides' on an appropriate response. If the incoming information is of low importance the system will not modify its ongoing activity. In fact, the motor system can still control movement in the absence of incoming proprioceptive information – which can occur through neural damage, for example. However, the tasks that the motor system can execute under these circumstances are ones that were pre-learned before the loss of proprioception. This means that the motor system would be incapable of controlling fine or new learned movements, or of improving these movements.

Lederman, 1997

Motor patterning has been discussed earlier in the text, and many of us use our limbs in subtly different ways, with slightly differing outcomes for the biomechanical efficiency of the limb/body area involved. This situation seems to be a consequence of how we learn the differing locomotor tasks through life. There is also a hypothesis within the manipulative professions that soft tissue injury and damage to the joints may lead to altered patterning. They consider empirically that this is the case. It would be logical in the short term to avoid further injury to the area but, when the injury heals and perhaps leaves some scarring or shortening of muscles and long-term disruption to ligaments and fascial sheaths around the muscles, does this then lead to a long standing adaptation of motor patterning? If so, it would then lead to a slight shift in whole-body movement control to accommodate the altered movement of the affected part, which might have diverse effects on the stresses and strains that the other parts of the body must accommodate during normal movement.

Manipulation to the affected joint or muscle/ligament/soft tissue structure of the area is thought to influence the proprioceptive system so that it eventually leads to a re-adaptation of the motor control of movement, and to re-adjustment of neural patterning. There have been questions as to whether this in fact can occur, and if so, which type of manipulation is the most effective for this purpose. Lederman's work suggests that many of the passive manipulations (i.e. where the practitioner moves the affected joint or soft tissue for the patient) are not as effective as getting the person to actively contract various muscles as part of the manipulation.

There are three stages of motor learning: cognitive, associative and autonomous.

Cognitive learning is what occurs during voluntary tasks that are being performed for the first time. The tasks are unfamiliar to the nervous system, and so require the recruitment of many sensory systems, such as sight, as well as proprioceptive feedback in order to become established. When one first learns a task, such as driving a car, only one or two aspects of the task can be concentrated on at a time. Gradually as the person becomes familiar with the simpler components of the task, the nervous system is moving into the **associative phase**, where less 'active' monitoring and concentration is required to execute them. In this state, more components of the task can be added to the earlier ones, and so the whole execution of the task can become more coordinated. Finally, through familiarization and repetition, the nervous system moves into the **autonomous phase**, when the movements within the task become largely unconscious, leaving the majority of the nervous system 'free' to monitor other factors, such as fast-approaching trees!

If one is trying to learn a new task, or adapt an old one, or relearn how to move a limb/body part in a different way, then this process must be gone through in order to achieve lasting change within the neural control mechanisms. Active contraction of muscles, under the particular guidance of the practitioner, is designed to get the person to engage the muscle in a particular task or phase of motion that has become unfamiliar to them. This engages the cognitive phase of motor learning, which is considered the most powerful/important phase for neuro-rehabilitation purposes.

This seems to be the role of the muscle energy techniques that Mitchell advocated. In this way, the Mitchell model provides a very powerful method of 'correction' of pelvic torsions/lesions/misalignments.

However, the model's major drawback is that, when coupled with the palpation of the bony landmarks, it takes time to monitor all components, decide upon the torsion pattern and affected muscle groups and decide exactly how the technique should be performed.

Historical perspective
Very possibly for this reason, as we saw with models of spinal movement, this model was somewhat revised in some parts of the profession.

However, when moving away from such models as Fryette, Mackinnon and Mitchell, one should acknowledge that they did at least indicate the immense complexity of pelvic motion, a concept that is easy to forget in the drive for simplicity.

Revised 'models' of pelvic torsion
As the osteopathic profession developed, various practitioners searched for a more easily assimilable model for assessing and treating pelvic problems. These people went back to considering the diverse soft tissues (muscles, ligaments and fascial structures) that attached to the bony parts of the pelvis, lumbar spine and lower limb, and considered how they could influence the basic 'springy' mobility of the pelvic articulations, thus compromising function, without the perceived need to categorize the torsions in such a dictatorial way (involving so many different variations of misalignment).

This revised approach does not give a 'model' in the sense of the ones previously discussed and should be considered more an approach to evaluation (and subsequent treatment) than a set descriptive model of possible movement/relation permutations. The assessment within this was designed to be more a dynamic and realistic comparison of what was happening in that area during activity and locomotion than a static 'snapshot'.

This approach centres on the dynamic motion testing of articulations and the responses of the surrounding soft tissues, which was previously described in the section on spinal mechanics as the revised model of spinal evaluation. As stated in the spinal section, this method of assessment will be discussed in a separate chapter. As such, it freed the practitioner from a prescriptive model and allowed them to take a three-dimensional view of the pelvic motion based on responses to passive movement of the articulation/area.

It is a method that is used throughout the body, which is why it will be described separately within the chapter on evaluation.

SUMMARY SO FAR

Spinal movement has been introduced as a complex dynamic of interplay of tensions within a multicurved and multisectional column. Motion within one part of the spine has been shown to be influential to other parts of that column. Next, the motion within the pelvis has been discussed, with respect to local torsions and movement restrictions and the influence that these can have upon the spinal mechanics and balance. These need to be placed in context with the mechanics of the lower limb. Before that, however, some other considerations of the pelvis within osteopathic practice need to be briefly introduced.

THE OBSTETRIC PELVIS

There are particular considerations for pelvic motion in the obstetric patient, and obstetric osteopathy is a large subject in its own right. These, however, cannot be discussed in much detail because of limited space. During the case-history section, though, these ideas will be briefly discussed in the management of a patient with pelvic pain who presented for treatment prior to and during her pregnancy.

The osteopathic perspective on obstetrics has two main exponents – Renzo Molinari and Stephen Sandler. Both run clinics for expectant mothers in the teaching clinics of their respective

schools, and both have made their contributions to this subject. However, it is thanks to Renzo Molinari that much of the information below is included.

Obstetrics has long been a subject of interest to osteopaths, but again, much of the osteopathic perspective is not referenced, not least because it is legally and ethically difficult for non-medical practitioners to be actively involved in the care of pregnant women up to and during delivery. There are many relative and absolute contra-indications for osteopathic intervention during obstetric care. But the profession has much to offer the pregnant woman and her baby, and with careful respect on all sides of the healthcare system osteopathy should be well placed to help this most wonderful aspect of human life. (The same can be said of osteopathic contributions to the subject of infertility, which will be touched upon in Chapter 9.)

The ideas outlined below (which represent a very small window on to the osteopathic vision of obstetric care) should indicate the large possibilities for properly guided and supported research into this field.

The pelvis in the non-pregnant female

This, as we have discussed, is a springy, integrated device that functions in a three-dimensional pattern, allowing complex interactions between the torso, pelvis and lower limbs. Visceral functions within the pelvis occur in among this dynamic, such as defecation, micturition and sexual function. The pelvis, acting as a container with a mobile muscular floor/internal basin, will gently massage the internal structures/organs of the pelvis. This helps to promote good circulation, with the pelvic floor structures (the levator ani muscle and the perineum) playing an accessory role in pelvic organ function.

The pelvis in the pregnant female

This has not only to perform all the functions listed above, it must do so under constantly changing load-bearing conditions, where the spine and abdominopelvic cavities change

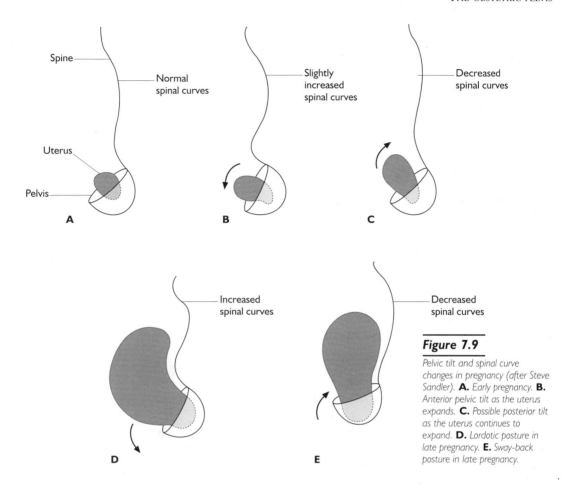

Spine
Normal spinal curves
Uterus
Pelvis

A

Slightly increased spinal curves

B

Decreased spinal curves

C

Increased spinal curves

D

Decreased spinal curves

E

Figure 7.9

Pelvic tilt and spinal curve changes in pregnancy (after Steve Sandler). **A.** *Early pregnancy.* **B.** *Anterior pelvic tilt as the uterus expands.* **C.** *Possible posterior tilt as the uterus continues to expand.* **D.** *Lordotic posture in late pregnancy.* **E.** *Sway-back posture in late pregnancy.*

shape, often dramatically. This is shown in Figure 7.9.

With these adaptations to the spine and abdomen, force-transference mechanisms alter, which changes pelvic motion parameters, and the development of a lordotic or sway-back posture affects sacral inclination, with further subsequent changes in pelvic joint motion – all of this occurring under a changing hormonal environment that leads to a relaxation of pelvic integrity, and possibly pelvic pain and joint instability as a result.

Spinal biomechanics during pregnancy

As indicated, spinal biomechanics change during the pregnancy, and often how much pain and discomfort the woman suffers seems to depend upon how smoothly her spine adapts to her changing pregnant posture. If we look at the changing spinal curves during pregnancy then we can see that several areas need to be flexible at different stages of the pregnancy, as indicated in Figure 7.9.

There could well be painful consequences if some areas of the spine were restricted/twisted at the beginning of the pregnancy and did not allow a smooth and fluidic change in curve shape to occur. Osteopaths would look throughout the spine (and lower limbs/rib cage and so on) to find and release as many areas of restriction as possible, to allow a more efficient changing of curve shape through the pregnancy. Muscular evaluation around the pelvic girdle, hips and pelvic floor are also important, as an efficient system of muscular support can help prevent pelvic instability syndromes, or at least limit them to some degree.

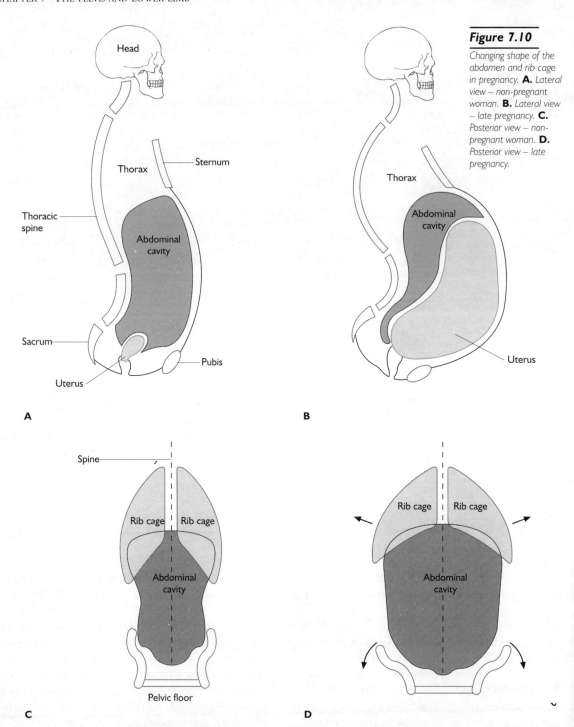

Figure 7.10

Changing shape of the abdomen and rib cage in pregnancy. **A.** Lateral view – non-pregnant woman. **B.** Lateral view – late pregnancy. **C.** Posterior view – non-pregnant woman. **D.** Posterior view – late pregnancy.

Rib cage mechanics and elasticity of the diaphragm are also important, and this allows a better and more even expansion of the abdominal cavity as the uterus expands. Visceral displacement and rib cage elasticity are necessary for the uterus to expand in a midline position and to help reduce/manage problems of breathlessness, oesophageal reflex and other visceral signs/symptoms of compression (Figure 7.10).

Uterine expansion

Another factor that will influence pelvic function is the direction of growth and expansion of the uterus, which is not always uniform. The ligamentous supports of the uterus pull increasingly (and often unevenly) on the bony parts of the pelvis they are attached to (with particular reference to the uterosacral ligaments) and, if the uterus expands unevenly, this can cause torsion within the pelvic bowl. According to the osteopathic perspective there are several determinants of uterine orientation, including other visceral compliance, elasticity within the abdominal walls and the shape of the bony pelvis and spine. In among this, one factor seems quite relevant – that of psoas tension/bulk.

The psoas muscles are thought by Molinari to act as guides for the vertical expansion of the uterus, and if they are of uneven bulk or tension, or the spine is not oriented evenly, then there may be differing pressure acting upon either side of the expanding uterus, causing it to deviate slightly to one side as it expands vertically. In practice this leads to a sidebending and rotation torsion of the uterus.

Expansion of the uterus in an even manner is desirable, both for the mother and for the baby. There are increasing numbers of hypotheses about what effects uterine wall tension can have on the developing fetus, and certainly undue tension either in small areas or in general is not an ideal situation for the baby to be exposed to. Specially trained osteopaths may end up working with uterine torsion patterns to relieve symptoms that the mother might have, but also to relieve stress upon the baby.

Engagement

Some biomechanical torsion patterns are also thought to be relevant to the process of engagement, although it has to be said that there are no documented cases of non-engagement due to lumbosacral joint stiffness. However, the cervix of the uterus is a very reflex-rich structure, and is sensitive to its environment. As the cervix descends into the pelvis, the orientation of the uterus, the tension of the muscles around the uterus and the amount of pelvic torsion or lumbosacral extension are thought by various osteopaths and midwives to be factors that could reflexly affect the process of engagement. Clearly other factors are involved, such as the size of the baby's head in relation to the mother's pelvis (with problems occurring if the head is 'too small' or 'too large').

Delivery

The pelvis and the pelvic floor structures must help maintain the integrity of normal visceral functioning of the pelvis, but must also be adaptable for the birth. The elasticity of the pelvic floor and perineum is vital if the descent of these structures is going to be allowed with the minimum of distress. The flexibility of the sacrococcygeal joint is also very important, as, if fixed into a flexion position it can either cause pressure on the descending fetal head (as can the ischial spines) or end up being damaged, or the coccyx being fractured in some instances. Many osteopaths can work in advance of the delivery to try to ensure that the pelvic floor muscles are supple and that the coccyx is mobile, to limit potential problems during the delivery. This work is often carried out as an adjunct to the pelvic floor exercises the woman should already be doing herself.

Rotatory forces during delivery

There are other considerations within the osteopathic perspective on the mechanisms of delivery that are interesting. These follow on from the alignment of the uterus by external pressures, and relate to the spiralling motion the baby performs as he/she moves down and through the birth canal. This is shown in Figure 7.11. Most births occur with the baby oriented into one direction – which is shown in Figure 7.12.

The shape of the pelvis allows the baby's head to align most easily along one of two axes, about

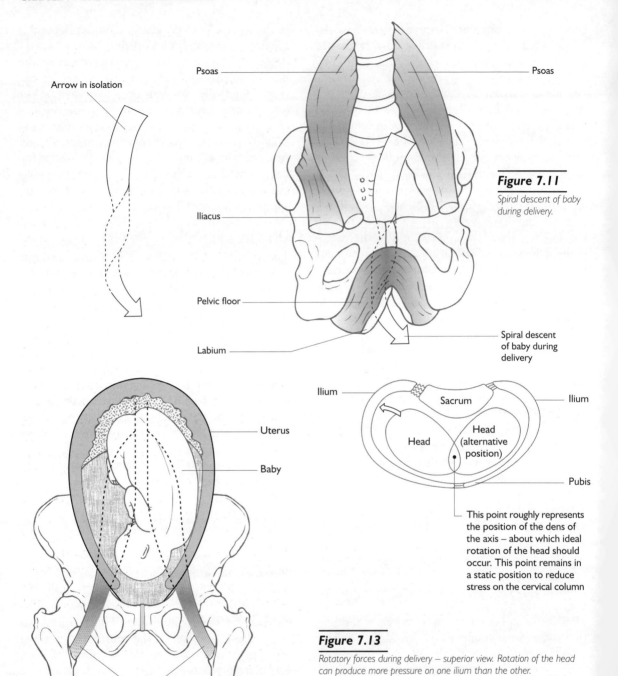

Arrow in isolation

Psoas

Psoas

Iliacus

Pelvic floor

Labium

Figure 7.11

Spiral descent of baby during delivery.

Spiral descent of baby during delivery

Uterus

Baby

Psoas

Figure 7.12

Fetal orientation at term – 94% of deliveries are in this position.

Ilium

Sacrum

Ilium

Head

Head (alternative position)

Pubis

This point roughly represents the position of the dens of the axis – about which ideal rotation of the head should occur. This point remains in a static position to reduce stress on the cervical column

Figure 7.13

Rotatory forces during delivery – superior view. Rotation of the head can produce more pressure on one ilium than the other.

which the head and body will then rotate. Rotatory forces are shown in Figure 7.13.

During descent and rotation, pressure will act on one ilium more than the other, and so one sacroiliac joint often has to open more than the other to allow easy delivery. In a case of a torsioned or relatively restricted pelvis, then this may mean that forces are directed unevenly both to the mother's head and also back on to the fetal skull, meaning that both mother and baby may suffer mechanical strains as a result.

The pelvic floor

In addition to the comments made above, the pelvic floor is thought to play a special role in delivery – actively helping the rotatory mechanics of the uterus to aid fetal descent in the easiest manner possible. Damage to the pelvic floor may be reduced if the mechanics of the whole pelvis are as optimal as possible before delivery, and the function of the pelvic floor may be aided for subsequent deliveries if such things as episiotomy scars are treated to improve overall muscle function in advance of the delivery. Of course, there are many reasons why delivery may become complicated and require the use of various forms of intervention; however, preparation of the tissues could be the key to easier deliveries in some women.

Postpartum

Of course, many deliveries can be very efficient and result in little strain to the maternal pelvis. However, in the case of episiotomy, the use of forceps, prolonged second stage, or some other factor/complication in the birth process, strain and injury can occur, which the osteopath is well placed to try to resolve in the postpartum period.

Summary

That concludes a very brief look at the osteopathic perspective on obstetrics. Now it is time to continue the picture of whole-body movement, by considering the influence of the lower limbs on pelvic motion and consequently spinal motion (and through that, the converse relations).

THE LOWER LIMB

The biomechanical arrangement of the lower limb has several important functions to perform.

It must help the dissipation of weight-bearing forces from above to be transmitted evenly through to the ground; it must help to coordinate the stability of the pelvis during static posture and locomotion, to preserve the stability of the pelvic girdle for effecting spine and trunk motion (Allum *et al.*, 1995); it must help counter moments of force induced by upper limb movements; and it must also provide an effective force-generating system to move the body during locomotion; all without placing strain upon its component parts.

The neural control of motion that we have been discussing so far clearly has many potentially conflicting demands to resolve, which we will mention briefly. Also, the arrangement of the ligamentous structures in the lower limb joints and the role of the connective tissue structures and tendons will be reviewed as they are important for the smooth transmission of force and the dissipation of strain within the lower limb.

The way that these components support the bony structures and the articular integrity is very important, and is oriented along the concepts within the tensegrity models that we discussed in a previous chapter. These allow for minimal stress to be placed upon individual components of the structure, and if we consider the ankle joint – one of the joints in the body that has to bear the most weight – we can see that the myofascial arrangements of the lower limb are very efficient as the ankle joint has very low incidences of degenerative osteoarthritis – a condition commonly associated with compression. Thus, compressive forces in the lower limb are somehow dissipated through the action and interaction of the myofascial system.

Osteopathic models concerned with lower limb motion

These centre on integrated neuronal control and how it might become disturbed, and also on the examination of the 'tensegrity integrity' of the lower limb, reflecting on the consequences that this will have for joint stress and strain, and articular and other soft tissue fatigue and injury.

Thus, the models are more similar to orthodox biomechanical reflections than some previous models, but because they reflect on the whole limb and how that is balanced to whole-body motion, they have additional perspectives that are not currently reflected in orthodox thinking.

If there is dysfunction within the lower limb, one must consider whether there are any problems throughout the rest of the body (including the upper limb) that might be directing force through to the pelvis and into the lower limb and might be compromising function there. After these components have been recognized, the manifestations of that dysfunction within the lower limb can be more reasonably addressed. Local injury to the lower limb, such as football or tennis traumas, can be managed efficiently, as the osteopath can look at ways of reducing the strain that passes through the injured and recovering part as a powerful adjunct to the healing process. This method also aims to reduce the long-term consequences of residual dysfunction from lower limb injury to the biomechanical arrangement of the rest of the body (Milan, 1994).

To explore these inter-relations, we must look at how the lower limb muscles work with the axial skeleton, and how the lower limb works within itself.

Influence of the lower limb in relation to the axial skeleton

As already indicated, during such actions as gait and standing on one leg, there is a requirement for the whole pelvis to move on the femur. Thus activity of the lower limb and hip girdle muscles can play a significant role in pelvic motion.

This activity must be coordinated through both limbs at once, and studies (Dietz, 1993) show that both limbs act in a cooperative manner, activity in each limb affecting the strength of muscle activation and time–space behaviour of the other. This interlimb coordination is believed to be mediated by the spinal interneuronal circuits within the propriospinal system that we discussed previously. The proximal lower limb muscles seem to be more important in controlling the centre of mass with respect to whole-body motion than the distal ones – a point that was made in a study that looked at multijoint movement strategies in the lower limb. Here it was found that musculoskeletal mechanics dictate that independent control of joints is relatively difficult to achieve. When one joint is restricted, the muscles controlling the other joints must work harder in order to control centre-of-mass accelerations. They also found that if the hip remains freer than more peripheral joints (e.g. the ankle) this expended less energy in general movement than if the ankle was free but the hip restricted (Kuo and Zajac, 1993). This seems to indicate that proximal articulations are more fundamental to controlling the centre of mass than more peripheral articulations.

The above interplay of muscular activity has particular relevance for the hip joint.

The hip

In order to permit the great range of motion that is available within the hip joint, its structure has been adapted from one that is very stable (a deep ball and socket arrangement) to one that is less so (a shallow socket). Through many motions of the hip, the position of the femoral head within the ilial socket depends on ligamentous integrity and muscular support.

In the standing position, the head of the femur is projecting forwards, and its position is guarded only by soft tissue integrity. The spiral arrangement of the ligaments of the hip, coupled with the action of the hip muscles – which can be thought of as a rotator cuff of the same type as the shoulder girdle rotator cuff – helps to keep the femoral head in reasonable contact with the acetabulum. The psoas and iliacus muscles are thought to be particularly important as an anterior support to the hip joint (Andersson *et al.*, 1995) and the forces acting between the hip joint and the femur can be indicated by the need for a synovial bursa between the psoas and the anterior surface of the joint to reduce them. This muscular arrangement is shown in Figure 7.14.

Certain positions lead to a slackening of the ligamentous support of the hip, one of which is flexion of the hip (which can come about

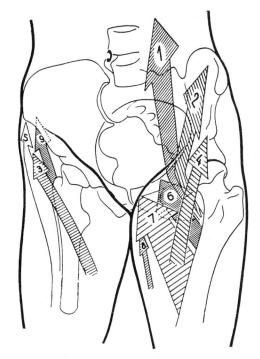

Figure 7.14

A. *Anterior view of the 'rotator cuff' muscles of the hip. 1 = psoas; 2 = iliacus; 3 = sartorius; 4 = rectus femoris; 5 = tensor fasciae lata; 6 = pectineus; 7 = adductor longus; 8 = gracilis; 9 = gluteal muscles.* **B.** *Posterior view of the 'rotator muscles' of the hip. 1, 1 ' = gluteus maximus; 2 = gluteus medius; 3 = gluteus minimus; 4 = biceps femoris; 5 = semitendinosus; 6 = semimembranosus; 7 = adductor magnus. (Reproduced with the permission of Churchill Livingstone from* The Physiology of Joints, *Vol. 3, Kapandji, 1974.)*

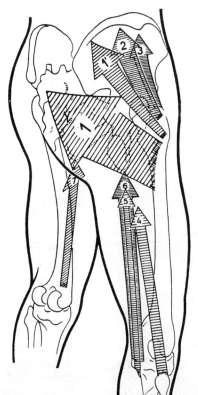

through poor posture, for example, with the person not standing with the hips sufficiently extended); the other is medial rotation of the lower limb. When we discuss the foot and ankle, we shall see that many articular problems in that area lead to a softening of the medial longitudinal arch, allowing the tibiotalar joint to shift medially and, through the torsion this induces within the tibia, to medially rotate the whole lower limb. The consequences for this at the level of the hip may be the aforementioned slackness. Even without such a situation developing, the manner of heel-strike during walking and the style of shoes one wears can also have a direct action on load-bearing forces within the hip (Bergmann *et al.*, 1995) and within the lower limb in general (Barnes and Smith, 1994).

Such situations are thought to lead to a relative loss of articular integrity, with some minor joint 'play' during motion. This, over time, can lead to stress within the articular surface of the hip and compromise the health of the cartilage. This is thought to be an important element in degenerative conditions of the hip joint.

Consequences for the pelvis (and its relation to the axial skeleton), and the rest of the lower limb

As we mentioned earlier, the proximal muscles of the lower limb (the hip muscles) are of prime importance in the neural control of balanced posture (and the control of the body's centre of mass) and integrated limb function. Disruption of hip mechanics will lead to increasing recruitment of the more distal muscles of the lower limb in an attempt to control whole-body stability. This places greater strain on the structures of the knee, ankle and foot.

The knee

The architectural arrangement of the knee is quite complex (Dye, 1996) and must withstand enormous force during motion, as it is required to be stable in many extreme positions. There must be support all around the knee, and there must be integrated function of all the ligaments of the knee, including those relating to the superior tibiofibular joint, for knee stability to be maintained (Veltri *et al.*, 1995, 1996). Stability during many movements, including axial torsion of the lower limb, is aided by meniscal mechanics and structural integrity. The menisci are shown in Figure 7.15.

The menisci act as mobile sensate bearings in the knee, which, together with the articular surfaces, muscles and ligaments of the joint, must accept, transfer and dissipate loads generated at the ends of the long mechanical levers of the tibia and femur (Bessette, 1992). The ability of the menisci to perform these tasks is based on the intrinsic material properties of the menisci as well as their gross anatomic structure and attachments (Fithian *et al.*, 1990). The menisci often work in concert with the anterior and posterior cruciate ligaments to ensure this dissipation of forces and prevent injury (Miller *et al.*, 1993; Woo *et al.*, 1992).

Additionally, the muscles acting around the knee and through the lower limb must be carefully coordinated with ligamentous activity for strain at the level of the knee to be minimized (Collins and O'Connor, 1991). This can be appreciated if one examines a complex motor task in the lower limb, such as pedalling a bicycle.

Here the limb activities may be quite complex – in that although the leg is trying to force the pedal downwards, parts of the leg/foot may be moving in directions not exactly in the plane of the desired force, and thus control of the overall process requires coactivation of monoarticular agonists and their biarticular antagonists, which provides a unique solution for these conflicting requirements: biarticular muscles appear to be able to control the desired direction of the external force on the pedal by adjusting the relative distribution of net moments over the joints while monoarticular muscles appear to be primarily activated when they are in a position to shorten and thus to contribute to positive work (van Ingen Schenau *et al.*, 1992).

Looking at the pictures opposite one can see that, in addition to effective neural control, the relations between bony position and relative

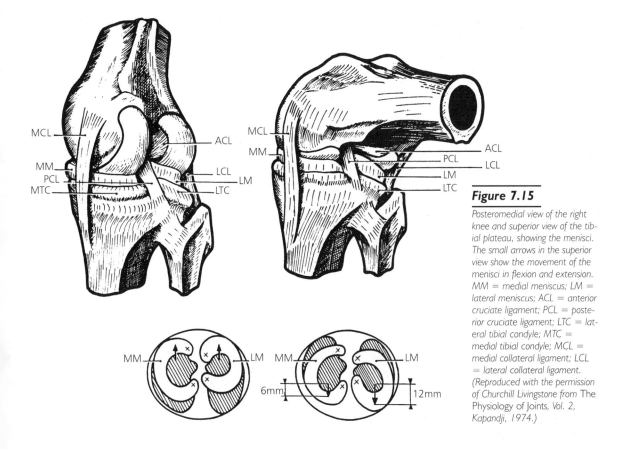

Figure 7.15

Posteromedial view of the right knee and superior view of the tibial plateau, showing the menisci. The small arrows in the superior view show the movement of the menisci in flexion and extension. MM = medial meniscus; LM = lateral meniscus; ACL = anterior cruciate ligament; PCL = posterior cruciate ligament; LTC = lateral tibial condyle; MTC = medial tibial condyle; MCL = medial collateral ligament; LCL = lateral collateral ligament. (Reproduced with the permission of Churchill Livingstone from The Physiology of Joints, Vol. 2, Kapandji, 1974.)

tension in the surrounding soft tissue structures are very important for knee integrity.

Clinically, any torsion that passes through the lower limb could disrupt these relative bony positions through the action of altered tension in the soft tissues influencing limb balance (Eckhoff, 1994). The pelvic torsions and hip positions that were discussed before could lead to an adapted orientation of the femur, thus compromising the integrity of the articular structures of the knee (Eckhoff *et al.*, 1994). Such torsions may only need to be slight, but acting over a period of time, and during all knee movements, strain could accumulate at the level of the knee, leading to inflammation, tissue injury (around and within the knee, including the menisci) and ultimately joint instability and damage. This can be seen in an analysis of gait adaptations and dynamic joint loading (Noyes *et al.*, 1992) and where alteration of the Q angle (both increase and decrease) increases contact stress in the patellofemoral joint (Pinar *et al.*, 1994; Brossmann *et al.*, 1993; Hirokawa, 1991).

Clinical relevance

Many 'orthopaedic' conditions of the knee might be more effectively managed from this wider perspective. For example, slight meniscal injuries and tears, chondromalacia patellae, Osgood–Schlatter's disease, degenerative and other arthritic conditions, bursitis around the knee and many cases of knee instability through ligamentous disruption can all be considered to be influenced by the wider biomechanical influences discussed here (Hirokawa, 1993).

Resolution of the dysfunction within the knee requires management of these other 'predisposing' and 'maintaining' factors for knee torsion.

If there is dysfunction at the knee, then this can disrupt the function of the pelvis and spine, as movement in the peripheral components of the lower limb is transmitted centrally during walking. In this way the orientation of the knee and also the fibular and foot articulations can have a bearing on hip girdle and pelvic motion. This is amply illustrated by Inman *et al.* (1981; see also Lehmann, 1993 and Chao *et al.*, 1994).

The foot

As will hopefully become evident (if it has not already), one cannot discuss lower limb torsion (or whole-body mechanics) without reference to the foot. The foot can influence more central structures such as the knee and hip–pelvic girdle, as well as being influenced by them.

The human foot is an intricate mechanism that cushions the body and adapts to uneven surfaces (Kotwick, 1982). It provides traction for movement, awareness of joint and body position for balance and leverage for propulsion (Chan and Rudins, 1994). Many practitioners feel that, in order for the spine to be balanced, one must start at the foot and work upwards, removing any restrictions and biomechanical problems from the bottom upwards. (The science of orthotics has made much of the influence of the foot on whole-body movement and control of posture.)

The role of the foot in neural control mechanisms of whole-body movement is important (Lepers and Breniere, 1995) in that the general function of proprioceptive reflexes involved in the stabilization of posture depends, in part, upon the presence of contact forces opposing gravity. In this context load receptors in the foot extensors are thought to signal changes of the projection of the body's centre of mass with respect to the feet (Dietz *et al.*, 1992). If there is disruption in the plantar fascia, for example, this can, through distortion of proprioceptive feedback, influence locomotion, as seen in functional biomechanical deficits in running athletes with plantar fasciitis (Kibler *et al.*, 1991).

The role of muscles acting in concert with fascia/connective tissue structures within lower limb mechanics

As discussed at the beginning of this section on the lower limb, we introduced the function of the lower limb as a force generator and a force distributor. Many biomechanical considerations within the foot, and hence back through the rest of the lower limb to the axial skeleton, depend upon the balanced integration of soft tissue structures involved in these two processes.

So, before discussing the foot in more detail, this component of lower limb function needs to be reviewed.

Coordinated muscle activity helps load transfer

During activity muscles acting over two joints function such that proximal action is transferred to the distal part, and thus movement is aided and mechanical energy is dissipated through the limb (Prilutsky and Zatsiorsky, 1994). The inter-coordination of muscle activity helps to dissipate the mechanical energy of the body and thus lessen the force applied to each individual part by the proximal muscles 'taking some of the work' of the distal muscles by transferring to them a part of the generated mechanical energy. In various studies limb muscles were tested and observed during the shock-absorbing phase of certain actions performed, such as squat thrusts. There emerges a relationship between proximal and distal muscles. Proximal muscles are used in such a way that they help dissipate forces acting throughout the limb during shock absorbency, whereas the more distal muscles are more concerned with the fine orientation of the individual joints of the limb during the activity.

The tendinous structures of the lower limb, including the tensor fascia lata, the Achilles tendon, the plantar fascia and the tendons of the long muscles moving the foot, play an important role in this transference.

Tensile properties of tendons aid force transference

The tensile strength of tendons is similar to bone, and tendons are slightly elastic and slightly

Figure 7.16

The arches of the foot. A–C = medial arch; A–B = transverse arch; B–C = lateral arch. (Reproduced with the permission of Churchill Livingstone from The Physiology of Joints, *Vol. 2, Kapandji, 1974.)*

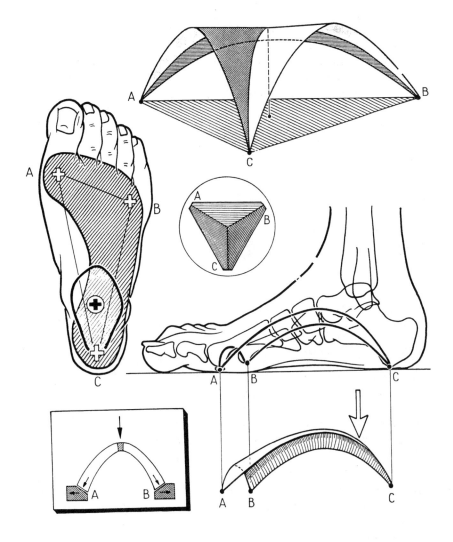

extendible. Because of this they can transfer considerable elastic energy from the muscle contractions that act upon them to the bones they themselves attach to. Tendons also exhibit viscosity, which allows them a degree of adaptation to strain. If the force acting through the tendon is very great, the point of insertion on to bone can often be the first place where that force overcomes the anatomical structure – with tendon avulsion resulting. Tendon rupture can also occur, a common site being the Achilles tendon in the calf. (The role of tendons and fascia in posture will be discussed after the upper limb has been introduced into the picture.)

Clinical relevance

Perhaps, in someone with an old tendon injury, the tendons may not be capable of applying the same transference, because of scarring and fibrous replacement of the elastic collagen content at the site of injury. In this case the general absorptive properties and dissipation of energy of normal limb function are diminished, perhaps placing strain on other (muscular) components that are less well designed to accommodate such forces over time. Also, if the limb is under a degree of torsion, this may compromise even healthy tendons, as applied force may be in a slightly different direction from the collagen

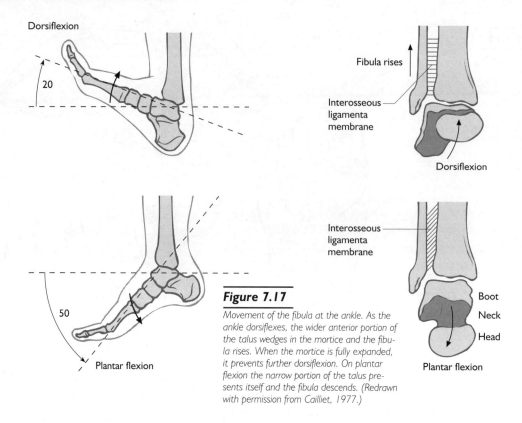

Figure 7.17

Movement of the fibula at the ankle. As the ankle dorsiflexes, the wider anterior portion of the talus wedges in the mortice and the fibula rises. When the mortice is fully expanded, it prevents further dorsiflexion. On plantar flexion the narrow portion of the talus presents itself and the fibula descends. (Redrawn with permission from Cailliet, 1977.)

fibres within that structure. This may also diminish their action in the integrative activity of force transference within the limb (whether lower or upper; Loren and Lieber, 1995).

The architecture of the foot

The architectural arrangement of the foot also aids in force transference and dissipation.

The foot is composed of a series of arches: the medial, lateral, transverse and anterior arches, which are shown in Figure 7.16.

The distribution of stresses during varied motion and the resistance of static distortions of the plantar vault depend on the integrity of these arches.

The relation between the tibia, fibula, their intraosseous membrane and the foot

The orientation of the tibiofibular articulations, under the influence of various muscles, will in-

fluence the orientation of the talus, and from that the rest of the foot (Xenos *et al.*, 1995). The converse relation also applies. Distortion and pressures within the foot will influence the other structures of the lower limb (Oatis, 1988).

Fibular mechanics and the action of the intraosseous membrane

During dorsiflexion and plantar flexion, the lower tibiofibular joint moves apart, and the fibula also moves superiorly and inferiorly. Figure 7.17 shows the fibular movements at the level of the ankle.

If the motion of the fibula is compromised (for example, by restriction at the level of the knee, by the action of muscles in the thigh inserting upon it, or by ligamentous disruption following ankle injury), this will lead to altered biomechanics at the level of the ankle and disrupt foot integrity (Wang *et al.*, 1996).

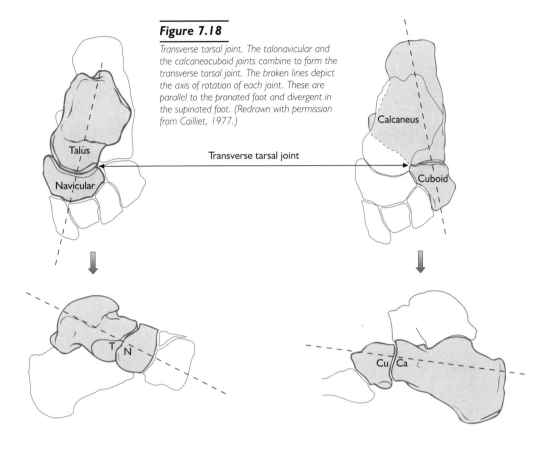

Figure 7.18

Transverse tarsal joint. The talonavicular and the calcaneocuboid joints combine to form the transverse tarsal joint. The broken lines depict the axis of rotation of each joint. These are parallel to the pronated foot and divergent in the supinated foot. (Redrawn with permission from Cailliet, 1977.)

The subtalar joint influences supination and pronation within the foot

The orientation of the talus is important for the function of the subtalar joint (Perry, 1983). The calcaneum rolls, pitches and rocks underneath the talus like a ship in choppy water. Any torsion acting from above, through the tibia, will influence talar movement and thus the relationship between the talus and the calcaneum (Sarrafian, 1993). If the subtalar joint cannot accommodate this, then the forces transferred to the rest of the foot will be greater than normal. Conversely, if the rest of the foot is restricted and normal force transference cannot be passed through the medial arch, for example, then the subtalar joint may need to adapt its motion to accommodate this. This action will have consequences up the lower limb to the knee and hip-pelvic girdle, as we discussed before.

The subtalar joint can also be responsible for a lot of heel pain, which may be an accumulation of tensions from the whole foot acting at the level of the calcaneum/plantar fascia (Bordelon, 1983).

The transverse tarsal joint

This is composed of the talonavicular joint and the calcaneocuboid joint and is shown in Figure 7.18.

These articulations help the torsioning forces acting through the foot during its complex movements and in load-bearing situations to be smoothly transferred to the anterior and transverse arches. Load-bearing causes several changes in the foot, including a rotation movement within all the tarsal articulations (Kitaoka *et al.*, 1995). Restriction or altered motion within these articulations (often as a result of dys-

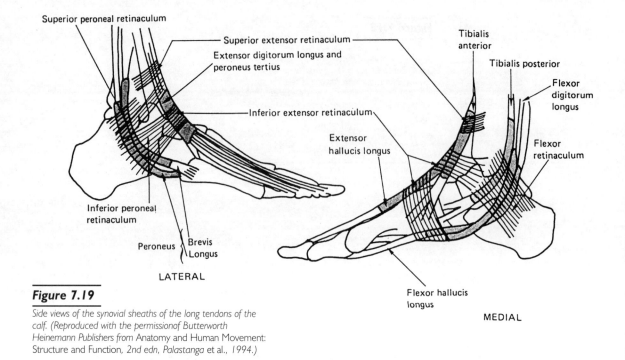

Figure 7.19

Side views of the synovial sheaths of the long tendons of the calf. (Reproduced with the permission of Butterworth Heinemann Publishers from Anatomy and Human Movement: Structure and Function, *2nd edn, Palastanga et al., 1994.)*

function in the articulations discussed above) will affect the integrity of the medial and lateral arches, and so overall foot function (again, with a reciprocal relationship operating; Rodgers, 1988).

The midtarsal articulations and the forefoot
The relations and motions of the cuneiform bones, the metatarsal and the tarsals depend on the orientation provided by the transverse tarsal articulations and the even transference of force from these joints (and from all factors influencing them).

Clinical relevance
The torsions and restrictions that can arise through disturbed mechanics acting on and within the foot can have implications for the forefoot. Many painful conditions associated with these joints could be addressed by resolving the biomechanical disturbances throughout the foot and lower limb. They should be seen as a final culmination of disturbed forces through the body, acting upon the foot (without forgetting the

influence of the toes on the rest of the foot and gait; Carrier *et al.*, 1994).

Conditions such as metatarsalgia, hallux valgus, Morton's neuroma, march fracture, interdigital neuritis, painful heel, plantar fasciitis and hammer toes can all be related to this process (Martorell, 1981).

Additionally, one should not forget the tendon sheaths acting around the ankle joint. These synovial sheaths are designed to reduce friction and strain upon the tendons running through them during locomotion. The tendon sheaths are shown in Figure 7.19.

Under ideal biomechanical situations, where all forces acting through the foot are balanced, the retinaculi and the synovial sheaths will be properly aligned and the forces produced by tendon action will be within tolerable limits. If there are any torsions such as those discussed throughout this section, this could lead to stress and irritation within these sheaths. This will not only lead to a variety of painful situations but also compromise foot function and the efficient function of related muscles.

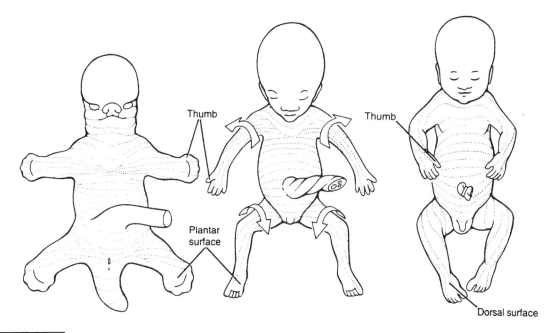

Thumb

Thumb

Plantar
surface

Dorsal surface

Figure 7.20

Rotation of the limbs. The dramatic medial rotation of the lower limbs during the sixth to eighth weeks of life causes the mature dermatomes to spiral down the limb. (Reproduced with the permission of Churchill Livingstone from Human Embryology, Larson, 1993.)

Compartment syndrome

The role of foot mechanics in the regulation of lower limb dynamics will continuously and variably distort the fascial compartments of the anterior and posterior lower leg. However, if these articulations become restricted, or torsioned, the compartments may become less elastic, leading to various types of compartment syndrome (Gerow *et al.*, 1993).

Stability and the lower limb

Before leaving the lower limb, we should consider the need for stability from birth right through to full bony maturation within the lower limb.

From birth, through infancy to childhood, the lower limb is subjected to a variety of stresses. When born, an infant's legs have been held in a flexed and externally rotated position and need to continue their medial rotation to take up the normal postnatal orientation of the lower limbs (Figure 7.20).

The limbs are also non-weight-bearing structures *in utero*. Both these facts are relevant for the eventual efficient function of the lower limbs.

The rotation of the limbs is influenced in part by muscular tensions. Muscular tensions acting in infancy may influence the appropriate 'unfolding' of the lower limb. In addition to this, as the child starts to stand and walk, the limbs undergo other positional changes, as the limb adapts to weight-bearing forces. This gradual change in function must not be hindered by any restrictions or general postural imbalance, as the muscular coordination of the limb and, very importantly, the final development of the bony architecture of the limbs might be compromised.

Ossification within the lower limbs

We have discussed osseous formation in a previous chapter, but it is useful to have a brief reminder here, to help expand on the points above.

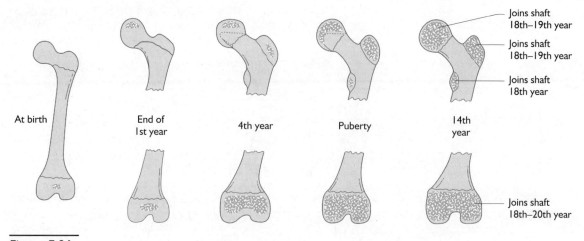

Joins shaft
18th–19th year

Joins shaft
18th–19th year

Joins shaft
18th year

At birth

End of
1st year

4th year

Puberty

14th
year

Joins shaft
18th–20th year

Figure 7.21

Stages of ossification within the femur. (Redrawn with the permission of Churchill Livingstone from Gray's Anatomy, 36th edn, Williams and Warwick, 1980.)

At birth, the diaphyses or shafts of the limb bones (consisting of a bone collar and trabecular core) are completely ossified, whereas the ends of the bones, called the epiphyses, are still cartilaginous. After birth, secondary ossification centres develop in the epiphyses, which gradually ossify. However, a layer of cartilage called the epiphyseal cartilage plate (growth plate) persists between the epiphysis and the growing end of the diaphysis. Continued proliferation of the chondrocytes in this growth plate allows both the diaphysis to lengthen and the final adult shape of the bones to emerge. The ossification centres of the lower limb are shown in Figure 7.21.

This process occurs throughout the body but is of particular clinical relevance here, because of the high weight-bearing and other forces that act upon the limb during this process. The changing rotation within the lower limbs and the changing varus/valgus relationships within the knees as the child grows will cause differing compressive loads within the developing bones (Frost, 1997). These often 'balance themselves out' over time, so that the limb develops normally, but if the malalignments are large, then the process of compression and bony adaptation is self-encouraging, and the knee can become quite compromised.

Uneven, unbalanced or slightly disrupted biomechanics throughout the body and lower limb

may eventually lead to a moderate adaptation of the final architectural structure of the bones, which could lead to the articular surfaces being oriented in a less than optimum direction. Trabeculae within the pelvis are shown in Figure 7.22, as an illustration.

Now it is time to incorporate the upper limb and thorax into our overall picture. This next chapter will include further analysis of gait and discuss the integration between the pelvis and the torso during locomotion, and will therefore add to the information already given in this chapter.

REFERENCES

Allum, J. H., Honegger, F. and Acuna, H. (1995) Differential control of leg and trunk muscle activity by vestibulo-spinal and proprioceptive signals during human balance corrections. *Acta Oto-Laryngologica*, 115, 124–129.

Andersson, E., Oddsson, L., Grundstrom, H. and Thorstensson, A. (1995) The role of the psoas and iliacus muscles for stability and movement of the lumbar spine, pelvis and hip. *Scandinavian Journal of Medicine and Science in Sports*, 5, 10–16.

Barnes, R. A. and Smith, P. D. (1994) The role of footwear in minimizing lower limb injury. *Journal of Sports Sciences*, 12, 341–353.

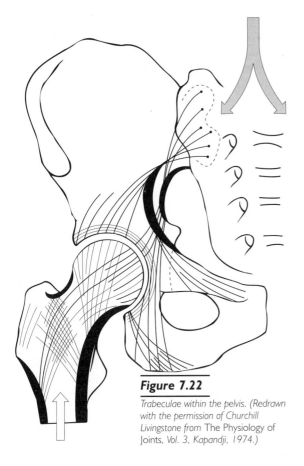

Figure 7.22

Trabeculae within the pelvis. (Redrawn with the permission of Churchill Livingstone from The Physiology of Joints, *Vol. 3, Kapandji, 1974.)*

Barral, J.-P. and Mercier, P. (1988) Visceral manipulation. In: *Visceral Manipulation*, Eastland Press, Seattle, WA.

Bergmann, G., Kniggendorf, H., Graichen, F. and Rohlmann, A. (1995) Influence of shoes and heel strike on the loading of the hip joint. *Journal of Biomechanics*, **28**, 817–827.

Bessette, G. C. (1992) The meniscus. *Orthopedics*, **15**, 35–42.

Bordelon, R. L. (1983) Subcalcaneal pain. A method of evaluation and plan for treatment. *Clinical Orthopaedics and Related Research*, **177**, 49–53.

Bowen, V. and Cassidy, J. D. (1981) Macroscopic and microscopic anatomy of the sacroiliac joint from embryonic life until the eighth decade. *Spine*, **6**, 620–628.

Brossmann, J., Muhle, C., Schroder, C. *et al.* (1993) Patellar tracking patterns during active and passive knee extension: evaluation with motion-triggered cine MR imaging. *Radiology*, **187**, 205–212.

Brunner, C., Kissling, R. and Jacob, H. A. (1991) The effects of morphology and histopathologic findings on the mobility of the sacroiliac joint. *Spine*, **16**, 1111–1117.

Cailliet, R. (1977) *Soft Tissue Pain and Disability*, F. A. Davis, Philadelphia, PA.

Carrier, D. R., Heglund, N. C. and Earls, K. D. (1994) Variable gearing during locomotion in the human musculoskeletal system. *Science*, **265**, 651–653.

Chan, C. W. and Rudins, A. (1994) Foot biomechanics during walking and running. *Mayo Clinic Proceedings*, **69**, 448–461.

Chao, E. Y., Neluheni, E. V., Hsu, R. W. and Paley, D. (1994) Biomechanics of malalignment. *Orthopedic Clinics of North America*, **25**, 379–386.

Collins, J. J. and O'Connor, J. J. (1991) Muscle–ligament interactions at the knee during walking. *Proceedings of the Institute of Mechanical Engineers*, **205**,11–18.

Dalstra, M. and Huiskes, R. (1995) Load transfer across the pelvic bone. *Journal of Biomechanics*, **28**, 715–724.

Dananberg, H. J. (1995) Lower extremity mechanics and their effect on the lumbo-sacral junction. *Spine*, **9**, 389–405.

Daum, W. J. (1995) The sacroiliac joint: an under-appreciated pain generator. *American Journal of Orthopedics*, **24**, 475–478.

Dietz, V. (1993) Gating of reflexes in ankle muscles during human stance and gait. *Progress in Brain Research*, **97**, 181–188.

Dietz, V., Gollhofer, A., Kleiber, M. and Trippel, M. (1992) Regulation of bipedal stance: dependency on 'load' receptors. *Experimental Brain Research*, **89**, 229–231.

Dontigny, R. L. (1995) Functional biomechanics and management of pathomechanics of the sacroiliac joints. *Spine*, **9**, 491–508.

Dorman, T. A. (1995) Elastic energy in the pelvis. *Spine*, **9**, 365–379.

Dorman, T. A. and Vleeming, A. (1995) Self-locking of the sacroiliac articulation. *Spine*, **9**, 407–418.

Dye, S. F. (1996) The knee as a biologic transmission with an envelope of function: a theory. *Clinical Orthopaedics and Related Research*, **325**, 10–18.

Eckhoff, D. G. (1994) Effect of limb malrotation on malalignment and osteoarthritis. *Orthopedic Clinics of North America*, **25**, 405–414.

Eckhoff, D. G., Kramer, R. C., Alongi, C. A. and Van Gerven, D. P. (1994) Femoral anteversion and arthritis of the knee. *Journal of Pediatric Orthopedics*, **14**, 608–610.

Ekberg, O., Sjoberg, S. and Westlin, N. (1996) Sports-related groin pain: evaluation with MR imaging. *European Radiology*, **6**, 52–55.

Fithian, D. C., Kelly, M. A. and Mow, V. C. (1990) Material properties and structure–function relationships in the menisci. *Clinical Orthopaedics and Related Research*, **252**, 19–31.

Friberg, O. (1991) Instability in spondylolisthesis. *Orthopedics*, **14**, 463–465.

Frost, H. M. (1997) Biomechanical control of knee alignment: some insights from a new paradigm. *Clinical Orthopaedics and Related Research*, **335**, 335–342.

Fryette (1954) *Principles of Osteopathic Technique*, American Academy of Osteopathy, Newark, NJ.

Gerlach, U. J. and Lierse, W. (1992) Functional construction of the sacroiliac ligamentous apparatus. *Acta Anatomica*, **144**, 97–102.

Gerow, G., Matthews, B., Jahn, W. and Gerow, R. (1993) Compartment syndrome and shin splints of the lower leg. *Journal of Manipulative and Physiological Therapeutics*, **16**, 245–252.

Hanson, P. and Sonesson, B. (1994) The anatomy of the iliolumbar ligament. *Archives of Physical Medicine and Rehabilitation*, **75**,1245–1246.

Hirokawa, S. (1991) Three-dimensional mathematical model analysis of the patellofemoral joint. *Journal of Biomechanics*, **24**, 659–671.

Hirokawa, S. (1993) Biomechanics of the knee joint: a critical review. *Critical Reviews of Biomedical Engineering*, **21**, 79–135.

Inman, V. T., Ralston, H. J. and Todd, F. (1981) *Human Walking*, Williams & Wilkins, Baltimore, MD, pp. 22–117.

Kapandji, I. A. (1974) *The Physiology of the Joints*, 2nd edn, Churchill Livingstone, New York.

Kibler, W. B., Goldberg, C. and Chandler, T. J. (1991) Functional biomechanical deficits in running athletes with plantar fasciitis. *American Journal of Sports Medicine*, **19**, 66–71.

Kissling, R. O. and Jacob, H. A. (1996) The mobility of the sacroiliac joint in healthy subjects. *Bulletin/Hospital for Joint Diseases*, **54**, 158–164.

Kitaoka, H. B., Lundberg, A., Luo, Z. P. and An, K. N. (1995) Kinematics of the normal arch of the foot and ankle under physiologic loading. *Foot and Ankle International*, **16**, 492–499.

Kotwick, J. E. (1982) Biomechanics of the foot and ankle. *Clinics in Sports Medicine*, **1**,19–34.

Kuchera, W. A. and Kuchera, M. L. (1992) *Osteopathic Principles in Practice*, 2nd edn, Kirksville College of Osteopathy, Kirksville, MO.

Kuo, A. D. and Zajac, F. E. (1993) Human standing posture: multi-joint movement strategies based on biomechanical constraints. *Progress in Brain Research*, **97**, 349–358.

Larson, W. J. (1993) *Human Embryology*, Churchill Livingstone, New York.

Lederman, E. (1997) *Fundamentals of Manual Therapy: Physiology, Neurology and Psychology*, Churchill Livingstone, Edinburgh.

Lehmann, J. F. (1993) Push-off and propulsion of the body in normal and abnormal gait. Correction by ankle–foot orthoses. *Clinical Orthopaedics and Related Research*, **288**, 97–108.

Leong, J. C., Luk, K. D., Chow, D. H. and Woo, C. W. (1987) The biomechanical functions of the ilio-lumbar ligament in maintaining stability of the lumbo-sacral junction. *Spine*, **12**, 669–674.

Lepers, R. and Breniere, Y. (1995) The role of anticipatory postural adjustments and gravity in gait initiation. *Experimental Brain Research*, **107**, 118–124.

Levin, S. M. (1995) The sacrum in three dimensional space. *Spine*, **9**, 381–388.

Loren, G. J. and Lieber, R. L. (1995) Tendon biomechanical properties enhance human wrist muscle specialization. *Journal of Biomechanics*, **28**, 791–799.

Maclennan, A. H. and Maclennan, S. C. (1997) Symptom-giving pelvic girdle relaxation of pregnancy, postnatal pelvic joint syndrome and developmental dysplasia of the hip. *Acta Obstetrica et Gynaecologica Scandinavica*, **76**, 760–764.

Martorell, J. M. (1981) Hallux disorder and metatarsal alignment. *Clinical Orthopaedics and Related Research*, **157**, 14–20.

Mens, J. M., Vleeming, A., Stoeckart, R. *et al.* (1996) Understanding peripartum pelvic pain. Implications of a patient survey. *Spine*, **21**, 1363–1369.

Milan, K. R. (1994) Injury in ballet: a review of relevant topics for the physical therapist. *Journal of Orthopaedic and Sports Physical Therapy*, **19**, 121–129.

Miller, M. D., Johnson, D. L., Harner, C. D. and Fu, F. H. (1993) Posterior cruciate ligament injuries. *Orthopaedic Review*, **22**, 1201–1210.

Mitchell, F. L. (1965) Structural pelvic function. *Academy of Applied Osteopathy Year Book*, **2**, 178–199.

Mitchell, F. L. and Mitchell, P. (1995) *The Muscle Energy Manual*, MET Press, East Lansing, MI.

Noyes, F. R., Schipplein, O. D., Andriacchi, T. P. *et al.* (1992) The anterior cruciate ligament-deficient knee with varus alignment. An analysis of gait adaptations and dynamic joint loadings. *American Journal of Sports Medicine*, **20**, 707–716.

Oatis, C. A. (1988) Biomechanics of the foot and ankle under static conditions. *Physical Therapy*, **68**, 1815–1821.

Palastanga, N., Field, D. and Soames, R. (1994) *Anatomy and Human Movement*, 2nd edn, Butterworth-Heinemann, Oxford.

Perry, J. (1983) Anatomy and biomechanics of the hindfoot. *Clinical Orthopaedics and Related Research*, **177**, 9–15.

Pinar, H., Akseki, D., Karaoglan, O. and Genc, I. (1994) Kinematic and dynamic axial computed tomography of the patello-femoral joint in patients with anterior knee pain. *Knee Surgery, Sports Traumatology, Arthroscopy*, **2**, 170–173.

Prilutsky, B. I. and Zatsiorsky, V. M. (1994) Tendon action of two-joint muscles: transfer of mechanical energy between joints during jumping, landing, and running. *Journal of Biomechanics*, **27**, 25–34.

Proby, J. (1930) *Mackinnon Technique*. Privately published.

Putz, R. and Muller-Gerbl, M. (1992) [Anatomic characteristics of the pelvic girdle]. *Unfallchirurg*, **95**, 164–167.

Rodgers, M. M. (1988) Dynamic biomechanics of the normal foot and ankle during walking and running. *Physical Therapy*, **68**, 1822–1830.

Sarrafian, S. K. (1993) Biomechanics of the subtalar joint complex. *Clinical Orthopaedics and Related Research*, **290**, 17–26.

Sgambati, E., Stecco, A., Capaccioli, L. and Brizzi, E. (1996) Morphometric evaluation of the symphysis pubis joint. *Italian Journal of Anatomy and Embryology*, **101**, 195–201.

Snijders, C. J., Vleeming, A., Stoeckart, R. *et al.* (1995a) Biomechanical modeling of sacroiliac joint stability in different positions. *Spine*, **9**, 419–432.

Snijders, C. J., Slagter, A. H., Van Strik, R. *et al.* (1995b) Why leg crossing? The influence of common postures on abdominal muscle activity. *Spine*, **20**, 1989–1993.

Takayama, A. (1990) [Stress analysis and movement in sacroiliac joints]. *Nippon Ika Daigaku Zasshi – Journal of the Nippon Medical School*, **57**, 476–485.

Van Ingen Schenau, G. J., Boots, P. J., de Groot, G. *et al.* (1992) The constrained control of force and position in multi-joint movements. *Neuroscience*, **46**, 197–207.

Veltri, D. M., Deng, X. H., Torzilli, P. A. *et al.* (1995) The role of the cruciate and posterolateral ligaments in stability of the knee. A biomechanical study. *American Journal of Sports Medicine*, **23**, 436–443.

Veltri, D. M., Deng, X. H., Torzilli, P. A. *et al.* (1996) The role of the popliteofibular ligament in stability of the human knee. A biomechanical study. *American Journal of Sports Medicine*, **24**, 19–27.

Vleeming, A., Snijders, C. J., Stoeckart, R. and Mens, J. M. (1995a) A new light on back pain: the self-locking mechanism of the sacro-iliacs and its implication for sitting, standing and walking. In: *Second World Interdisciplinary Congress on Low Back Pain, San Diego, CA*, pp. 149–168.

Vleeming, A., Stam, H. J. and Stoeckart, R. (1995b) Integration of the spine and legs: influence of hamstring tension on lumbo-pelvic rhythm. In: *The Integrated Function of the Lumbar Spine and Sacro-iliac Joints*, ECO, Rotterdam, pp. 111–121.

Vleeming, A., Pool-Goudzwaard, A. L., Hammu-doghlu, D. *et al.* (1996) The function of the long dorsal sacroiliac ligament: its implication for understanding low back pain. *Spine*, **21**, 556–562.

Vukicevic, S., Marusic, A., Stavljenic, A. *et al.* (1991) Holographic analysis of the human pelvis. *Spine*, **16**, 209–214.

Walker, J. M. (1992) The sacroiliac joint: a critical review. *Physical Therapy*, **72**, 903–916.

Wang, Q., Whittle, M., Cunningham, J. and Kenwright, J. (1996) Fibula and its ligaments in load transmission and ankle joint stability. *Clinical Orthopaedics and Related Research*, **330**, 261–270.

Wilder, D. G., Pope, M. H. and Frymoyer, J. W. (1980) The functional topography of the sacroiliac joint. *Spine*, **5**, 575–579.

Willard, F. H. (1995) The anatomy of the lumbosacral connection. *Spine*, **9**, 333–355.

Woo, S. L., Livesay, G. A. and Engle, C. (1992) Biomechanics of the anterior cruciate ligament. ACL structure and role in knee function. *Orthopaedic Review*, **21**, 835–842.

Wood, KB., Schendel, M. J., Olgilvi, J. W. *et al.* (1996) Effects of sacral and iliac instrumentation on strains in the pelvis: a biomechanical study. *Spine*, **21**, 1185–1191.

Xenos, J. S., Hopkinson, W. J., Mulligan, M. E. *et al.* (1995) The tibiofibular syndesmosis. Evaluation of the ligamentous structures, methods of fixation, and radiographic assessment. *Journal of Bone and Joint Surgery (American Volume)*, **77**, 847–856.

8 COMPARISONS AND CONTRASTS IN BIOMECHANICAL MODELS: THE UPPER LIMB AND THORAX

IN THIS CHAPTER:

- Upper limb coordination with trunk/pelvis–lower limb function
- Neural mechanisms coordinating upper and lower limb activity
- Neural mechanisms within the upper limb
- The shoulder girdle
- The role of fascia in upper limb mechanics
- The elbow, forearm and wrist
- Rib cage mechanics
- General thoracic cage movement
- The diaphragm
- The stomatognathic system (including the anterior throat, hyoid and mandible)

The upper limb, as well as functioning as a relatively independent structure, is associated with trunk and lower limb-pelvis function. The upper limb is connected to the axial skeleton via the shoulder girdle, which is carefully arranged to allow coordinated function with the rest of the body. The shoulder girdle works as a whole to ensure that scapula position is orientated in an optimal way to accommodate various activities of the upper limb. Through the shoulder girdle, there are many interactions between the upper limb and thorax, and between it and the cervical spine, neck and jaw.

Many problems within the upper limbs come about as a result of quite distant problems, and even many wrist and hand strains, injuries and problems can benefit from treatment throughout the body. This may seem strange but, as the chapter unfolds, the reasons for this should become apparent.

We will look briefly at most of the links (neural and mechanical) that the upper limb has with the rest of the body, and we will start by considering its relations with the lower limb and pelvis.

UPPER LIMB COORDINATION WITH TRUNK/PELVIS–LOWER LIMB FUNCTION

Upper limb activity is coordinated with that of the lower limb and pelvis. This occurs in many movements, particularly walking and running. During gait, as the legs swing, the pelvis moves and the centre of mass of the body is shifted. This is counterbalanced by trunk torsion and movement (Van Emmerik and Wagenaar, 1996) and swinging of the upper limbs (which occurs contralaterally with respect to the legs). For this counterbalancing to be efficient, there needs to be a 'whole-body' strategy (MacKinnon and Winter, 1993) within neural control systems. These strategies include the role of the spine, and are adjusted by feedback from proprioceptors throughout the body. To appreciate these strategies, two components must be considered:

- force transference mechanisms between the upper and lower limb girdles;
- the neural coordination of muscle activity.

Force transference mechanisms

In a previous chapter we discussed the role of connective tissues (fascial structures) in aiding muscular activity and in posture. By using various fascial structures, the activity within the limb and trunk muscles can be made more efficient by passing force into the fascial system, which it stores as elastic energy. This means that the inherent recoil properties of these 'elastic tissues' can help propel movement and act as a break to

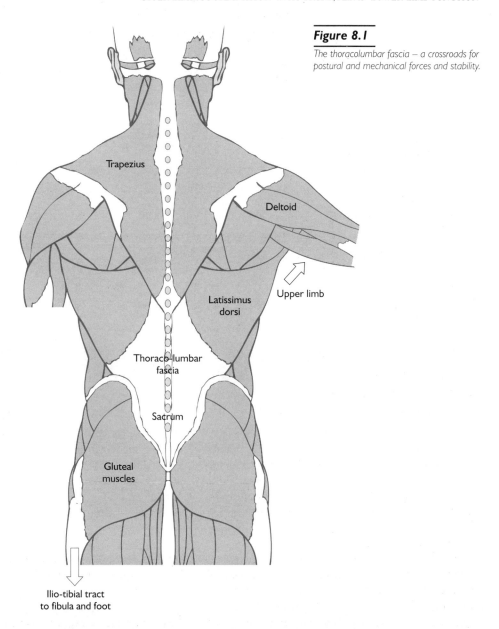

Figure 8.1

The thoracolumbar fascia – a crossroads for postural and mechanical forces and stability.

momentum, thus improving muscular efficiency and limiting strain.

Force transference between the upper and lower limbs is mediated through the thoracolumbar fascia. This is a large, diamond-shaped structure that connects the upper limb to the lower limb. Muscles that are normally described as hip, pelvic and leg muscles will interact with so-called arm and spinal muscles via the thoracolumbar fascia. This arrangement allows for effective load transfer between the spine, pelvis, legs and arms (Vleeming *et al.*, 1995). All muscles attaching to the thoracolumbar fascia should be thought of as forming an integrated system of leverages. The thoracolumbar fascia and muscles relating to it are shown in Figure 8.1.

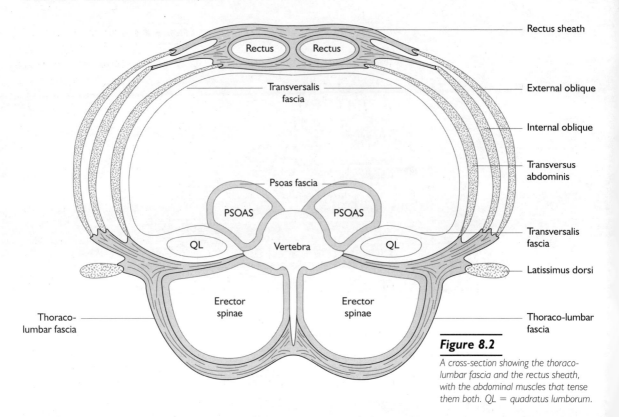

Figure 8.2

A cross-section showing the thoraco-lumbar fascia and the rectus sheath, with the abdominal muscles that tense them both. QL = quadratus lumborum.

The important inter-relation between the pelvic, lower limb and upper limb muscles means that there is a dynamic relation between efficient function of the lower and upper limbs, and provides a mechanism whereby dysfunction in one limb may be directly influential on another (especially its contralateral/superior–inferior opposite limb).

The integrity of the thoracolumbar fascia, and hence its ability to act as a load transfer system, depends in part upon the activity of the abdominal muscles. The abdominal muscles help to tense the thoracolumbar fascia (and also the rectus sheath), and this tension helps the fascia to dissipate force (Adams and Dolan, 1995). The tension in the thoracolumbar fascia induced through abdominal muscle action also enables the thoracolumbar fascia to provide a stable insertion point for many muscles involved with locomotion and the control of posture (e.g. erector spinae, the glutei and latissimus dorsi). The rectus sheath and abdom-inal muscles that tense the thoracolumbar fascia are shown in Figure 8.2. Through this link, poor abdominal muscle activity and tone may lead to inefficient action of the thoracolumbar fascia, and hence contribute to mechanical disturbance in the upper and lower limbs and the spine.

Fascial and tendinous action in posture

As introduced earlier, the above structures act as a mechanism for supporting the body during posture using the least muscular energy. For example, tension in the thoracolumbar fascia acts through the glutei muscles to the iliotibial tract, which engages the fibula. This then provides tension in the intraosseous membrane between the fibula and the tibia, forming an absorptive mechanism allowing the tibiotalar joint a degree of 'non-muscular' flexibility. These inferior connections (through the fibular and intraosseous membrane and associated muscles) blend with the plantar fascia. In this way they help to absorb weight-bearing forces and sway-motion forces during static and dynamic posture.

The thoracolumbar fascia also helps transfer the weight-bearing forces through the pelvis, where it helps to engage the ligamentous arrangement of the sacroiliac joints (especially the sacrotuberous ligaments and the fascial/ligamentous annular ring, which travels from the sacrotuberous ligaments to the ischial tuberosities and along the inferior pubic rami to the symphysis pubis). This provides an effective system for absorbing forces that would tend to nutate the sacrum (Chapter 7). Any inclination to anterior tipping of the pelvis is also offset by tension in the rectus sheath. Remember that both the rectus sheath and the thoracolumbar fascia act in concert through the action of transversus abdominis. This enables the thoracolumbar fascia to support the spine posteriorly up to the lower thoracic area, where the posterior convexity of the thoracic spine helps to maintain static posture with minimal effort. In the cervical region, the ligamentum nuchae helps to support the cervical column and the weight of the head.

Anterior support of the head and neck region is provided by the deep cervical fascia, which runs from the base of the skull along the front of the cervical column, over the anterior surface of the cervical muscles (longissimus colli and scalenes, for example) and inserts into the anterior longitudinal ligament of the spine. This layer of fascia is called the prevertebral fascia and supports the action of the anterior cervical muscles, especially the scalenes. The tension in the rectus sheath (which offsets pelvic torsion) is transmitted through the anterior rib cage via the sternum, and is in itself offset by the action of the scalene muscles on the upper ribs (which help to support the sternum).

If trunk and pelvic posture is correctly maintained, with the head ultimately in line with the anterior talus, the shoulder girdle becomes oriented so that the weight of the arms hangs slightly posterior to the head position. This enables the arm weight to act through the clavicle and to spread the anterior thorax, also offsetting the inferior pull by the rectus sheath.

This tension across the anterior chest reduces some of the tensile load on the prevertebral fascia in the cervical region, allowing a degree of freedom in neck motion that might not be possible if the prevertebral fascia was principally engaged in postural support. This inter-related dynamic was mentioned in Chapter 5 and illustrated in Figure 5.9. It is shown here in more detail in Figure 8.3.

Relationship to osteopathic models

The Littlejohn models of mechanics discussed whole-body posture on the basis of investigation of weight-bearing forces acting through the body (which were discussed before) and how force is dissipated through the above system of linkages. Other models look purely at the anatomical links discussed above to consider how action in one part of the body is immediately transmitted to distant parts. Either way, the influence of altered postural balance, acting through these fascial planes, leads to a discussion of commonly occurring postural imbalances, which can become manifest in a variety of symptoms.

The early models, including Littlejohn mechanics, looked at the effects of weight-bearing that was a little too posterior or anterior. When the weight-bearing changes, whole-body dynamics alter, with the effect that anterior weight-bearing leads to different areas of strain from posterior weight-bearing. Not only are strains induced in various parts of the spine and limbs but the dynamics of the body cavities are also adapted, giving certain types of visceral dysfunction. Some visceral 'conditions' are thought to be associated more with anterior weight-bearing than with posterior weight-bearing. These patterns of changes are shown in Figure 8.4.

The revisionist models that we have been discussing had, in moving away from the mechanistic complexity of Littlejohn, somehow 'mislaid' the relevance of changes in local biomechanics to whole-body posture. Subsequently, the schools that put Littlejohn aside have had to 're-formulate' a picture of whole-body mechanics based upon anatomical first principles.

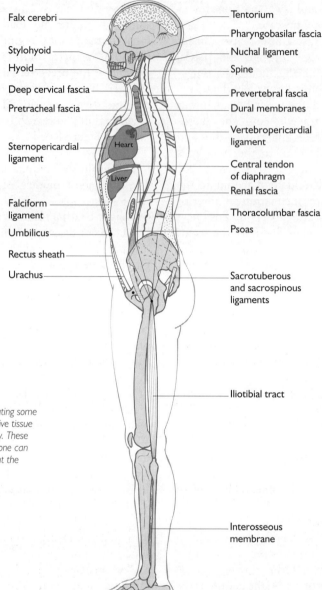

Figure 8.3

A lateral view of the body indicating some of the main fascial and connective tissue structures that support the body. These tissues are interconnected and one can observe them passing throughout the body as a continuous system.

'Revisionist osteopathic schools' and the modern orthodox study of biomechanics are now coming to a similar concept of whole-body mechanics and postural stability, through looking at how the body is arranged and how its structures can dissipate force, if the posture is well maintained. Eventually, we should all be speaking the same language!

Whole-body mechanics and upper limb function

For the purposes of this chapter, the point of the above discussion is to set the stage for the idea that the general posture of the person can be influential to shoulder girdle activity and hence upper limb function. For example, if trunk stability

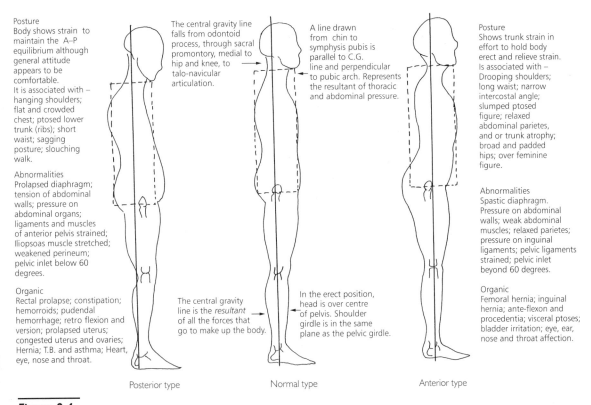

Posture
Body shows strain to maintain the A–P equilibrium although general attitude appears to be comfortable.
It is associated with – hanging shoulders; flat and crowded chest; ptosed lower trunk (ribs); short waist; sagging posture; slouching walk.

Abnormalities
Prolapsed diaphragm; tension of abdominal walls; pressure on abdominal organs; ligaments and muscles of anterior pelvis strained; Iliopsoas muscle stretched; weakened perineum; pelvic inlet below 60 degrees.

Organic
Rectal prolapse; constipation; hemorrhoids; pudendal hemorrhage; retro flexion and version; prolapsed uterus; congested uterus and ovaries; Hernia; T.B. and asthma; Heart, eye, nose and throat.

The central gravity line falls from odontoid process, through sacral promontory, medial to hip and knee, to talo-navicular articulation.

The central gravity line is the *resultant* of all the forces that go to make up the body.

A line drawn from chin to symphysis pubis is parallel to C.G. line and perpendicular to pubic arch. Represents the resultant of thoracic and abdominal pressure.

In the erect position, head is over centre of pelvis. Shoulder girdle is in the same plane as the pelvic girdle.

Posture
Shows trunk strain in effort to hold body erect and relieve strain. Is associated with – Drooping shoulders; long waist; narrow intercostal angle; slumped ptosed figure; relaxed abdominal parietes, and or trunk atrophy; broad and padded hips; over feminine figure.

Abnormalities
Spastic diaphragm. Pressure on abdominal walls; weak abdominal muscles; relaxed parietes; pressure on inguinal ligaments; pelvic ligaments strained; pelvic inlet beyond 60 degrees.

Organic
Femoral hernia; inguinal hernia; ante-flexon and procedentia; visceral ptoses; bladder irritation; eye, ear, nose and throat affection.

Posterior type   Normal type   Anterior type

Figure 8.4

Different posture types with different weight-bearing patterns. Each posture places different strain throughout the body and produces an associated range of symptoms, both somatic and visceral.

is not maintained and the centre of mass shifts slightly, the torso may be thrust forwards a little or sunk 'posteriorly' (into thoracic kyphosis). This has the effect of altering shoulder girdle orientation, giving, for example, retraction or protraction of the scapulae, respectively. This will clearly affect the muscular action of the shoulder girdle and upper limb (which will be discussed later) and influence the neural mechanisms coordinating activity within the upper limb and its motion in relation to the lower limbs and trunk (which is discussed below).

Neural mechanisms coordinating upper limb and lower limb activity

During locomotion, whole-body balance is ensured by differing recruitment strategies in all limbs and within the axial skeleton. In the frontal plane, for example, balance is ensured by the centre of mass passing medial to the supporting foot, thus creating a continual state of dynamic imbalance towards the centre plane of progression (MacKinnon and Winter, 1993). Balance of the trunk and swing leg is maintained by active hip abduction activity, while accommodating the contribution of the passive accelerational moment passing through the thoracolumbar fascia. Posture of the upper trunk is regulated by the spinal lateral flexors and provides a stable base from which shoulder girdle muscles control upper limb swing, both to counter momentum-induced changes in body mass position and to load the thoracolumbar fascia to continue locomotion in an energy-efficient manner.

So, during locomotion, different body parts move in many directions simultaneously, requiring a complex monitoring system to ensure balanced progression of movement. These motions are indicated in Figure 8.5. This diagram shows that there is a lateral sway of the pelvis and torso during forward motion; that in a frontal plane, the shoulders and hips move either towards or away from each other during different stages of gait; and that from above, the hip and pelvic girdles rotate in opposite directions.

Even going up and down stairs requires different muscle activity to maintain stability: a study noted that there were subtle differences in body mass transfer between different activities such as going up stairs and going down stairs (Zachazewski *et al.*, 1993). This implies that the overall intercoordination of body movement needs to be quite an adaptable system!

Various studies have explored where the main proprioceptors involved in such a neural control system may be found. In one, a gain control mechanism for postural reflexes that is dependent on body weight was demonstrated, which led to the hypothesis that the receptors for this mechanism are distributed along the vertical axis of the body. It was suggested that these force-dependent receptors were pressure receptors within the joints and the vertebral column (Horstmann and Dietz, 1990). This implies that the role of spinal mechanics in the proprioceptive monitoring and adjustment of upper and lower limb activity during locomotion or other activities such as arm raising/load carrying (Vernazza *et al.*, 1996b) may be important (Vernazza *et al.*, 1996a). Clinically this might imply that restriction within the spine can affect lower and upper limb function.

In another study that looked at the regulation of bipedal stance, dependency on 'load' receptors was also noted (Dietz *et al.*, 1992). According to observations, the influence of body load has to be taken into account for the neuronal control of 'upright stance', in addition to the systems known to be involved in this regulation (e.g. efferent input from vestibular canals, visual and muscle stretch receptors). It was felt that these

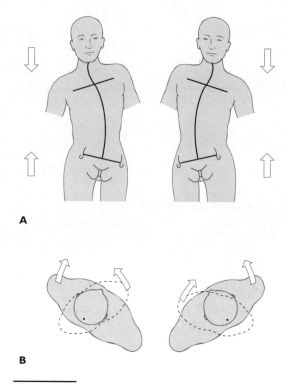

A

B

___

Figure 8.5

*Body torsion and oscillation during gait. **A.** In a frontal plane, the shoulders and hips incline towards or away from each other during different stages of gait. **B.** In a superior view, the shoulder girdle and the pelvis rotate in opposite directions. **C.** There is a lateral sway of the pelvis during forward motion.*

'newly acknowledged' afferent inputs probably arose from Golgi tendon organs (acting as load receptors activating postural reflexes) and represented a newly discovered function of these receptors in the regulation of stance and gait.

Thus injury to the tendinous structures of the lower limb may have more profound effects upon the neural control of posture and interlimb coordination than has previously been recognized.

Independent of gait, there appears to be a definite 'hip–ankle strategy' during shoulder movement (Aruin and Latash, 1995) that will help stabilize posture during arm movements. It seems that the patterning within the proximal limb muscles is fairly constant between individuals during postural adjustment, while patterning in distal muscles (which take care of fine adjustments) is more likely to vary across subjects. And, in situations where additional loads or complex postures are anticipated, the neural control unit may alter the muscle recruitment strategy, with the temporary goal of enhancing spinal stability beyond the normal requirements in order to accommodate the extra forces caused by using the arms under loaded conditions (Panjabi, 1992).

In conclusion, then, if there is any restriction of any of these parts – legs, pelvis, spine, trunk and arms – this swinging, oscillatory, intercoordinated balance, which occurs during walking and other activities, will be disturbed. This may result in distortion of any of the constituent parts, in an attempt to stabilize and correct the gait as a whole. Clinically, problems in one part of the body will thus influence the upper limbs and *vice versa*.

Having considered the relation of the upper limbs to whole-body movement and posture, it is now time to consider movement within the upper limb itself.

MOVEMENT PATTERNS WITHIN THE UPPER LIMB

Neural mechanisms within the upper limb

In general, the upper limb is different from the lower limb in that it is not always involved in weight-bearing. It is more concerned with such things as feeling, exploring, picking up objects and then moving these either away from or towards the body (movement of objects is often directed towards the face, as in eating, for example). Whether there is a degree of additional load inherent within these activities (such as picking up an object) or not, the upper limb itself is a load that needs to be stabilized at its point of contact with the axial skeleton (Brand, 1993).

Hence there is a hierarchy of control in that first the proximal limb is stabilized, then the middle portion of the limb (the elbow) and after that the wrist and hand can be orientated to finally execute the task required (as was mentioned above).

The activity in the proximal muscles (of the shoulder girdle) is coordinated closely with the action of axial muscles. During upper limb motion, the proximal articulations must first be stabilized in an appropriate orientation. This stabilized position can then form a base for progression of muscular activity (from proximal to distal) through the upper limb so that the hand and fingers are eventually properly positioned to perform the desired task. The different behaviours of proximal and distal muscles during anticipatory postural adjustments, particularly in preparation for fast arm movements (Aruin and Latash, 1995), is such that, without this proximal–axial stabilization, the more distal actions of the upper limb would be poorly controlled/ coordinated.

This has begun to be explored in relation to specific tasks of the upper limb, and in one study it was found that wrist movements were dependent upon elbow position and movements but the difference was not solely due to antagonist muscle activity – in other words, it was not simply the stretch in the extensors, for example, that altered the activity of the flexors; the difference arose on a more global level throughout the muscles of the upper limb (Virji-Babul and Cooke, 1995).

When the wrist/hand is loaded, there are feedback loops present that then help to guide the control of proximal structures in adaptation of the load. One study investigating this found that wrist muscle activation patterns and stiffness associated with stable and unstable mechanical loads were associated with clear differences in flexor muscle synergy in the presence and absence of co-contraction of other wrist/upper limb muscles (De Serres and Milner, 1991). This implies that stability of the wrist under load is maintained only through dynamic monitoring and the adaptability of contraction within the proximal muscles. The complexity of wrist movement is perhaps responsible for the quite extensive and involved interneuronal connections linking forearm and wrist muscles, which are being currently investigated (Aymard *et al.*, 1995a). Also, there seem to be different strategies

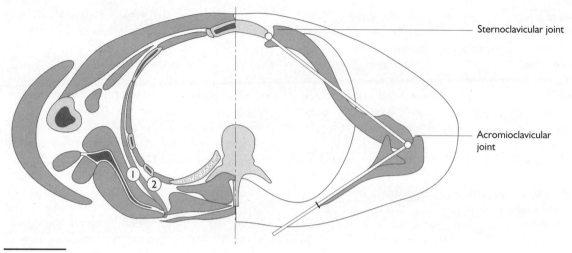

Figure 8.6

Superior view of the shoulder girdle, showing the scapulothoracic joint and the clavicular articulation. The scapulothoracic joint is 'formed' by the spaces between the scapula and the serratus anterior muscle (1) and between the chest wall and the serratus anterior muscle (2). (Redrawn from Kapandji, 1982.)

available within the forearm, as during muscle fatigue there are different reciprocal inhibitions operating from otherwise (Aymard *et al.*, 1995b).

Interlimb coordination

There are even cases where activity in one arm can influence the other, through mechanisms of reciprocal innervation that operate on a bilateral basis. (This realization arose from a case study of writer's cramp. Reciprocal innervation that this induced within the affected limb acted within not only that limb but also the asymptomatic one; Aruin and Latash, 1995.)

Clinically, the above means that dysfunction in the proximal upper limb affects activity in the distal portion. When symptoms arise in the distal limb, it is often as a result of restriction proximally.

Exploring the biomechanical relations within the shoulder girdle and upper limb will expand the picture of inter-relatedness that is reflected in the neural control of upper limb activity.

The shoulder girdle

From the above discussion (and the preceding one concerning the relations between the upper and lower limbs during gait) it is clear that the suspensory apparatus of the upper limb to the axial portion of the body must be able to be co-ordinated so that it moves in concert with the rest of the body. The 'articular' structures of the upper limb in this context are the scapulothoracic joint and the clavicular articulations (the sterno-clavicular and acromioclavicular joints). These joints are shown in Figure 8.6.

The shoulder girdle literally suspends the upper limb off the axial skeleton, and the points of attachment (through the joints mentioned above) and a variety of muscles, including trapezius, form a 'cape-like' arrangement of soft tissues that sits over the axial skeleton and rib cage, giving it an insertion that runs from the occiput to the iliac crest (via the thoracolumbar fascia). This implies that movement of the spine and thorax, for example, are particularly important for the 'base stability' of the upper limb.

The shoulder girdle is a very large structure, which is not easily appreciated unless one compares it with the body without its shoulder 'cape'. The difference in outline between the axial skeleton and the shoulder girdle shown in Figure 8.7 gives some impression of the number and size of the muscles involved with upper limb motion.

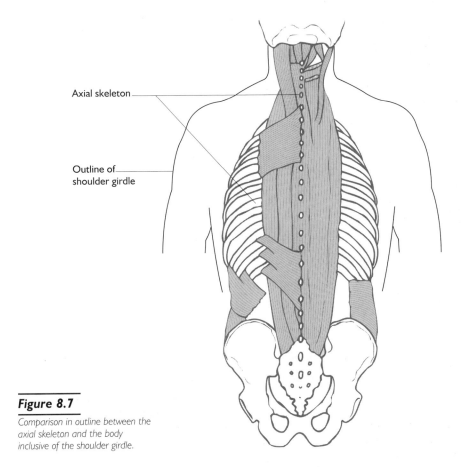

Axial skeleton

Outline of
shoulder girdle

Figure 8.7

*Comparison in outline between the
axial skeleton and the body
inclusive of the shoulder girdle.*

Muscles involved in proximal stability

The orientation of the upper limb itself is
governed by the position of the glenoid of the
scapula. This is governed by the scapulothoracic
joint and the clavicular attachments (Nicholson
et al., 1996). The muscles around the shoulder
girdle and the rotator cuff muscles of the
humerus are like a series of guy-ropes. These
must be evenly tensioned and balanced so that
the motion of the humeral head is always contained within the glenoid labrum (Soslowsky *et
al.*, 1997; Blasier *et al.*, 1997; Malicky *et al.*,
1996), although muscle activity is not so important for the glenohumoral joint at rest
(Matsen *et al.*, 1991). The importance of the
scapulothoracic joint is sometimes overlooked,
but it is vital for smooth function of the upper
limb as a whole (Culham and Peat, 1993).

Clinically, any altered tension or activity in
any of these muscles will lead to an altered
orientation of the glenoid, and hence humerus,
and this will have implications for the biomechanics of the glenohumoral joint and, subsequently, the rest of the upper limb (Warner *et al.*,
1996). Evaluation of shoulder, elbow, wrist and
hand pain or dysfunction therefore requires a
careful analysis and comparison of tension in all
of these muscles. The varied directions of 'pull'
ono the shoulder girdle by various muscles are
indicated in Figure 8.8.

Most osteopaths approach the management of
upper limb problems (such as 'tennis/golfer's
elbow', repetitive strain injury of the wrist and
some carpal tunnel problems) from the spine and
thorax first and then out into the upper limb
itself: if the humerus is not orientated properly,

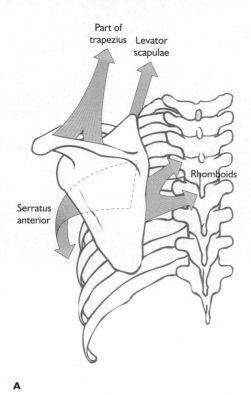

A

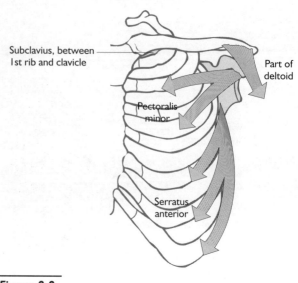

Figure 8.8

*Two views of the shoulder girdle (**A**, posterior; **B**, anterior), indicating the direction of pull of some of its muscles. Collectively, the muscles of the shoulder can align the glenoid in a number of ways. However, uneven muscular tension can lead to an adverse orientation of the glenoid.*

then the biomechanics of the rest of the arm cannot be optimal. Also, general body posture, and workplace ergonomic factors (Stock, 1991), can cause a shift in position of the shoulder girdle and therefore the upper limb. This shift in position can be relevant for many upper limb problems from the shoulder to the wrist.

Because of all of the above, clinical evaluation of the shoulder and its problems must include areas that are distant to the shoulder (Kibler, 1995).

The movements within the scapulothoracic joint are also influenced by the clavicular mechanics, which we will discuss below.

The clavicle

The clavicle is the only bony point of contact between the upper limb and the rest of the body. Its articulations, especially the sternoclavicular joint, are pivotal for efficient upper limb orientation and subsequent function (Soslowsky *et al.*, 1996). Clavicular mechanics are illustrated in Figure 8.9.

Torsions affecting the clavicle

Many osteopathic texts describe the most common subluxations of the clavicle as occurring at its medial end, in relation to sternoclavicular joint mechanics. Such subluxations can be:

- impaction medially;
- subluxation posteriorly (into the body).

Treatment of many cervicothoracic and upper limb problems can be aided by exploration and resolution of any clavicular restrictions or torsions.

The glenohumoral joint

This is a highly mobile joint (which can be relatively unstable; Soslowsky *et al.*, 1992) and, for reasons mentioned above and illustrated below, it is very vulnerable to damage (Neviaser, 1983).

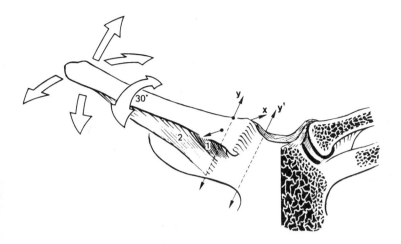

Figure 8.9

The movements of the clavicle at the sternoclavicular joint. When all the movements indicated by the arrows are combined, the medial end of the clavicle can swivel in a circular manner, pivoting around the fixed point of the subclavius muscle (indicated by the figures 1 and 2). (Amended with the permission of Churchill Livingstone from The Physiology of Joints, Vol. 1, Kapandji, 1974.)

Torsions affecting the glenohumoral joint and the rotator cuff muscles, including biceps tendinitis

These torsions have already been introduced. To reinforce the concepts discussed, some additional information may be useful. There is evidence that the gliding tendons of supraspinatus and biceps brachii show a normal functional adaptation in structure at frictional sites. Fibrocartilage is laid down and there is avascular tissue in the affected areas (Tillmann and Koch, 1995). When the shoulder girdle and glenohumoral joint are under tension, this adaptation of tendon structure may be more widespread, especially in conditions of unphysiological strain to the tendon, such as in some sports (McCann and Bigliani, 1994). This is thought to provide a focus point for inflammation, weakness and even rupture of the tendon involved.

The role of fascia in upper limb mechanics

As in our discussions of the rest of the body and the lower limbs, fascial and tendinous structures have an important role in upper limb function. This is particularly so with respect to loads carried in the hands and arms. There are various muscles that can help to stabilize arm motion during load carrying (Bigliani *et al.*, 1996), depending on the relative position of the arm with respect to the body. However, two are especially important, as their tendons are uniquely placed to help transfer load from the arm through into the scapulae and hence into the

main fascial load-bearing structures of the trunk. Trunk and thoracic spine stability is maintained through the mechanisms discussed before, allowing a firm base for the action of the scapulothoracic muscles (including trapezius and rhomboids) to stabilize scapular action.

The insertion of the long head of biceps and triceps on to the superior and inferior glenoid tubercles, respectively, allow load from the upper limb to be passed through to the scapula, so 'bypassing' the glenohumoral joint itself. The biceps brachii muscle also inserts into the posterior part of the radial tuberosity and into the bicipital aponeurosis. This is a fascial structure that passes around the upper forearm and inserts into the deep fascia of the forearm. Hence loads from the arm are supported by fascial structures within the forearm and pass through to the scapulae, via the biceps and triceps tendons, and into the trunk.

Clinical relevance

Any damage to these fascial structures or tendons (such as discussed above) could affect load transference within the upper limb, requiring greater muscular energy to achieve the same outcomes (in load-carrying situations). This leads to muscular fatigue, strain and injury. As stated, earlier, strain to the tendinous structures of the triceps and biceps could be limited by maintaining efficient whole-body posture and locomotor balance.

In particular, if the load transference mechanisms are inefficient, then greater strain will be placed at the level of the glenohumoral joint, requiring the rotator cuff muscles to work much harder to maintain the anatomical relationship of the head of the humerus to the glenoid labrum and cavity. Many rotator cuff problems could be seen as a failure of the load transference mechanisms.

Torsions affecting the elbow, forearm and wrist
The head of the radius is not as stable as the head of the fibula (its comparable lower limb structure) and the forces acting upon it through the action of the biceps brachii muscle mean that the superior radioulnar joint can become unstable. The radius and ulna move around each other, and the radius can move longitudinally to create a piston-like action (Linscheid, 1992). The action of biceps can often lead to an external rotation of the radius, leading to a relative posterior subluxation of the radial head. This places strain on the annular ligament, resulting in pain and instability. There are also a variety of muscle strains possible with different joint movements in different ranges and with different loads (Murray et al., 1995).

Any restriction in radial mobility will affect forearm mechanics (Kauer, 1992), which, especially when coupled with humeral torsion (as discussed above), may mean that both hand and forearm mechanics are vulnerable to compromise.

This often manifests itself in muscular problems (ischaemia, contracture and pain), as a result of their increased action to compensate for poorer articular mechanics. Lateral epicondylitis ('tennis elbow') is a good example of what can follow on from this tension.

Radial mechanics, the dynamics of the intraosseous membrane and the orientation of the radiocarpal (wrist) joint can affect carpal, metacarpal and digital orientation, and musculotendinous structures relating to the hand and fingers (Kauer and de Lange, 1987; Cobb et al., 1993). Many pain presentations, such as writer's cramp, and repetitive strain injuries of the wrist,

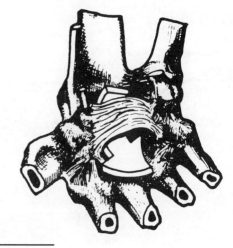

Figure 8.10
The carpal tunnel. The arrow indicates the passage of vascular, tendinous and neural structures through the tunnel. (Amended with the permission of Churchill Livingstone from The Physiology of Joints, Vol. 1, Kapandji, 1974.)

may be related to this mechanism. Workplace and sporting ergonomic factors (Rettig and Patel, 1995) such as keyboard positioning or tennis racket thickness/weight, and weight-bearing stresses, may also play a role (Schroer et al., 1996).

Dysfunction that arises at, or accumulates at the level of the wrist often constricts the carpal tunnel (Figure 8.10), through which all important vascular and nervous structures pass from the arm into the hand, although there are several mechanisms through which carpal tunnel syndrome can arise. Compression of these vascular and nervous structures can be a consequence of altered carpal tunnel mechanics due to local distortion only or arising as a result of upper limb torsion patterns (Skandalakis et al., 1992; Chen, 1995).

The carpus
This mechanism, consisting of two rows of intricately fitting bones, moves in quite a complex way (Kauer, 1986) and indeed, during different hand or forearm movements, each row of bones within the carpus can move with different strategies. The bones seem to move in a helical/spiral

Figure 8.11

The movements of the carpal bones in adduction and abduction of the wrist. The arrows indicate that a variety of movements of the individual carpal bones occur in different directions during these actions. (Amended with the permission of Churchill Livingstone from The Physiology of Joints, *Vol. 1, Kapandji, 1974.)*

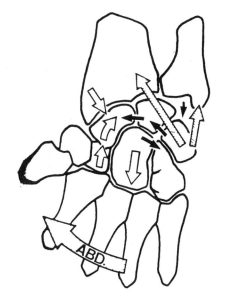
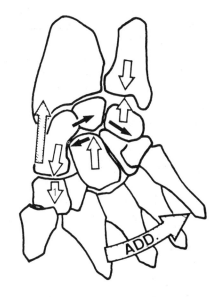

orientation with either flexion/extension or lateral deviation of the hand in relation to the forearm (Savelberg *et al.*, 1991, 1993). This means that there are many possibilities for minor but significant combinations of subluxation within the carpal arrangement, which could be relevant for many hand and forearm pain presentations. It may also mean that carpal restrictions could be highly relevant for limitations/adaptations in forearm movement dynamics. This is especially so if the intraosseous membrane becomes affected (Werner and An, 1994). The complex movements of the carpus are indicated in Figure 8.11, which shows the movements occurring during adduction and abduction of the wrist.

THE THORAX

Having looked in detail at the upper limb, it is now time to explore the thorax, which has so many connections with the upper limb. This is a very interesting area mechanically as, like the pelvis, it has to perform several different functions.

The thorax has a role to play in weight-bearing, as was discussed earlier in the section on fascial and tendinous action in posture. Any problems in whole-body posture may limit thoracic cage elasticity and compliance, and hence have an effect on other functions of the thoracic cage, such as respiration.

Osteopathic models of rib cage mechanics

Rib movements are classically described as being like those of a bucket handle and pump handle, relating to the orientation of the rib movement against the spinal column. Classically, the ribs move upwards in inspiration and downwards in expiration. These rib movements are shown in Figure 8.12.

Such rib movements gave rise to the idea that, when restricted, the ribs could become fixed, either in inspiration or expiration (the anterior ends of the ribs being held superiorly or inferiorly, respectively, and the posterior section of the ribs – the angles – being held inferiorly in inspiration and superiorly in expiration). There are many manipulative techniques that are designed to correct these malalignments, using thrust techniques or muscle energy techniques, for example. However, models considering rib movement have had to be expanded as knowledge of whole-rib cage mechanics has increased, alongside a greater understanding of the physiological components of rib cage movement.

Figure 8.12

Movement of the ribs at the costovertebral joints. The pictures show the amount of displacement that occurs along the length of the rib during inspiration and expiration movements. (Reproduced with the permission of Churchill Livingstone from The Physiology of Joints, Vol. 3, Kapandji, 1974.)

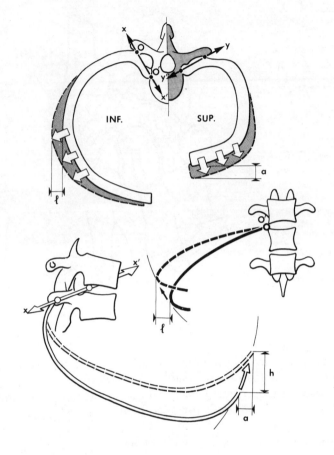

Rib movement

Rib movement has for a long time been considered in relation to the various muscle actions upon the ribs. For many years the intercostals were attributed with a very complex biomechanical effect, such that the internal intercostals were considered as expiratory muscles and the external intercostals inspiratory muscles (Kapandji, 1974). The way in which the intercostals organize these actions is now understood to be very complex (Epstein, 1994; Loring and Woodbridge, 1991) and these actions relate to air movement and also fluid movement within the thoracic cavity (De Troyer and Estenne, 1988). It appears that during inspiration and expiration there are cascades of action within the intercostal muscles, which start at one end of the rib cage and progress to the other to produce the required changes in rib cage shape. During inspiration the external intercostals activate segmentally from superior to inferior, and during (forced) expiration the intraosseous internal intercostal muscles activate segmentally from inferior to superior (De Troyer and Estenne, 1988).

This is interesting as it means that, during inspiration, the upper ribs must first be stabilized (for example, by the scalenes – De Troyer *et al.*, 1994) so that the ribs below can be moved by progressive intercostal contraction, which moves in an inferior wave. Then, during expiration, the inferior ribs must be stabilized (by quadratus lumborum and the arcuate ligaments, for example, which will be discussed below with the diaphragm) before a wave of muscle action can move the ribs above, by passing in a superior direction.

Note: The muscles and structures that stabilize the upper and lower ribs are also important, as any restriction that affects their movement might disturb the reflex control of these respiratory waves and so affect rib cage function, especially when one appreciates that the costovertebral joints are considered to have joint receptors that are capable of influencing inspiratory intercostal activity (De Troyer, 1997).

Clinically, restrictions and altered tension/movement patterns in any of these structures will disturb the normal 'flow' of respiration and can be related to respiratory system symptoms and pain in the musculoskeletal components of the thorax.

The changing shape of the thoracic cavity relates to physiological function

The physiological function of the thoracic cavity depends upon it being deformed by muscle action to create a difference in pressures, which then influences gaseous and fluid movement into and out of the thoracic organs. Different muscles change the shape of the thoracic cavity in different ways. Muscles at the side of the rib cage produce changes in the anteroposterior diameter, whereas muscles at the front and back of the rib cage cause changes in the transverse diameter (Loring, 1992). The diaphragm, which has a role in chest wall mechanics (Lichtenstein et al., 1992), will be discussed below. The changing shape of the thorax is also relevant to speech, and the intercostal muscles are involved in the control of appropriate airflow over the glottis to effect speech (Estenne et al., 1990; Zocchi et al., 1990).

Mechanical interface between the ribs and the thoracic organs

The parietal pleura and the fibrous pericardium play an interesting role between the skeletal components of the thorax and the thoracic organs. As the external components are moved, so the parietal pleura and fibrous pericardium are engaged. This influences thoracic organ function. In particular, when the parietal pleural layer is engaged, it passes force through the pleural fluid to the visceral pleura around the lung and causes the lung to expand by an induction of a relatively negative pressure between the two layers of pleura (Lai-Fook and Rodarte, 1991). Restriction of movement in sections of the rib cage and stiffness in parts of the parietal pleura may lead to unequal expansion of the lung tissue, with subsequent implications for respiratory function and efficiency.

The external rib cage (the bony and muscular components) must therefore be compliant in order to ensure an effective respiratory function. In other words, the rib cage must be elastic so that it can be deformed to change the shape of the thorax, and the lungs and pleural layers must be elastic enough to allow these changes in shape and volume (Stamenovic et al., 1990; Tucker and Jenkins, 1996). (Note: The term 'elastic' is equivalent to 'compliant'.)

Mechanical characteristics of the respiratory system

The mechanical characteristics of the respiratory system are relevant elements in the evaluation of lung function since any change in them is a prompt sign of impending problems (Avanzolini et al., 1995). The mechanical properties of the lung are important determinants of its efficiency as a gas-exchanging organ. Under normal circumstances the airways should offer very little mechanical impedance to airflow, allowing for almost effortless and uniform distribution of fresh gas throughout the lung (Bates, 1991). Local changes in lung tissue compliance may have an effect on air flow throughout the lung (Similowski and Bates, 1991), creating areas of turbulence where some areas of the lung do not expand at the same rate or experience the same mixing of gaseous elements as others (Kamm, 1995). Indeed inhomogeneity of gas distribution within the lungs is becoming increasingly recognized. The effects of this over time may be that this altered flow, creating different locally acting pressures on the lung tissue, may cause it to deform and adapt to that pressure. Its local compliance may change (become reduced where there is less airflow).

Generally, respiratory diseases are held to be responsible for changes in airway resistance that produce the inhomogeneity mentioned above. However, as the chest wall mechanics and compliance are so intimately related to lung compliance and airflow, it seems reasonable to question whether any resistance to movement in the somatic chest wall might not have a compromising effect upon lung compliance and airflow. This might be an important consideration if one accepts the premise that airway disease affects lung compliance, which leads to visceral and parietal irritation through the inflammation that accompanies these disorders (Dechman *et al.*, 1993; Ingram, 1990; Sahn, 1990). The effect of the inflammation on the pleura is to reduce its compliance and render it less elastic. In this state, the parietal pleura will not permit the external rib cage to accommodate the movement required from the action of the respiratory muscles. This could lead to two things: a limitation in the movement of the somatic components and reduced respiratory efficiency.

Thus, as well as the action of the intercostal muscles and other respiratory muscles, the parietal pleura may also have an effect upon rib motion. Any mechanical restrictions within the thoracic visceral and fascial structures can lead to a whole variety of musculoskeletal system restrictions, through their anatomical links and the physiological interdependence discussed above. Thoracic visceral restrictions can be very important when considering such things as cervicothoracic pain syndromes, brachial neuritis and many shoulder girdle, as well as spinal pain patterns. This concept is one that is little explored in other systems of manual medicine – and it is therefore an important osteopathic contribution to any debate on clinical biomechanics.

This concept means that, when exploring biomechanical restrictions within the thorax, the effects of the lungs and pleura cannot be overlooked; and also, when treating thoracic organ problems, external work to the somatic components to help organ compliance and so organ function must not be forgotten.

There are a variety of techniques within osteopathy to explore and treat restrictions within the whole thorax, which include not only the musculoskeletal components but the lungs and heart, with their associated pleura and pericardium, as well as the oesophagus, fascial and other structures within the mediastinum.

Further discussion of the internal mechanics of the thorax and their influence upon organ function will be undertaken in more detail in Chapter 9. For now, the discussion on the relationship between rib movement and the thoracic spine will be continued.

Rib mechanics in relation to the thoracic spine

Rib motion is considered necessary for efficient thoracic spine mobility (Oda *et al.*, 1996). The upper nine or ten ribs will attach to two adjacent vertebrae. In this way, if rib mechanics are affected, the action of the corresponding thoracic vertebrae will also be affected. This was discussed in Chapter 6, and the articulations between the ribs and thoracic vertebrae were illustrated in Figure 6.3.

Many long-standing thoracic spine restrictions that do not seem to respond to local work (i.e. manipulations directed only at the intervertebral articulations of the spine) may resolve if the rib mechanics are first released. There are other reasons why rib mechanics are considered important within osteopathy, though. These include a relation between rib movement and the function of the autonomic nervous system.

The autonomic nervous system

As has been discussed extensively in previous chapters, the autonomic nervous system and the somatic nervous system are linked in a particular way. Through these links, various intervertebral articulatory restrictions and their accompanying local soft tissue changes may well be related to organ dysfunction (either as cause or effect). Rib mechanics are important in this concept as they may relate not only to thoracic spine restriction (and therefore the presumed link this has with organ function) but also to the function of the paravertebral chain of ganglia (which is part of

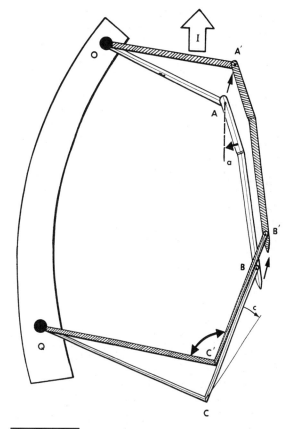

the sympathetic branch of the autonomic nervous system).

As will be discussed in Chapter 9, circulation within neural tissue is very important to its function. Rib movement may create a gentle 'massaging' action at the level of the sympathetic ganglia, passively aiding local tissue circulation. Rib restrictions may mean that circulation within this neural tissue is compromised through lack of this passive 'massaging' normally induced by rib movement.

Whatever the effects of rib restriction are, though, one needs to appreciate that rib mechanics do not only relate to activity within the posterior articulations of the ribs. Indeed, many restrictions within these posterior articulations only arise following adapted movement within the anterior rib cage components, which we will now discuss.

Anterior rib cage motion – other perspectives on rib mechanics

Anterior rib cage motion is composed of movement in the sternum, the manubrium and the costal cartilage articulations between these structures and the anterior parts of the ribs. There is an elastic coupling between the ribs and the manubriosternum, which is very important for overall thoracic function.

As discussed above, restriction in rib movement will reduce possible lung volumes, and this is thought to be due in part to the way that sternal restrictions affect rib cage mechanics. The elastic coupling between the ribs and the sternum (as provided by the costal cartilages) should allow a variety of different rib movements during sternal movement (De Troyer and Wilson, 1993). If sternal (or costal cartilage) mechanics are affected, this will alter the way the whole rib will move and may induce torsion and restriction within the posterior articulations of the ribs (and hence the thoracic spine).

Osteopathic models

Interest in the anterior rib cage has dwindled in some osteopathic models of thoracic cage mechanics, which might seem unusual. The

Figure 8.13

Side view of the movements of the sternum during inspiration. (Reproduced with the permission of Churchill Livingstone from The Physiology of Joints, Vol. 3, Kapandji, 1974.)

ethical considerations of working on the anterior rib cage may be one reason for this, but should not be a bar to working in this very important area. Fortunately, this 'lack of interest' in the mechanics of the anterior rib cage is now being overturned. Sternal and costal cartilage movements are illustrated in Figure 8.13.

The clinical implications of anterior rib cage restriction are many and varied, and could give rise to many symptoms in and around the thorax and even in distant parts of the body. The anterior rib cage is implicated in all the movements we have discussed so far. These are revised below.

General considerations

The motion of the anterior rib cage, coupled with compliance in the intercostal section of the rib cage (discussed above), is necessary for global movements of the thorax and torso. The need for global movement has been discussed in the section on the function of the upper limb, as has the role of the thorax in whole-body movement. Additionally, we have stated that one cannot discuss the respiratory role of the thorax without remembering the extensive links that the thorax has with upper limb structures and parts of the axial skeleton, many of which are mediated through muscular attachments on to the anterior rib cage. As we have seen, these relationships are complex, and when we include the diaphragm (see below) they become more so. Diaphragmatic mechanics strongly influence movements within the anterior rib cage. Thus the mechanics of the anterior rib cage are important to all the things we have discussed so far.

When viewed as a whole, the thorax, including its anterior components, should act as a compliant and three-dimensionally elastic structure.

For global movements, such as those used in sports, reaching over the back seat of the car, doing the housework and all manner of combined movement tasks, the thorax must ideally be fully elastic in all ranges. Many global movements can be restricted because the thorax is not mobile to an appropriate degree, or in sufficient directions. The thorax, then, should be quite distortable, which does seem to be the case (Chihara *et al.*, 1996; Kenyon *et al.*, 1997; Closkey *et al.*, 1992).

The forces acting within the thorax are quite strong and, if elasticity in one or more components is restricted, this can place strain on other parts of the thorax. Trying to use the torso in combined movements when some parts of the rib cage are not sufficiently compliant may lead to a number of minor sprains and strains within the thorax, and even stress fractures of the ribs (Lin *et al.*, 1994).

Scoliosis

This distortability must operate within a balanced system of forces, such that the thorax as a whole remains oriented in a neutral midline position at rest: a balanced system of muscular forces acting around the thorax is necessary for uniform spinal stability (Pal, 1991). Disruption of these forces is one of the factors thought to be associated with scoliosis formation, which can in itself have consequences for respiratory function (Culham *et al.*, 1994; Upadhyay *et al.*, 1995). Other forces may act upon the thorax affecting rib cage mechanics. Posture, which has to be maintained against gravity, is an important consideration, as gravity appears to have quite an effect on rib cage mechanics (Liu *et al.*, 1991; Estenne *et al.*, 1992).

In considering these global movements, it is appropriate to consider how the thorax moves as a unit. This will allow us to see more clearly some of the normal movements of the anterior rib cage and to appreciate the implications of restriction in this area.

General thoracic movement

Accessory rib motion during thoracic cage rotation

As well as the bucket handle and pump handle (inspiratory and expiratory) movements of the ribs, osteopaths consider that there is an additional rib movement that occurs passively, during general torso movement (in rotation). This 'additional' movement is where the rib heads move either anteriorly or posteriorly during rotation of the thorax, which will be explained in a moment.

This concept is one that has yet to feature much within orthodox considerations. However, within osteopathy it is considered very important both for function of the rib cage during locomotion and other biomechanical activity, as well as with respect to thoracic organ function. This motion is shown in Figure 8.14, which shows a superior view of the rib cage and draws an analogy between the rib articulations with the vertebrae, and a series of cogwheels.

If one twists to the right (as shown in Figure 8.14), there will be a series of movements induced in the posterior rib articulations, as soft tissue 'slack' is taken up. In twisting to the right,

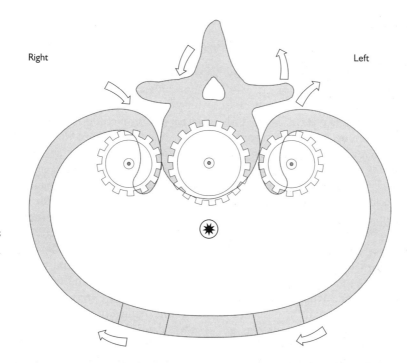

Figure 8.14

Superior view of movements at the costovertebral joints, represented as a series of cog-wheels. The star represents the axis about which general rotation of the torso occurs (in this case, to the right, as indicated by the arrows). See text for further discussion.

Right

Left

the rib on the right will rotate so that the rib head moves anteriorly against the vertebra. The cog-wheel analogy means that, as this occurs, the vertebra will rotate so that the spinous process moves to the right. This movement is very slight, and stops once all the 'slack' in the ligaments and soft tissues around the costovertebral articulations of the right rib has been taken up. As the vertebra rotates in the manner described, the left rib also moves. The head of the left rib moves posteriorly, because of the cogwheel arrangement shown. The whole of the rib rotates, with the effect that the anterior end of the left rib moves to the right – which is exactly what should happen during general thoracic rotation to the right. Hence, we come full circle, having followed rib movement all around the chest. The opposite movements occur when rotating to the left.

Axes of motion within the thoracic cage
When all the above is put together, we can have an idea of the position of the axis around which the thorax moves as a whole. This allows us to reflect upon the consequences for thoracic

motion if any component part is not sufficiently mobile/compliant. It also reinforces the opinion that movement within the anterior rib cage is essential for thoracic spine biomechanics.

This view of thoracic cage motion will be returned to in Chapter 9. There we will describe how, through the attachments of the pleura and pericardium on to the internal surfaces of the ribs and intercostal muscles, this general rotatory motion is passed through into the visceral and other fascial structures of the thorax. Pleural and pericardial restrictions limit thoracic cage mobility, and *vice versa*, which leads to a variety of clinical considerations, some of which we can begin to consider below.

Clinical application
Several techniques have now been developed to examine and treat restrictions in motion of the anterior rib cage. Apart from the relations of anterior chest pain mechanics to the thoracic spine and surrounding area function, treatment to the anterior/general rib cage may be necessary in a number of different situations (including orofacial pain; Hruska, 1997). This point will be

better explained later in this chapter, in the section on the stomatognathic system.

Road traffic trauma, especially in relation to seat-belt injuries, can be particularly helped by considering the subsequent function of the anterior rib cage. Most patients suffer chronic pain in the chest following this type of injury, and because they have often been told that 'it is bruising' that will 'go eventually' they do not think to request further treatment (as they might with neck pain injury associated with whiplash and road traffic accidents). Hence they often suffer for longer than is necessary.

Treatment can also be useful following surgical procedures to the chest or axilla. For example, many people suffer postsurgical pain as restriction in mobility following thoracic surgery, which is not unexpected. Procedures such as mastectomy, organ biopsy, lung surgery through the chest wall and operations through the sternal route (as in many cardiac procedures) may leave much tension and scarring in the anterior chest. This can be reduced, and postoperative suffering eased, by gentle work on the muscles, fascia and articulations within the area. There are some very gentle mobilizations that are worlds away from the often-mentioned 'thrust techniques' – which would be inappropriate in a recovery situation – can be very safely used and are of much benefit. Some of these can be applied within days of the surgical intervention.

Other situations where anterior chest treatment may be considered are in conditions of the breast such as non-cyclical breast pain and some cases of mastitis. These types of condition are related to poor lymphatic drainage from the breast. Most of the breast lymph normally drains into the axillary glands, and tension in the pectoralis fascia might compromise such drainage. Such tension may be related to restrictions in anterior chest mechanics. Other situations include the consequences of soft tissue change following radiotherapy; following trauma to the rib cage such as blows to the chest; or strain following severe coughing or in association with long-standing respiratory conditions.

Anterior chest pain

In addition to the comments made above under 'clinical application' any dysfunction within the muscles of the thorax could influence rib cage motion, and could lead to stress and strain affecting the articulations of the anterior thorax. This latter situation could lead to many painful conditions that are evident in their own right, or be mistaken for pain of visceral origin. Many visceral pathologies refer pain to the chest and, while one needs to be very careful that one does not mistakenly pass over a serious visceral condition requiring medical intervention, the converse is also true. Many patients have unnecessary medical intervention following treatment for mechanical chest pain mistakenly attributed to visceral disease. Within the orthodox medical profession there is a poor understanding of thoracic cage mechanics and the role this could play in 'chest pain of unknown origin' (Selbst, 1990).

The special role of transversus thoracis

The role of the transversus thoracis muscle (shown in Figure 8.15) is very important to anterior chest mechanics, and it is often a forgotten but highly relevant muscle to consider following sternal trauma, respiratory problems and emotional distress.

Many of the sensations of tight chest that come on with shock and various emotions may be a physical tightening of this muscle. Many patients who are afraid/nervous/distressed develop, over time, chronic tension in this muscle, which clearly affects their thoracic mechanics and also acts as a maintaining feature for the emotional distress (sensation in this area reinforcing the emotional patterning connections within the central nervous system).

Ethical considerations

Clearly there are issues in relation to ethics, and differential diagnosis when working with the breast (as in any other body area) and the anterior chest. The patient must be quite sure of the reasons for any working on the area, and must have indicated their understanding for the technique, and given their consent.

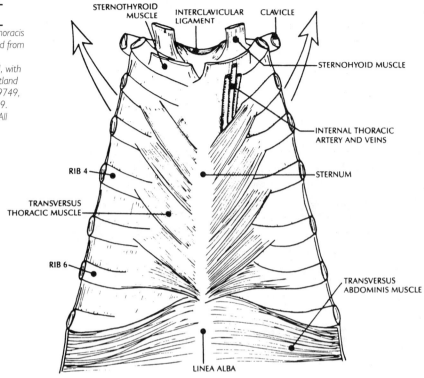

Figure 8.15

Appropriate work in this area, however, can result in great relief from a number of painful conditions affecting the anterior chest and breast, and should not be overlooked in general patient management.

THE DIAPHRAGM

This discussion of the anterior rib cage is not complete without reference to the diaphragm. The diaphragm is a very important structure and we shall see that it influences many things in addition to anterior rib cage mechanics.

As the diaphragm has extensive insertions and is involved in many different activities, it is useful to consider it in some detail. Ever since Galen (129–200 AD) made incredible and extensive experimental and clinical observations of the diaphragm (Derenne *et al.*, 1995), this structure has continued to fascinate and confound. The information discussed below is only a tiny con-

sideration of the possibilities for motion and physiology that it is involved with.

The varied functions of the diaphragm

The diaphragm is an important meeting place for forces and dynamics because of its action as a coupling between the thorax and the abdomen (Boynton *et al.*, 1999). As well as respiration, the diaphragm is involved in a number of bio-mechanical considerations.

The action of the diaphragm on the anterior rib cage

If one looks at the attachments of the diaphragm to the costal margin, as shown in Figure 8.16, one can see that tension in the diaphragm will influence directly the elasticity and compliance of the cartilage forming the costal margin.

Diaphragmatic tension can occur in a non-uniform pattern, which can lead to some sections of the costal margin being restricted while others

Figure 8.16

Inferior view of the diaphragm showing the crurae and the arcuate ligaments. (Reproduced with the permission of Novartis from Atlas of Human Anatomy, 2nd edn, Netter, 1997.)

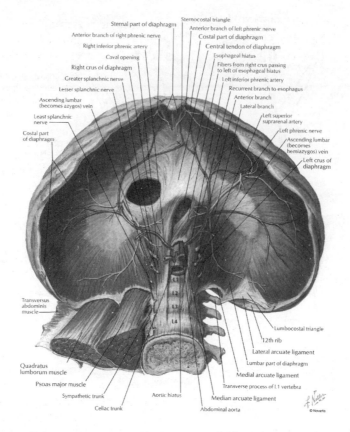

remain free. If one section of the costal margin is restricted, then the anterior ends of the ribs associated with it will also become restricted. This will affect rib mechanics in many ways (which we have already discussed). Tension in the diaphragm can also affect the movement of the sternum, with diverse effects.

The action of the diaphragm in providing a platform to aid trunk stability

The diaphragm acts with the abdominals and pelvic floor muscles to increase intra-abdominal pressure. This allows a greater leverage to be transmitted from the rectus sheath via the transversus abdominis to the thoracolumbar fascia and the fascial sheath around the erector spinae muscles. This increases the leverage potential of these muscles, while at the same time stabilizing individual lumbar vertebral motion. This role of the diaphragm in biomechanical considerations under load is illustrated by a study that showed

that the diaphragm is much more developed in weightlifters than in non-weightlifters (McCool *et al.*, 1997). It appears that you can train your diaphragm!

The role of the diaphragm in thoracolumbar mechanics

The role of the diaphragm in thoracolumbar mechanics is best appreciated by reflecting on the insertions that the posterior wall of the diaphragm has to the lumbar spine and the lower ribs, via the arcuate ligaments. These are also shown in Figure 8.16. The mid section of the posterior wall of the diaphragm attaches to the lumbar spine via the crurae of the diaphragm. The right crus attaches to the first three lumbar vertebrae and the left crus attaches to the first two lumbar vertebrae. The median arcuate ligament forms an arch between the two crurae, and forms a bridge over the aorta so that it can pass underneath the diaphragm without being compressed as the diaphragm contracts. The medial arcuate ligaments pass from the lateral aspects of the crurae to the tip of the transverse processes of the first lumbar vertebra (L1). (There are therefore two medial arcuate ligaments, one on either side.) The lateral arcuate ligaments pass from the tip of the transverse process of L1 to the tip of the 12th rib. (Again, there are two lateral arcuate ligaments, one on either side.) The medial arcuate ligaments form a bridge over the psoas muscles, and the lateral arcuate ligaments form a bridge over the quadratus lumborum muscles, so that they can function 'independently' of the diaphragm.

If there are any tensions within the posterior wall of the diaphragm or within the arcuate ligaments (such as might follow chest pathology, upper abdominal pathology or surgery, or poor breathing mechanics resulting in poor use of the diaphragm, for example), these will affect the mechanics of the upper lumbar spine and the 12th ribs and will lead to a variety of restriction patterns within the thoracolumbar junction. Evaluation of these structures is therefore important in any clinical situation where thoracolumbar mechanics are involved.

The role of thoracolumbar, lumbar and lower rib mechanics in diaphragm function

Through the above attachments, movement in the thoracolumbar and lumbar spine and the lower rib cage can be influential to diaphragmatic activity. Because of the torsions that act upon the upper lumbar spine and through the thoracolumbar region and lower rib cage during locomotion (and other normal biomechanical activities), the diaphragm during respiration is constantly contracting against a mobile base. The function of other muscles acting upon the lower ribs and the lumbar spine (such as quadratus lumborum, serratus posterior inferior and psoas) is to act in concert with the diaphragm in respiration to help stabilize the thoracolumbar area to ensure a firm base for diaphragmatic action. In this way there is a complex dynamic of inter-related forces acting in and around the diaphragm, so that it functions in the most optimal way in any given

movement or body position. Consequently, mechanical restriction and adverse muscle tension in any of these components will affect the diaphragm, leading to a variety of problems, including respiratory system dysfunction.

Clinical relevance

Many locomotor problems that are associated with thoracolumbar mechanical restriction (such as most cases of low back pain for example) may be relieved by releasing the diaphragm and ensuring elasticity within the crural attachments and the arcuate ligaments.

The diaphragm and respiration

The diaphragm is involved extensively with respiration, and works in a variety of ways to ensure changes in thoracic volume and pressure. It is useful to briefly mention the role of the diaphragm in respiration separately, as its functions in this respect are complex.

The diaphragm works in respiration by having a zone of apposition between the lungs, rib cage and the abdominal viscera. It works in concert with the rib cage and the abdominal muscles (Cala et al., 1993). The diaphragm shortens and thickens during inspiration (Cohn et al., 1997) and the lower rib cage widens (Gauthier et al., 1994; Petroll et al., 1990). The diaphragm does not necessarily work like a vertical piston, but more like a 'widening piston'. It does not work uniformly in all situations and there is quite a regional variation in deformation of the diaphragm during respiration (Pean et al., 1991). This may have implications where there are a variety of small factors affecting diaphragm motion that, while individually insignificant, collectively may have important respiratory consequences.

Osteopathic models and the diaphragm

As implied through all the above, it is very difficult to examine a person with respect to any symptom they might have without including the diaphragm in that consideration. The diaphragm is as central to osteopathic practice as it is within a person's anatomy.

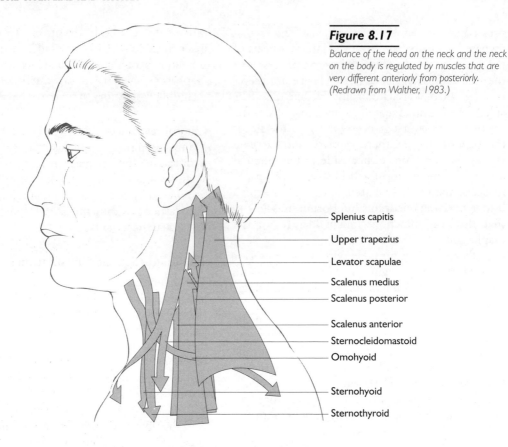

Figure 8.17

Balance of the head on the neck and the neck on the body is regulated by muscles that are very different anteriorly from posteriorly. (Redrawn from Walther, 1983.)

Splenius capitis

Upper trapezius

Levator scapulae

Scalenus medius

Scalenus posterior

Scalenus anterior

Sternocleidomastoid

Omohyoid

Sternohyoid

Sternothyroid

The mechanical influences of the diaphragm are enormous, and whole books could be devoted to their discussion. Sadly, there is insufficient room within this text to analyse them all. Suffice it to say that the diaphragm can influence the spine and thoracic cage (and from there the cervical spine and head relations), and through the abdominals the pelvis and lower limbs, and no assessment of the person with respect to their biomechanical status is complete without a thorough examination of this structure.

Other considerations of diaphragmatic function

The wide-ranging role of the diaphragm with respect to fluid dynamics (and so body physiology) will be discussed in Chapter 9. It is through this relationship with fluid movement that the action of the diaphragm aids tissue health and immune function and it is through the massaging of the abdominal organs (especially the upper gastro-intestinal tract and the kidneys) that the diaphragm helps visceral function in general.

The diaphragm is also related to emotions. Many emotions/tensions associated (by the patients) with the epigastric area are in reality found to be focused within the diaphragm when the person is examined physically (Keleman, 1985).

Releasing tension within the diaphragm and its bony relations, and improving diaphragmatic action through breathing retraining, will positively influence all the types of problem discussed above.

Finally, our discussion of the upper limb and thorax would not be complete without a review of their links with the stomatognathic system.

THE STOMATOGNATHIC SYSTEM

The stomatognathic system incorporates the head, neck and jaw. It includes the hyoid bone

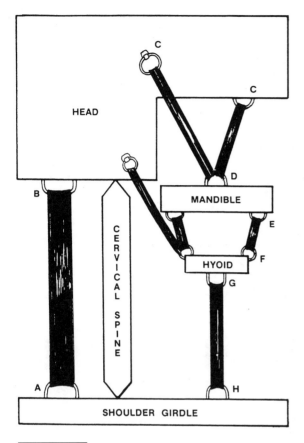

Figure 8.18

Block diagram of the closed kinematic chain of the stomatognathic system. The sternocleidomastoid muscle has been left out for clarity. (Reproduced from Applied Kinesiology, Vol. II, D. S. Walther, Systems DC. 1983, with permission.)

and the muscles connecting it to the manubrium, mandible and scapula, and it includes the fascial sheets within the anterior cervical region as well as other structures in the neck.

The inter-relatedness of parts within this system has been much discussed in various books, including one by Walther, an American chiropractor (1983). Figures 8.17 and 8.18, reproduced from this text, give some idea of these interconnections and show the way that many of the muscles in this region act in a dynamic, balancing way. The efficiency of this balancing system contributes to effective function of the mouth, throat, cervical spine and head, as well as the thorax and upper limb.

This system of balancing muscular action means that the orientation of the cervical column could be influenced as much by combined tensions within these muscles as by other areas of the spine and pelvis.

Hyoid, mandible and sternal relations

The hyoid is uniquely placed to monitor the diverse patterns of tension that can arise through this system of soft tissues during everyday activity (including locomotion, talking, eating and breathing). The hyoid and related muscles are shown in Figure 8.19.

This shows that the hyoid links the scapula, manubrium, mandible and cranial base. The hyoid is also attached to the pharynx (in which the eustachian tube and pharyngeal tonsils are embedded) and the tongue.

Any torsions within this area will have consequences for the anterior cervical fascia and the thyroid gland; and also for pharyngeal, eustachian tube, laryngeal, tongue and temporomandibular joint (TMJ) mechanics and the various tonsils within this region. They will also 'distort' the proprioceptive feedback essential for the control of whole-body posture. (The stomatognathic system should be viewed as a part of the balance control systems for the whole body; Walther, 1983.)

The tongue, TMJ and bite problems

The orientation of the jaw, and of the tongue between the hyoid and mandible, is another example of a functionally integrated system. Figure 8.20 shows the attachments of the tongue.

Swallowing mechanics, dental occlusion and a variety of other actions depend upon the smooth coordination of these bony structures, and of the head and neck mechanics in general. Dysfunction in these parts can therefore have widespread effects.

This will be relevant, for example, for suckling in babies and in learning good voice control (see below). The structures of the pharynx and larynx may in themselves be put under strain in an infant who is constantly mouth-breathing for some reason (such as chronic upper respiratory

Figure 8.19

Anterior view of muscular attachments to the hyoid. (Reprinted from Craniosacral Therapy II. Beyond the Dura by John Upledger, with permission of Eastland Press, P.O. Box 99749, Seattle, WA 98199, Copyright 1987. All rights reserved.)

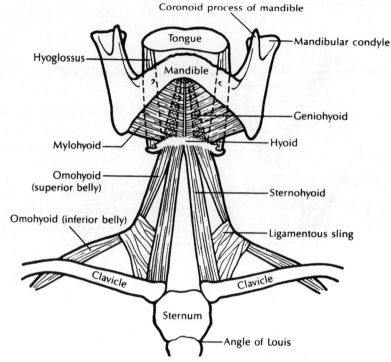

Figure 8.20

Lateral view of muscular attachments to the hyoid. (Reprinted from Craniosacral Therapy II. Beyond the Dura by John Upledger, with permission of Eastland Press, P.O. Box 99749, Seattle, WA 98199, Copyright 1987. All rights reserved.)

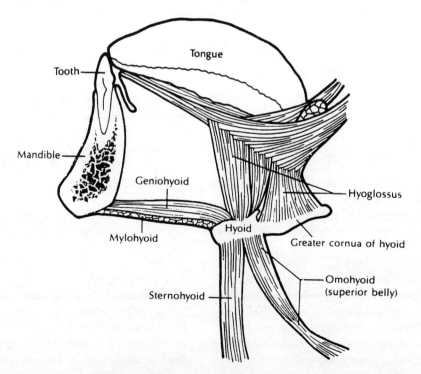

Figure 8.21

The nasopharynx, viewed from behind, showing the eustachian tube entering the upper pharyngeal area. (Reproduced with the persmission of Novartis from Atlas of Human Anatomy, *2nd edn, Netter, 1997.)*

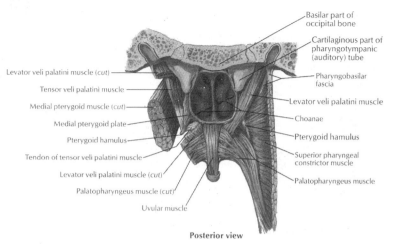

Posterior view

tract infection) and this will compromise function in the stomatognathic system as a whole.

The stomatognathic system, proprioception and the control of head posture

It is suggested by many practitioners within the manipulative professions that the role of the TMJ (and stomatognathic system) is as influential to the neural control of whole-body posture as the special senses of the eyes and ears. This has yet to be confirmed but nevertheless forms a substantial part of the therapeutic approach of sections of the osteopathic profession to such problems as dizziness, vertigo and certain eye problems. In addition to this it has even been suggested that shear forces on the teeth may be informative to the proprioceptive control of head orientation and whole-body posture (Trulsson and Johansson, 1996). (Certainly they would have influence on the action of the local muscles of the jaw and cervical region, which are intimately involved in the process of eating.) The clinical applications of these considerations have not been fully explored.

Pharyngeal mechanics, tonsillar function and the eustachian tube

Figure 8.21 shows the pharynx and some of its attachments.

Briefly, the pharynx is attached to the hyoid, the pterygoid plates of the sphenoid, the basi-occiput (just anterior to the foramen magnum)

and a variety of deep fascial structures in the upper portion of the anterior cervical region. The eustachian tube, pharyngeal tonsils and various lymphatic tissues attach to and drain into the pharynx. Their patency and ability to drain and function effectively depends upon a compliant pharynx (and therefore on good, integrated mobility within the stomatognathic system).

Tension and torsion through the soft tissues of the throat and anterior cervical spine will limit the general lymphatic drainage of these tissues and areas, thus compromising tissue health and reducing immune efficiency. Tensions around the upper pharynx are particularly important for the mechanics of the eustachian tube and middle ear drainage.

This has consequences for many ear, nose and throat conditions, especially in children. For example, much can be done to resolve the distress and irritation caused by the condition known as glue ear (related to otitis media). This is done by releasing tensions found within these tissues (and others, within the cranium for example), thus allowing greater tissue drainage and flexibility. This seems to reduce the incidence of ear infections and suffering among many children presenting to osteopathic practices who specialize in this area.

The voice

Voice production depends on laryngeal mechanics and the proper control of breath and air pressure over the vocal cords. The shaping of the air with-

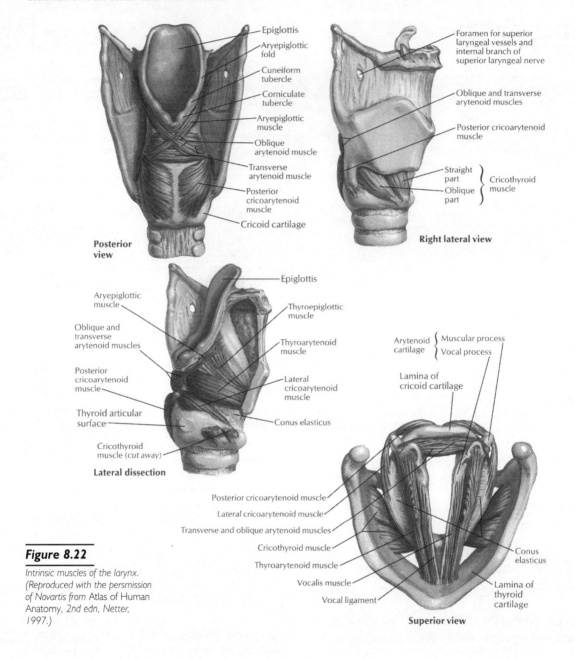

Epiglottis
Aryepiglottic fold
Cuneiform tubercle
Corniculate tubercle
Aryepiglottic muscle
Oblique arytenoid muscle
Transverse arytenoid muscle
Posterior cricoarytenoid muscle
Cricoid cartilage

Posterior view

Foramen for superior laryngeal vessels and internal branch of superior laryngeal nerve
Oblique and transverse arytenoid muscles
Posterior cricoarytenoid muscle
Straight part
Oblique part
} Cricothyroid muscle

Right lateral view

Epiglottis
Aryepiglottic muscle
Oblique and transverse arytenoid muscles
Posterior cricoarytenoid muscle
Thyroid articular surface
Cricothyroid muscle (*cut away*)
Thyroepiglottic muscle
Thyroarytenoid muscle
Lateral cricoarytenoid muscle
Conus elasticus

Lateral dissection

Arytenoid cartilage { Muscular process / Vocal process
Lamina of cricoid cartilage

Posterior cricoarytenoid muscle
Lateral cricoarytenoid muscle
Transverse and oblique arytenoid muscles
Cricothyroid muscle
Thyroarytenoid muscle
Vocalis muscle
Vocal ligament
Conus elasticus
Lamina of thyroid cartilage

Superior view

Figure 8.22

Intrinsic muscles of the larynx. (Reproduced with the persmission of Novartis from Atlas of Human Anatomy, 2nd edn, Netter, 1997.)

in the mouth and pharynx is important only after the other factors have produced the volume of air for the mouth to 'mould'. The larynx is shown in Figure 8.22.

Speech therapists within orthodox practice work with the tensions in these areas by exercise, retraining of the voice and sound production. Osteopaths can greatly facilitate this process by physically working on these tissues, allowing them to participate in a physiological manner within voice production, and by working with posture so that the head and neck are balanced evenly upon the thorax, thus minimizing torsion within the anterior throat (Lieberman, 1997).

Osteopaths would also look at the state of the abdominal muscles (and associated structures), as these are important for producing correct air pressure at the level of the larynx.

SUMMARY

This chapter should have given some insight to the osteopathic perspectives of upper limb and thoracic motion and their inter-relations throughout the rest of the body.

It is now time to consider the role of fluid dynamics, as it is governed by body movement.

REFERENCES

Adams, M. A. and Dolan, P. (1995) *Posture and Spinal Mechanics During Lifting.*

Anetzberger, H. and Putz, R. (1996) The scapula: principles of construction and stress. *Acta Anatomica (Basel)*, **156**, 70–80.

Aruin, A. S. and Latash, M. L. (1995) Directional specificity of postural muscles in feed-forward postural reactions during fast voluntary arm movements. *Experimental Brain Research*, **103**, 323–332.

Avanzolini, G., Barbini, P., Cappello, A. and Cevenini, G. (1995) Influence of flow pattern on the parameter estimates of a simple breathing mechanics model. *IEEE Transactions on Biomedical Engineering*, **42**, 394–402.

Aymard, C., Chia, L., Katz, R. *et al.* (1995a) Reciprocal inhibition between wrist flexors and extensors in man: a new set of interneurones? *Journal of Physiology (London)*, **487**, 221–235.

Aymard, C., Katz, R., Lafitte, C. *et al.* (1995b) Changes in reciprocal and transjoint inhibition induced by muscle fatigue in man. *Experimental Brain Research*, **106**, 418–424.

Barral, J.-P. (1991) *The Thorax*, Eastland Press, Seattle, WA.

Bates, J. H. (1991) Lung mechanics – the inverse problem. *Australasian Physical and Engineering Sciences in Medicine*, 14,197–203.

Bigliani, L. U., Kelkar, R., Flatow, E. L. *et al.* (1996) Glenohumeral stability. Biomechanical properties of passive and active stabilizers. *Clinical Orthopaedics and Related Research*, **330**, 13–30.

Blasier, R. B., Soslowsky, L. J., Malicky, D. M. and Palmer, M. L. (1997) Posterior glenohumeral subluxation: active and passive stabilization in a biomechanical model. *Journal of Bone and Joint Surgery (American Volume)*, **79**, 433–440.

Boynton, B. R., Barnas, G. M., Dadmun, J. T. and Fredberg, J. J. (1999) Mechanical coupling of the rib cage, abdomen, and diaphragm through their area of apposition. *Journal of Anatomy*, in press.

Brand, P. W. (1993) Biomechanics of balance in the hand. *Journal of Hand Therapy*, **6**, 247–251.

Cala, S. J., Edyvean, J. and Engel, L. A. (1993) Abdominal compliance, parasternal activation, and chest wall motion. *Journal of Applied Physiology*, **74**, 1398–1405.

Chen, W. S. (1995) Median-nerve neuropathy associated with chronic anterior dislocation of the lunate. *Journal of Bone and Joint Surgery (American Volume)*, **77**, 1853–1857.

Chihara, K., Kenyon, C. M. and Macklem, P. T. (1996) Human rib cage distortability. *Journal of Applied Physiology*, **81**, 437–447.

Closkey, R. F., Schultz, A. B. and Luchies, C. W. (1992) A model for studies of the deformable rib cage. *Journal of Biomechanics*, **25**, 529–539.

Cobb, T. K., Dailey, B. K., Posteraro, R. H. and Lewis, R. C. (1993) Anatomy of the flexor retinaculum. *Journal of Hand Surgery (American Volume)*, **18**, 91–99.

Cohn, D., Benditt, J. O., Eveloff, S. and McCool, F. D. (1997) Diaphragm thickening during inspiration. *Journal of Applied Physiology*, **83**, 291–296.

Culham, E. and Peat, M. (1993) Functional anatomy of the shoulder complex. *Journal of Orthopaedic and Sports Physical Therapy*, **18**, 342–350.

Culham, E. G., Jimenez, H. A. and King, C. E. (1994) Thoracic kyphosis, rib mobility, and lung volumes in normal women and women with osteoporosis. *Spine*, **19**, 1250–1255.

De Serres, S. J. and Milner, T. E. (1991) Wrist muscle activation patterns and stiffness associated with stable and unstable mechanical loads. *Experimental Brain Research*, **86**, 451–458.

De Troyer, A. (1997) Role of joint receptors in modulation of inspiratory intercostal activity by rib motion in dogs. *Journal of Physiology (London)*, **503**, 445–453.

De Troyer, A. and Estenne, M. (1988) Functional anatomy of the respiratory muscles. *Clinics in Chest Medicine*, **9**, 175–193.

De Troyer, A. and Wilson, T. A. (1993) Sternum dependence of rib displacement during breathing. *Journal of Applied Physiology*, 75, 334–340.

De Troyer, A., Cappello, M. and Brichant, J. F. (1994) Do canine scalene and sternomastoid muscles play a role in breathing? *Journal of Applied Physiology*, 76, 242–252.

Dechman, G., Sato, J. and Bates, J. H. (1993) Effect of pleural effusion on respiratory mechanics, and the influence of deep inflation, in dogs. *European Respiratory Journal*, 6, 219–224.

Derenne, J. P., Debru, A., Grassino, A. E. and Whitelaw, W. A. (1995) History of diaphragm physiology: the achievements of Galen. *European Respiratory Journal*, 8, 154–160.

Dietz, V., Gollhofer, A., Kleiber, M. and Trippel, M. (1992) Regulation of bipedal stance: dependency on 'load' receptors. *Experimental Brain Research*, 89, 229–231.

Epstein, S. K. (1994) An overview of respiratory muscle function. *Clinics in Chest Medicine*, 15, 619–639.

Estenne, M., Zocchi, L., Ward, M. and Macklem, P. T. (1990) Chest wall motion and expiratory muscle use during phonation in normal humans. *Journal of Applied Physiology*, 68, 2075–2082.

Estenne, M., Gorini, M., Van Muylem, A. *et al.* (1992) Rib cage shape and motion in microgravity. *Journal of Applied Physiology*, 73, 946–954.

Gauthier, A. P., Verbanck, S., Estenne, M. *et al.* (1994) Three-dimensional reconstruction of the in vivo human diaphragm shape at different lung volumes. *Applied Physiology*, 76, 495–506.

Horstmann, G. A. and Dietz, V. (1990) A basic posture control mechanism: the stabilization of the centre of gravity. *Electroencephalography and Clinical Neurophysiology*, 76, 165–176.

Hruska, R. J. Jr (1997) Influences of dysfunctional respiratory mechanics on orofacial pain. *Dental Clinics of North America*, 41, 211–227.

Ingram, R. H. Jr (1990) Physiological assessment of inflammation in the peripheral lung of asthmatic patients. *Lung*, 168, 237–247.

Kamm, R. (1995) Shear-augmented dispersion in the respiratory system. *Symposium of the Society for Experimental Biology*, 49, 277–295.

Kapandji, I. A. (1974) The thoracic vertebral column. In: *The Physiology of the Joints*, Vol. 3, Churchill Livingstone, New York, pp. 128–169.

Kauer, J. M. (1986) The mechanism of the carpal joint. *Clinical Orthopaedics and Related Research*, 202, 16–26.

Kauer, J. M. (1992) The distal radioulnar joint. Anatomic and functional considerations. *Clinical Orthopaedics and Related Research*, 275, 37–45.

Kauer, J. M. and de Lange, A. (1987) The carpal joint. Anatomy and function. *Hand Clinics*, 3, 23–29.

Keleman, S. (1985) *Emotional Anatomy: The Structure of Experience*, Centre Press, Berkeley, CA.

Kenyon, C. M., Cala, S. J., Yan, S. *et al.* (1997) Rib cage mechanics during quiet breathing and exercise in humans. *Journal of Applied Physiology*, 83, 1242–1255.

Kibler, W. B. (1995) Biomechanical analysis of the shoulder during tennis activities. *Clinics in Sports Medicine*, 14, 79–85.

Lai-Fook, S. J. and Rodarte, J. R. (1991) Pleural pressure distribution and its relationship to lung volume and interstitial pressure. *Journal of Applied Physiology*, 70, 967–978.

Lichtenstein, O., Ben-Haim, S. A., Saidel, G. M. and Dinnar, U. (1992) Role of the diaphragm in chest wall mechanics. *Journal of Applied Physiology*, 72, 568–574.

Lieberman, J. (1997) In: *The Voice Clinic Handbook* (eds T. Harris *et al.*), Whurr, London.

Lin, H. C., Chou, C. S. and Hsu, T. C. (1994) Stress fractures of the ribs in amateur golf players. *Chung Hua I Hsueh Tsa Chih (Taipei)*, 54, 33–37.

Linscheid, R. L. (1992) Biomechanics of the distal radioulnar joint. *Clinical Orthopaedics and Related Research*, 275, 46–55.

Liu, S. B., Wilson, T. A. and Schreiner, K. (1991) Gravitational forces on the chest wall. *Journal of Applied Physiology*, 70, 1506–1510.

Loring, S. H. (1992) Action of human respiratory muscles inferred from finite element analysis of rib cage. *Journal of Applied Physiology*, 72, 1461–1465.

Loring, S. H. and Woodbridge, J. A. (1991) Intercostal muscle action inferred from finite-element analysis. *Journal of Applied Physiology*, 70, 2712–2718.

McCann, P. D. and Bigliani, L. U. (1994) Shoulder pain in tennis players. *Sports Medicine*, 17, 53–64.

McCool, F. D., Conomos, P., Benditt, J. O. *et al.* (1997) Maximal inspiratory pressures and dimensions of the diaphragm. *American Journal of Respiratory and Critical Care Medicine*, 155, 1329–1334.

MacKinnon, C. D. and Winter, D. A. (1993) Control of whole body balance in the frontal plane during human walking. *Journal of Biomechanics*, 26, 633–644.

Malicky, D. M., Soslowsky, L. J., Blasier, R. B. and Shyr, Y. (1996) Anterior glenohumeral stabilization factors: progressive effects in a biomechanical model. *Journal of Orthopaedic Research*, **14**, 282–288.

Matsen, F. A. III, Harryman, D. T. II and Sidles, J. A. (1991) Mechanics of glenohumeral instability. *Clinics in Sports Medicine*, **10**, 783–788.

Murray, W. M., Delp, S. L. and Buchanan, T. S. (1995) Variation of muscle moment arms with elbow and forearm position. *Journal of Biomechanics*, **28**, 513–525.

Netter, F. H. (1997) *Atlas of Human Anatomy*, 2nd edn, Novartis, East Hannover, NJ.

Neviaser, R. J. (1983) Painful conditions affecting the shoulder. *Clinical Orthopaedics and Related Research*, **173**, 63–69.

Nicholson, G. P., Goodman, D. A., Flatow, E. L. and Bigliani, L. U. (1996) The acromion: morphologic condition and age-related changes. A study of 420 scapulas. *Journal of Shoulder and Elbow Surgery*, **5**, 1–11.

Oda, I., Abumi, K., Lu, D. *et al.* (1996) Biomechanical role of the posterior elements, costovertebral joints, and rib cage in the stability of the thoracic spine. *Spine*, **21**, 1423–1429.

Pal, G. P. (1991) Mechanism of production of scoliosis. A hypothesis. *Spine*, **16**, 288–292.

Panjabi, M. M. (1992) The stabilizing system of the spine. Part I. Function, dysfunction, adaptation, and enhancement. *Journal of Spinal Disorders*, **5**, 383–389; discussion 397.

Pean, J. L., Chuong, C. J., Ramanathan, M. and Johnson, R. L. Jr (1991) Regional deformation of the canine diaphragm. *Journal of Applied Physiology*, **71**, 1581–1588.

Petroll, W. M., Knight, H. and Rochester, D. F. (1990) Effect of lower rib cage expansion and diaphragm shortening on the zone of apposition. *Journal of Applied Physiology*, **68**, 484–488.

Rettig, A. C. and Patel, D. V. (1995) Epidemiology of elbow, forearm, and wrist injuries in the athlete. *Clinics in Sports Medicine*, **14**, 289–297.

Sahn, S. A. (1990) The pathophysiology of pleural effusions. *Annual Review of Medicine*, **41**, 7–13.

Savelberg, H. H., Kooloos, J. G., de Lange, A. *et al.* (1991) Human carpal ligament recruitment and three-dimensional carpal motion. *Journal of Orthopaedic Research*, **9**, 693–704.

Savelberg, H. H., Otten, J. D., Kooloos, J. G. *et al.* (1993) Carpal bone kinematics and ligament lengthening studied for the full range of joint movement. *Journal of Biomechanics*, **26**, 1389–1402.

Schroer, W., Lacey, S., Frost, F. S. and Keith, M. W. (1996) Carpal instability in the weight-bearing upper extremity. *Journal of Bone and Joint Surgery (American Volume)*, **78**, 1838–1843.

Selbst, S. M. (1990) Chest pain in children. *American Family Physician*, **41**, 179–186.

Similowski, T. and Bates, J. H. (1991) Two-compartment modelling of respiratory system mechanics at low frequencies: gas redistribution or tissue rheology? *European Respiratory Journal*, **4**, 353–358.

Skandalakis, J. E., Colborn, G. L., Skandalakis, P. N. *et al.* (1992) The carpal tunnel syndrome: Part III. *American Surgeon*, **58**, 158–166.

Soslowsky, L. J., Flatow, E. L., Bigliani, L. U. and Mow, V. C. (1992) Articular geometry of the glenohumeral joint. *Clinical Orthopaedics and Related Research*, **330**, 181–190.

Soslowsky, L. J., An, C. H., DeBano, C. M. and Carpenter, J. E. (1996) Coracoacromial ligament: in situ load and viscoelastic properties in rotator cuff disease. *Clinical Orthopaedics and Related Research*, **330**, 40–44.

Soslowsky, L. J., Carpenter, J. E., Bucchieri, J. S. and Flatow, E. L. (1997) Biomechanics of the rotator cuff. *Orthopedic Clinics of North America*, **28**, 17–30.

Stamenovic, D., Glass, G. M., Barnas, G. M. and Fredberg, J. J. (1990) Viscoplasticity of respiratory tissues. *Journal of Applied Physiology*, **69**, 973–988.

Stock, S. R. (1991) Workplace ergonomic factors and the development of musculoskeletal disorders of the neck and upper limbs: a meta-analysis. *American Journal of Industrial Medicine*, **19**, 87–107.

Tillmann, B. and Koch, S. (1995) [Functional adaptation processes of gliding tendons]. *Sportverletzung Sportschaden*, **9**, 44–50.

Trulsson, M. and Johansson, R. S. (1996) Encoding of tooth loads by human peridontal afferents and their role in jaw motor control. *Progress in Neurobiology*, **49**, 267–284.

Tucker, B. and Jenkins, S. (1996) The effect of breathing exercises with body positioning on regional lung ventilation. *Australian Physiotherapy*, **42**, 219–227.

Upadhyay, S. S., Mullaji, A. B., Luk, K. D. and Leong, J. C. (1995) Relation of spinal and thoracic cage deformities and their flexibilities with altered pulmonary functions in adolescent idiopathic scoliosis. *Spine*, **20**, 2415–2420.

Upledger, J. E. (1987) *Craniosacral Therapy II. Beyond the Dura*, Eastland Press, Seattle, WA.

Van Emmerik, R. E. and Wagenaar, R. C. (1996) Effects of walking velocity on relative phase dynamics in the trunk in human walking. *Journal of Biomechanics*, **29**, 1175–1184.

Vernazza, S., Cincera, M., Pedotti, A. and Massion, J. (1996a) Balance control during lateral arm raising in humans. *Neuroreports*, **7**, 1543–1548.

Vernazza, S., Alexandrov, A. and Massion, J. (1996b) Is the center of gravity controlled during upper trunk movements? *Neuroscience Letters*, **206**, 77–60.

Virji-Babul, N. and Cooke, J. D. (1995) Influence of joint interactional effects on the coordination of planar two-joint arm movements. *Experimental Brain Research*, **103**, 451–459.

Vleeming, A., Pool-Goudzwaard, A. L., Stoeckart, R. *et al.* (1995) The posterior layer of the thoracolumbar fascia. Its function in load transfer from spine to legs. *Spine*, **20**, 753–758.

Walther, D. S. (1983) *Applied Kinesiology, vol. II: Head, Neck and Jaw Pain and Dysfunction – The Stomatognathic System*, Systems DC, Colorado.

Warner, J. J., Lephart, S. and Fu, F. H. (1996) Role of proprioception in pathoetiology of shoulder instability. *Clinical Orthopaedics and Related Research*, **330**, 35–39.

Werner, F. W. and An, K. N. (1994) Biomechanics of the elbow and forearm. *Hand Clinics*, **10**, 357–373.

Zachazewski, J. E., Riley, P. O. and Krebs, D. E. (1993) Biomechanical analysis of body mass transfer during stair ascent and descent of healthy subjects. *Journal of Rehabilitation Research and Development*, **30**, 412–422.

Zocchi, L., Estenne, M., Johnston, S. T. *et al.* (1990) Respiratory muscle incoordination in stuttering speech. *American Review of Respiratory Disease*, **141**, 1510–1515.

9 FLUID DYNAMICS AND BODY MOVEMENT

INTRODUCTION

The importance of fluid dynamics within osteopathic practice cannot be overestimated.

An interest in fluid dynamics is extremely useful in many cases. Many clinical symptoms and situations can be associated with disrupted fluid flow. A few examples of when osteopaths would consider fluid dynamics include:

- oedema associated with a sprained ankle, damaged wrist or constricted intervertebral foramen;
- helping to reduce pain and swelling in cases of rheumatoid arthritis or carpal tunnel syndrome by dispersing fluid build-up;
- chronic pelvic pain associated with pelvic venous congestion;
- cerebrospinal fluid dynamics in children for a variety of reasons, including birth trauma and some neurological disorders;
- soft tissue injury and irritation.

Osteopaths recognize many areas of clinical need where improvement of fluid dynamics would have a positive therapeutic effect. As with all clinical interventions, each must be analysed with respect to possible benefit against possible risk in mobilizing body fluids. Broad clinical training and an understanding of physiology and pathology are all vital to this analytical process.

This chapter builds upon the information given previously concerning the architectural arrangement of the body and how movement is thought to aid fluid dynamics. This chapter will discuss those elements that have not already been covered – fluid flow in the body cavities: the abdomen, pelvis and thorax, the cranium and spinal column and the intervertebral foramen. It will also introduce the subject of organ motion, including the general biomechanics of the abdominopelvic and thoracic organs, and will discuss the central and peripheral nervous systems as 'a complete organ' with its own system of biomechanics, necessary to its health. Within this it will also discuss the idea of motion (both 'voluntary' and 'involuntary' – these terms will be clarified within the text), and introduce the concept of the 'involuntary mechanism', which is a dynamic shifting of forces throughout the body, leading to harmonious integration of function.

This chapter will make the point that one does not need to work with the involuntary mechanism to use the concept of the central and peripheral nervous systems as an organ, and that one can look at their biomechanics in a 'conventional way' through general biomechanical principles. It will also discuss the concept of balanced ligamentous tension and its relevance to motion throughout the head, spine and the rest of the body.

Note: While many of the physiological relations discussed are well accepted, some of the following ideas and reflections on the therapeutic relations discussed are not currently fully clinically evaluated or validated. Indeed, some of them are considered somewhat controversial. However, they represent physiological perspectives based on the vision of human movement and its relations that osteopaths have developed, which they use within their practice and hope to investigate and develop further.

One further aim of this chapter is to give anatomical examples of areas of the body that may affect various aspects of fluid flow, in order to provide a foundation for the osteopathic clinical management of a variety of conditions. (The underlying mechanisms to these relations have been discussed, including the idea of microbiomechanics and interstitial circulation. This latter point is clearly relevant to all tissues in the body in whatever organ or structure, and underlies all discussions on fluid movement.)

We will start by discussing general (systemic) blood and lymph circulation.

SYSTEMIC (BLOOD AND LYMPH) CIRCULATION

The point has been made previously that, because the internal environment of the body is largely a fluid medium, the preservation of the volume and composition of the body fluids is absolutely vital to circulatory status and to the management of the extraordinarily complicated functions of

the human body (Hill, 1990). Complex feedback control mechanisms exist to ensure homeostasis or equilibrium in the body fluids (and therefore tissues) and include participation by the kidneys, lungs, gastrointestinal tract, circulatory system, endocrine system and central nervous system.

In normal circumstances, the time taken for the total volume of the blood to be circulated once around the body is in fact quite small, considering the distance that it has to travel. Circulation time (i.e. the time taken for blood to travel from the right atrium, through the pulmonary circulation, back to the left ventricle, through the systemic circulation down to the foot and back to the right atrium) is usually about 23 seconds, from around 28 heart beats (Tortora and Anagnostakos, 1981). That is a lot of blood to move, carrying a lot of information. To maintain this flow, and the tissue perfusion rates associated with it (and hence all subsequent physiological processes), an adequate blood pressure is necessary.

Physiological determinants of blood flow

The forces or mechanisms that determine blood flow can be divided into two: those that control flow input (driving pressure gradient) and those that control flow output (resistance to flow; Colbert, 1993). These are shown in Figure 9.1.

As Figure 9.1 illustrates, there are many factors influencing the flow of blood and blood pressure. Circulation is a closed circuit, and the action of one part of the system will influence the rest. Although there are constant fluctuations in cardiac preload caused by the effects of respiration and changes in posture on venous return to the heart, arterial blood pressure remains remarkably constant (Triedman and Saul, 1994). Thus the system is quite adaptable and can compensate for variations within it, although it may not be able to completely compensate for all situations. If one part of the equation falters or is sufficiently compromised, then this places a strain on the other parts, which might seriously compromise overall circulatory efficiency.

The following discussions on the relationship between the musculoskeletal system, body move-

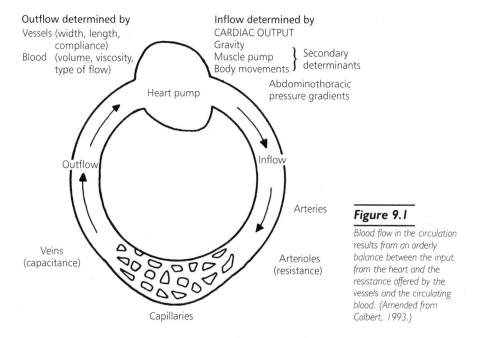

Outflow determined by
Vessels (width, length,
      compliance)
Blood (volume, viscosity,
      type of flow)

Inflow determined by
CARDIAC OUTPUT
Gravity
Muscle pump } Secondary
Body movements } determinants
Abdominothoracic
pressure gradients

Heart pump

Outflow

Inflow

Arteries

Veins
(capacitance)

Arterioles
(resistance)

Capillaries

Figure 9.1

Blood flow in the circulation results from an orderly balance between the input from the heart and the resistance offered by the vessels and the circulating blood. (Amended from Colbert, 1993.)

ment and circulation will concentrate upon the inflow part of the equation, as this is where the 'passive' and massaging effects of musculoskeletal action are most relevant. Factors relating to the outflow part of the equation have been briefly discussed in Chapter 4 (as these factors relate to the neural control of vasoconstriction/dilation within the arterial tree and the relative distribution of blood volume through the various 'parts' of the vascular tree such as the upper limbs, the lower limbs, the abdominal organs and so on).

Later on we will also review the action of the musculoskeletal system on other body fluid movements, such as the peritoneal and pleural fluids and the cerebrospinal fluid.

The relation of body movement to venous and lymphatic fluid dynamics

There are many influences on circulation, both neural and chemical, but one factor is particularly interesting to osteopaths: the influence of the musculoskeletal system and body movement on venous return and also on lymph circulation. And as we shall see, there are specific areas throughout the body where musculoskeletal system activity is thought to directly aid/influence fluid transport.

Clinically, this implies that, where there are some types of circulatory disorder, then certain biomechanical restrictions may be partly or wholly related to these disorders; and also that restoration of mobility/change of use of various body parts and articulations may result in a certain degree of improvement of circulatory efficiency, even if the musculoskeletal factors did not cause the fluid disruption in the first place.

Many diseases and pathophysiological conditions are complicated by poor fluid dynamics and impaired lymphatic flow, and it may be that reducing biomechanical stress on various key structures will reduce limitations to fluid flow in the body and therefore help the body's own self-regulating and self-healing mechanisms to manage the disorder more effectively. (Note: As already stated before, there are various relative contraindications for this type of intervention strategy, which one needs a sound pathological training to appreciate.)

Different body areas affect gross fluid movement

Some of the main 'mechanical' aids to venous return are the calf pumps and the actions of the thoracic diaphragm. The action of the thoracic diaphragm itself is aided by the combined actions of the abdominal wall muscles and the pelvic floor muscles (pelvic diaphragm). Two sites in the body are particularly important for lymphatic circulation. These are the cisterna chyli, situated just underneath the diaphragm, and the thoracic ducts, in the thoracic inlet.

These areas will now be discussed, with reference to how mechanical restriction in the above-mentioned areas can conflict with fluid dynamics and flow.

Calf pumps

Pumps are formed where the calf muscles act as a 'squeezing' influence upon the deep veins within the calf. This 'squeezing' is a very important aid to fluid movement and, although fluid will circulate without its influence, the amount moved in a certain time will be decreased. The deep venous system is an integrated group of veins beginning in the deep venous plexus of the foot and terminating in the lower pelvis. Following contraction of the foot, calf and thigh muscles the blood flows from a multitude of high-pressure veins to a single low-pressure one (Tretbar, 1995). Valves prevent back-flow of fluid into the area just 'drained'.

Clinical relevance

The condition of varicose veins in the lower limbs may be related to poor calf pump mechanics, as well as perhaps a genetic predisposition to weaker connective tissue of the blood vessels.

Osteopaths would say that you need good movement in the articulations of all the lower limb joints, and to a lesser degree those of the pelvis and low back, for the calf pumps to be effective. Osteopaths would consider that there would be a minor decrease in efficiency of the pumping ability within a limb that had suffered, for example:

- repeated strain to the ankle mechanism, such that its movements are permanently affected;
- other traumas to the limb, which may lead to chronically scarred and contracted muscular and fascial components of the limb, leading to a less effective pump mechanism.

However, such factors may have a less detrimental effect on circulation if the function of those muscles/related fascial compartments are somewhat improved by physical therapeutics and exercise/rehabilitation. Care must be taken when working within the mechanics of the lower limb, as direct mobilization of thrombi within blood vessels (a common complication of varicosities) is clearly a risk if soft tissue techniques are carried out unadvisedly. Thus direct mobilization of the calf muscles may not always be carried out in some cases, but work can still be directed at the surrounding articulations and biomechanical factors to have some influence on the situation.

Note: Soft tissue support of the axillary and subclavian veins may also aid venous return from the upper limb. The attachments of the axillary vein are shown in Figure 9.2 to illustrate this. The mechanics of the thoracic inlet are reviewed later.

The calf pumps also aid lymph fluid movement in fascial compartments in the lower limb. Body movement in general aids lymph movement in fascial compartments elsewhere.

Details concerning fluid movement in fascial compartments have already been alluded to in Chapter 3, but are revised and given a little more analysis here.

Where the mechanism governing fluid movement between compartments fails, for whatever reason, there is an immediate and often serious consequence for the function of the part of the body concerned. Increases in intracompartmental tissue pressure result from increases in fluid pressure plus the contributions of cells, fibres, gels and matrices, all limiting drainage of the increased pressure of fluid. The result is an increased venous (and lymphatic) pressure that

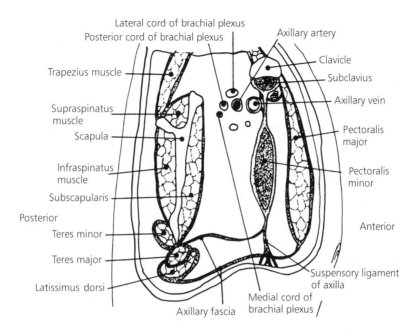

Figure 9.2

Lateral cord of brachial plexus
Posterior cord of brachial plexus
Axillary artery
Trapezius muscle
Clavicle
Subclavius
Supraspinatus muscle
Axillary vein
Scapula
Pectoralis major
Infraspinatus muscle
Pectoralis minor
Subscapularis
Posterior
Anterior
Teres minor
Teres major
Suspensory ligament of axilla
Latissimus dorsi
Axillary fascia
Medial cord of brachial plexus

lowers the arteriovenous pressure gradient, resulting in decreased local blood flow (Mabee and Bostwick, 1993).

One of the most common presentations of failure of fluid movement in the compartments of the body is known as 'compartment syndrome', where pressure builds up within the compartments (Gerow *et al.*, 1993). This leads to an ischaemic condition of the muscles within the affected compartment, and can commonly affect the anterior calf muscles (tibialis anterior) and the multifidus muscles in the lumbar spine, for example.

Another common presentation is where poor compartment dynamics lead to poor fluid drainage, resulting in local tissue oedema. For example, in cases of sprained ankle, there may be tight or injured muscles through the calf area and the calf pumps are likely to be less effective than normal. Also, the compartments of the lower limb may be slightly constrained, as a result of altered mechanics distorting the shape of these structures. All this may mean that the oedema created by the ligamentous injury in the ankle may not drain very efficiently through the restricted compartments and may not be aided by a reduced efficiency of the calf pumps. The

longer the oedema remains, the less effective the tissue healing is, local to the site of damage.

Other sites are also prone to this sort of problem. These include synovial sheaths, the carpal tunnels of the wrist and the tarsal tunnels of the foot.

Altered biomechanics might contribute to tissue strain and irritation, and to an altered shape of some of these compartments that might be constraining to fluid flow. If oedema does build up, this can have increasing clinical significance for related neural and tendon structures, manifesting in carpal tunnel syndrome, for example. The carpal tunnel is illustrated in Figure 9.3.

In fact, any site of tissue injury anywhere in the body, where inflammation and oedema arise, can benefit from therapeutic measures that release surrounding soft tissue tensions to aid local fluid dynamics. Mobilizing the areas and tissues involved is thought to be very beneficial in these cases.

The thoracic diaphragm – its relationship to venous flow

One of the biggest aids to venous flow is the action of the diaphragm, through the cyclical

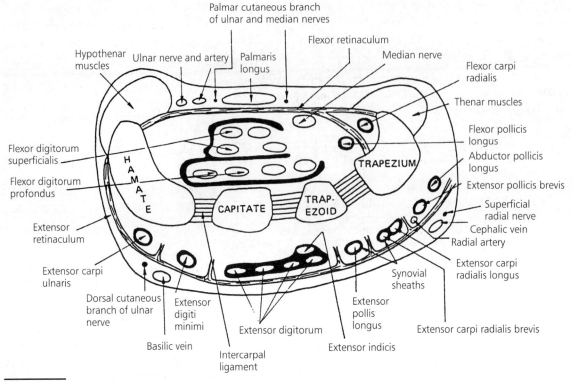

Figure 9.3

Transverse section through the wrist region showing the relationship of the various structures that pass into the hand. (Reproduced with the permission of Butterworth Heinemann Publisahers from Anatomy and Human Movement: Structure and Function, *2nd edn, Palastanga et al., 1994.)*

difference in pressure between the thoracic and abdominal cavities. Diaphragmatic action has influence upon blood circulation, venous return and lymphatic return (as well as influencing peritoneal and pleural fluid movement, as will be discussed later). The diaphragm was illustrated in Figure 8.16.

Treatment of the diaphragm must be one of the most consistent aspects of an osteopath's work, as this structure can influence so many other parts of the body and its effect on biomechanics, physiology and homeostasis is potentially enormous. The diaphragm is one of the most remarkable areas of the body in that it has so much influence and the consequences of its dysfunction can manifest anywhere from the head to the toes.

Many structures are involved with breathing

mechanics, and also in regulating the dynamics of the abdominal wall and the thoracic and pelvic diaphragms, which all work together to ensure effective central venous blood flow. Breathing mechanics have been discussed in Chapter 8, and the point to remind readers of here is that mechanical restriction in the articulations of the thorax and upper lumbar spine may influence diaphragmatic action and so potentially limit its efficiency as a regulator of central venous flow. Physically manipulating the body in an attempt to restore the mechanical function of these various structures and muscular diaphragms may improve venous return.

The thoracic diaphragm aids the calf pump mechanics to maintain somatic venous drainage, but may also influence visceral venous drainage.

Venous circulation within the abdominal cavity

The visceral-abdominal cavity is drained mostly through the portal venous system of veins (although there are some connections between the systemic system of veins and veins coming from the lower part of the intestinal tract).

Any condition that compromises portal circulation, such as many liver pathologies, can lead to back pressure within the portal venous system, which then affects the venous plexi of the intestines. This can often manifest itself in conditions such as oesophageal varicosities and haemorrhoids (rectal varicosities).

Some types of varicosity (such as haemorrhoids) are traditionally considered by osteopaths to also be related, in a number of cases, to poor breathing mechanics. The concept is that poor posture, poor abdominal tone and inefficient pelvic floor and thoracic diaphragm mechanics may affect abdominal venous return to such a degree that varicosities result.

As stated, the thoracic diaphragm works in concert with the abdominal wall muscles and the pelvic floor/diaphragm, which aids pelvic venous drainage. It is worthwhile looking a little more closely at venous drainage within the pelvis, as several factors combine to influence its efficiency.

Pelvic floor mechanics and pelvic venous drainage

Being the most inferiorly placed of the body cavities makes fluid drainage from the pelvis more complex than in other body areas. For this reason, the different parts and tissues of the pelvis must all work together to promote fluid dynamics. In particular the mechanics of the pelvic floor muscles and urogenital diaphragm are increasingly being studied, and are thought to have a considerable role to play in the circulation of the pelvic bowl.

As well as many neurological conditions (such as those arising following childbirth, due to pudendal nerve damage) which affect the function of the pelvic muscles, articular restrictions throughout the pelvis are thought to interfere with effective pelvic floor muscular function. In particular, the sacrococcygeal articulation is considered by osteopaths to affect pelvic floor action if it is damaged. Coccygeal damage is very common, and many patients have at some stage fallen on to their behinds and suffered injury to this region, causing long-term compromised activity within the pelvic floor muscles.

Other factors within the musculoskeletal system that might contribute to inefficient pelvic articular function and poor pelvic floor activity include the mechanics of the lumbosacral joints (as this relates to sacral and sacrococcygeal movement, and general pelvic orientation) and the mobility of the ilia (all of which were discussed in Chapter 7).

Other factors influencing fluid flow in this region include the dynamics of the soft tissues of the internal pelvis. Visceral movement and biomechanics, as we shall see later, are thought to play a role in fluid dynamics within the body cavities as a whole; and within the pelvis, drainage from its deeper parts is aided by a general elastic movement within and around the organs of the pelvis. Organ biomechanics is a 'new concept' for orthodox practitioners and the study of the combined function of the different components of the visceral pelvis can be a fraught one. Many orthodox practitioners still consider the pelvic organs to be unrelated structures, and do not have a concept of integrated movement influencing fluid dynamics. The lack of communication between specialists of the various organs and disorders of the (internal) pelvis was amply illustrated by Wall and DeLancey's parody of the 'hole' pelvis or the 'whole' pelvis, in an article in *Perspectives in Biology and Medicine* (Wall and DeLancey, 1991). There is still much work to be done before an inclusive vision of fluid dynamics and functional organ inter-relations within the pelvis is achieved.

However, any problems with the dynamics of the articular and soft tissue structures of the pelvis, including the organs, can eventually lead to pelvic venous congestion, and releasing/treating these mechanical factors may improve fluid dynamics and therefore tissue health.

Pelvic venous congestion can manifest itself in a number of different ways, such as chronic pelvic pain and internal and external pelvic varices. (Apparently, pelvic venous congestion is a frequently overlooked cause of chronic pelvic pain; Gupta and McCarthy, 1994.) It may also complicate conditions such as prostatitis.

Management
There are various ways of improving venous congestion and the subsequent pain syndromes, but one of the simplest is by performing pelvic floor exercises. Kegel first described the use of exercises (for improving the function of the pelvic floor, which may help to improve pelvic venous drainage) in the 1940s, and various regimens of exercise have now been employed by physiotherapists and others, including osteopaths, for many years (Wallace, 1994).

Osteopaths also have other clinical approaches to improving pelvic floor action (to aid venous circulation) through direct and indirect work to the levator ani muscles and the perineum, and other components within the articular pelvis, and in some cases to the internal soft tissues and organs of the pelvis. There are a number of techniques (internal and external) that could be employed in this region. These must always be employed with sensitivity and respect for the patient.

Local work on the pelvic floor is also necessary in cases of scarring and restricted mobility (following childbirth, for example), which can lead to many other painful conditions and problems with pelvic organ function. Unfortunately there is not the scope to discuss these ideas fully, but some of the case studies will include details of this concept.

The diverse mechanical inter-relations of the somatic pelvis have been discussed in detail in Chapter 7, and the reader should not forget that, to maintain freedom of movement within the pelvic bowl, other parts of the body may have to be treated, to achieve an overall improvement in biomechanical efficiency.

General lymph drainage

Most aspects of this relationship have been discussed before, in relation to compartment dynamics. The fluid from all body compartments is directed to various regional lymph nodes, which collect together and eventually form the thoracic ducts, which return the lymph into the venous circulation at the level of the thoracic inlet. The lymphatic system is shown in Figure 9.4.

Respiration and lymph flow
The lymph effluent from lymph glands and residua from capillary filtrates, along with newly absorbed solvent water, join the blood circulation during pulmonary inspiration in volumes proportional to the volume of air inspired with each breath (Shields, 1992).

Thus, if the rib cage cannot expand well or the diaphragm is not working very efficiently, then lymph return may be compromised. Any restriction in the articulations and their accompanying soft tissues (muscular and ligamentous) of the rib cage and associated spinal articulations could have a degree of influence on tidal volume of air moved during respiration (Tucker and Jenkins, 1996) and hence affect lymph flow at the same time.

Respiratory mechanics can influence three particular structures that are very important for lymphatic drainage throughout the body. These are the cisterna chyli and the two thoracic ducts.

The thoracic ducts
The two thoracic ducts allow all lymph within the body to return to the venous and therefore the systemic circulation, and so find its way to all the regulatory organs that determine the chemical constituents of all body fluids. The thoracic ducts enter the venous circulation by opening into the junction between the jugular vein and the brachiocephalic vein, on each side of the body. Osteopaths regard this entry point as a bit of a design fault in that the vessels passing through the thoracic inlet are prone to compression by the muscular and/or bony elements that make up the thoracic inlet. The thoracic ducts are shown in Figure 9.5.

The thoracic inlet
Because of the above, the thoracic inlet is in need of special consideration in relation to fluid

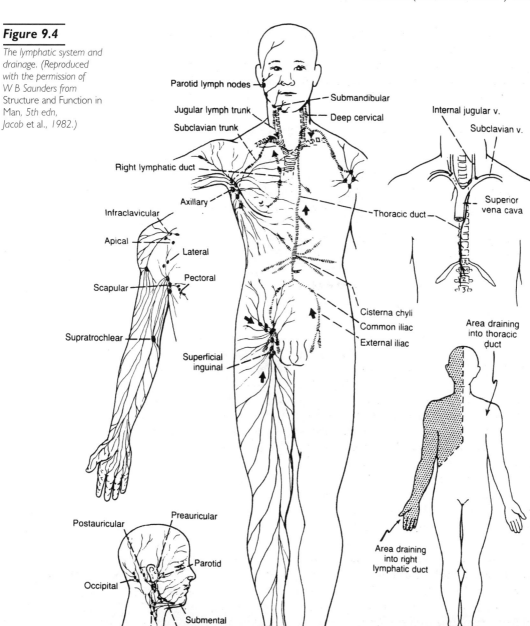

Figure 9.4

The lymphatic system and drainage. (Reproduced with the permission of W B Saunders from Structure and Function in Man, 5th edn, Jacob et al., 1982.)

dynamics. The anatomical complexity of this region leads to very intricate and inter-related biomechanics between the neural, fascial, muscular, visceral and vascular structures that run through this area. This complexity makes the consequences of mechanical distortion very interesting to analyse. The thoracic inlet is shown in Figure 9.6.

Figure 9.5

The left and right thoracic ducts. (Reproduced with the permission of Churchill Livingstone from Gray's Anatomy, 36th edn, Williams and Warwick, 1980.)

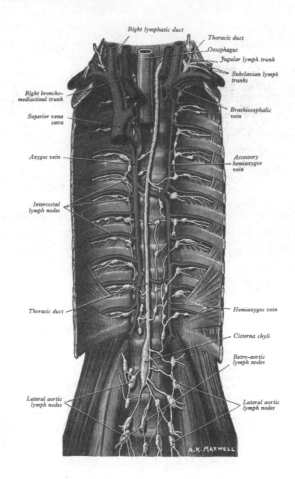

Clinical application

Any physical restriction within and around the thoracic inlet is perceived to limit/reduce lymph circulation and entry into the systemic circulation. Thoracic inlet mechanics can also compromise venous return from the upper limb (Blanchard *et al.*, 1992; see again Figure 9.2) and contribute to symptoms of swelling, heaviness, fatigue and cyanosis in the upper limb (Liebenson, 1988). This condition is commonly known as 'thoracic outlet syndrome' (or 'inlet syndrome', depending on how you view it!). This syndrome includes vascular events as described and also peripheral neuropathy of the brachial plexus as it passes through this region.

Freedom of movement at this level is essential for the health of the whole body because of its influence on general lymphatic circulation and hence immunity. This occurs because not only can the vascular and neural components become constricted and irritated, so too can the thoracic ducts, as they enter the venous system in this region. If the thoracic ducts are constricted in any way, this will affect lymphatic drainage, with resultant compromise in general lymphatic flow, compromising health and immunity. Even tissues quite distant from the thoracic inlet might end up with a type of 'lymphatic varicosity and congestion' due to pressure at the level of the thoracic inlet. This might influence the progression of or recovery from a variety of disorders, ranging from sinusitis to fractured wrist, stomach ulcer or any tissue irritation/damage that can be thought to be indirectly influenced by maintaining

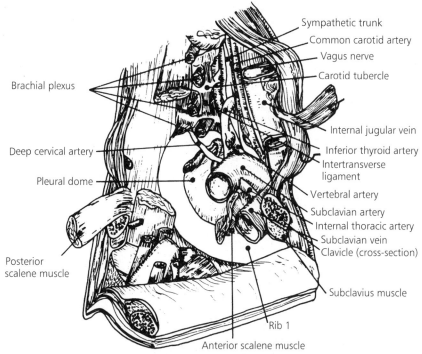

Figure 9.6

Sympathetic trunk
Common carotid artery
Vagus nerve
Carotid tubercle
Brachial plexus
Internal jugular vein
Inferior thyroid artery
Intertransverse ligament
Deep cervical artery
Vertebral artery
Pleural dome
Subclavian artery
Internal thoracic artery
Subclavian vein
Clavicle (cross-section)
Subclavius muscle
Posterior scalene muscle
Rib 1
Anterior scalene muscle

adequate lymph movement at the level of the thoracic inlet (according to osteopathic theory).

Osteopathic perspective
Osteopaths would argue that, before massaging a local area to promote fluid movement, it is necessary to look at the major drainage sites first (such as the thoracic inlet and the thoracolumbar junction of the spine and diaphragm, to influence the cisterna chyli) and then move 'backwards' (peripherally), releasing structures that were found to be restricted in some way and therefore promoting lymph flow from the initial lymphatics back to the systemic circulation. Releasing local fluids only to have their passage blocked or impeded by tension in more central areas makes little therapeutic sense.

The shoulder girdle
When considering the thoracic inlet in general and locally, for the drainage of the upper limb and axillary region (and therefore also the breast), the orientation of the upper limb and

shoulder girdle cannot be overlooked in the clinical evaluation of lymph and venous drainage. Figure 9.2 showed the attachments of the axillary vein. Mechanical torsion in the region of the shoulder girdle may well adversely affect fluid dynamics in this and neighbouring vessels.

Dysfunction within the biomechanics of the shoulder girdle can lead to alterations in clavicular orientation and restrictions of the first rib, scalenes and many other tissues that make up the thoracic inlet. As the mechanics of the shoulder girdle also influence the mechanics of the anterior throat, there is also the possibility the restriction here (at the shoulder) will influence the drainage of the head and neck region (mediated through the thoracic inlet area) and therefore influence the progress of such things as sinusitis, chronic nasopharyngeal infection/irritation, chronic tonsillitis, and so on. Some of the case studies will highlight this point.

The torsional factors within the biomechanics of the shoulder, neck and throat regions have been discussed in Chapter 8, and readers are referred back to that chapter for further clinical insights.

The cisterna chyli

The diaphragm and other structures of the thoracic cage are also important as they influence the cisterna chyli, which is the meeting point for the lymphatic drainage of all structures below the diaphragm – both visceral and somatic (including the lower limbs). Some of this abdominal lymph drains directly into the thorax via the thoracic ducts but these structures are also clearly influenced by diaphragmatic action. The position of the cisterna chyli can be seen in Figure 9.5. However, this did not include its relations to the diaphragm, which are shown in Figure 9.7.

The diaphragm can influence the activity of the cisterna chyli by several means. These include the ability of a diaphragm that is 'too tight' to physically constrict the cisterna and inhibit the easy flow of lymph through into the thoracic duct. Associated with this is the idea that any reduced movement of the diaphragm will contribute to tension in the fascia overlying the anterior lumbar spine and associated structures, and that this can further 'constrict' the cisterna. Long-term reduced movement of the thoracolumbar and upper lumbar regions of the spine eventually means that there is also little 'external massaging' of the cisterna, thus reducing the pump to relying only on its own motility. This concept can be expanded by considering torsion at the thoracolumbar region and how tightness in the psoas or quadratus muscles may affect the orientation of this region and of the 12th rib. These factors can adversely affect the tension in the arcuate ligaments of the diaphragm, further compromising the drainage of the cisterna as it passes lymph through these areas to the thoracic ducts.

Therefore, improving mobility and reducing tension and restriction in all the above mentioned regions may improve the drainage from the abdominopelvic cavity and the lower limbs, and so aid tissue health and recovery in these areas.

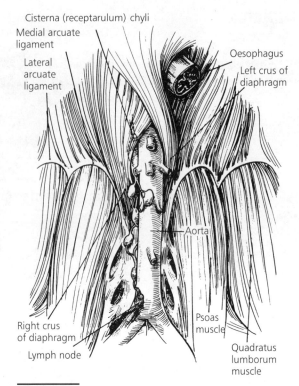

Figure 9.7

The diaphragm and related structures, showing especially the relationship of the cisterna chyli to the crura. (Reproduced with the permission of Sutherland Cranial Teaching Foundation, Inc. from Teaching in the Science of Osteopathy, Sutherland, 1990.)

THE FLOW OF OTHER FLUID SYSTEMS WITHIN THE BODY CAVITIES

That musculoskeletal function is necessary for both venous and lymph return is a well-established principle. What is not so well explored is the influence of body movement on the dynamics of other fluids in the body.

Osteopaths consider, for example, that body movement influences fluid dynamics (to a greater or lesser extent) within the peritoneal and pleural cavities (Ahrenholz and Simmons, 1988; Negrini *et al.*, 1994) and to a lesser degree it may also influence the circulation of the cerebrospinal fluid, although this is less certain (Flanagan, 1988). It will be of interest to explore this mechanical relation to the fluid flow within the body cavities, to appreciate the rationale for osteopathic manipulation of the body to aid various disease and disorders within these cavities (and their organs).

The physiological and pathophysiological role of fluid flow within the body cavities

Organ health is in part maintained by the flow of the serous fluids of the body: the peritoneal, pleural and pericardial fluids. There is a fine balance between production of these fluids and their drainage, in order to keep cavity fluid dynamics in equilibrium. There are a variety of mechanisms and disorders that can disrupt fluid flow in these areas and lead to disequilibrium in the fluid dynamics, and we will be discussing those related to the mechanics of the body.

An important point was made in an earlier chapter: that if there is restriction to fluid flow this may compromise tissue health and predispose to disease. Also, if an organ becomes diseased for whatever reason, various restrictions in relevant parts of the musculoskeletal system may limit recovery potential in the diseased organ, as continued oedema and poor fluid dynamics within the tissues are maintained by poor movement in the musculoskeletal system.

In the event of organ disease becoming established, there is often an increase in fluid quantities within the cavities (inflammation, for example, causes exudation of fluids and contributes to oedema). Additionally, this fluid is not always most effectively drained, and so oedema in the tissues builds up and increased fluid pressure in the serous spaces can result. Depending on the cause of fluid build-up, there is sometimes the need for this to be surgically released, or addressed through pharmacological means. However, in general, maintaining good lymph drainage by mechanical means is essential to the eventual restoration of normal fluid levels.

As the disease process continues, or subsides, fluid flow often remains disturbed. This may mean that there is a chronic oedematous state, in the lungs of asthmatics or chronic bronchitics, for example, or long-standing oedema in the tissues consequent to chronic inflammation, e.g. in the wall of the bladder in interstitial cystitis, the intestinal wall in Crohn's disease or the wall of the bile duct and gall-bladder in biliary dyskinesia, and many other conditions. In these situations, the presence of the oedema itself may be a partial maintaining factor for the disease process in that organ, as reduced flow rate of the serous fluid, and lymph flow in general, is compromising to immune function and to the normal chemical environment at a cellular level. These factors can encourage the ongoing disease state.

There are several ways to address this, but the one we will concern ourselves with here is the role of the musculoskeletal system in cavity fluid dynamics and the concept of visceral articulations (motion between the organs in the cavities) as an aid to effective fluid dynamics.

Peritoneal circulation

Fluid is both filtered into and absorbed from the peritoneal space through the peritoneum. Numerous large lymphatic channels lead from the peritoneal surface of the diaphragm. With each diaphragmatic excursion significant quantities of lymph flow out of the peritoneal cavity into the thoracic duct (diZerega and Rodgers, 1992). Fluid also flows into the mesenteries and from there into the mesenteric lymph nodes, before draining into the cisterna chyli, from there to the thoracic duct and ultimately to the venous circulation. The peritoneal fluid within the peritoneal cavity migrates/drains along several 'routes' defined by the shape and orientation of the folds of the peritoneum, as illustrated in Figure 9.8.

The influence of organ mobility

It is recognized that the mobility of the small bowel tends to limit the accumulation of fluid in the central portion of the peritoneal cavity under normal circumstances (Ahrenholz and Simmons, 1988) and it may be that there is some physiological advantage in ensuring good mobility between the abdominal organs to help fluid movement. The clinical relevance of this is still to be explored, and the general subject of visceral articulations will be discussed a little later.

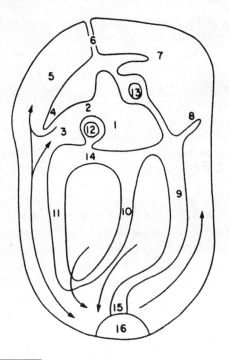

Figure 9.8

Direction of flow of the peritoneal fluid. (Reproduced with the permission of Springer Verlag from The Peritoneum, *DiZerega and Rodgers, 1992.)*

Thoracic diaphragm influence on peritoneal fluid movement

Movement in the subdiaphragmatic part of the peritoneal cavity is very important for peritoneal fluid movement (Williams and Warwick, 1980). At one time there was thought to be an increased rate of absorption at the subdiaphragmatic portion of the diaphragm attributed to small 'slits'/apertures in the diaphragmatic peritoneum. These supposedly allowed movement of peritoneal fluid into the lymphatic vessels of the diaphragm, and postoperatively people would be inclined slightly so that any infectious or other noxious material would not enter the systemic circulation by being allowed to pool in the subdiaphragmatic region as it might if the patient was laid supine. This explanation of increased absorption was at one time discredited when anatomists decided that the slits were in fact small breaks in the peritoneum due to damage

caused by autopsy and dissection. However, there are now scanning electron microscope pictures of similar structures – stomata – indicating a direct route for the drainage of peritoneal fluid into the diaphragmatic lymphatics (diZerega and Rodgers, 1992). Therefore there *are* direct drainage routes associated with the diaphragm but it is probably also the fact of the large area of peritoneum found in the subdiaphragmatic region, rather than just these stomata, that gives the impression of increased drainage rates at this level.

That said, movement of the diaphragm and lower rib cage is clearly important to subdiaphragmatic lymph/peritoneal fluid drainage, as when it is reduced the drainage becomes impaired.

Other factors

Although peritoneal fluid does indeed enter the diaphragmatic initial lymphatics during expiration (Aukland and Reed, 1993), this is not the only way that lymph transport can be facilitated: stretching of tissues containing the initial lymphatics seems to increase fluid transport tenfold and it seems reasonable to hypothesize that gross body movement passing through the torso, coupled with respiration and the relative movement of one organ against its neighbour during these activities, would gently stretch and mobilize the peritoneum in that region, aiding fluid movement into the mesenteric lymphatics.

This aspect may well have a practical clinical application, in that external mobilization of the thorax and abdomen, and mobilizing the organs to ensure their relative mobility, may aid peritoneal drainage/promote fluid movement. Visceral biomechanics are discussed below.

Peritoneal fluid movement is complicated by adhesion formation

Any adhesion within the abdominopelvic cavity will affect the relative mobility of the organs and, depending on its site and extent, may limit the overall flow of peritoneal fluid. Adhesion formation is a complicated subject, but an osteopathic hypothesis is outlined below where reduced movement and flow of the peritoneal fluid is thought to be related to adhesion formation.

Adhesion formation: a hypothesis
One exciting aspect would be to evaluate the usefulness of gentle mobilizing of the abdomen postoperatively to evaluate whether this seemed to have any effect on the occurrence of adhesion formation, which is very disabling (in some cases) for the patient and an expensive complication (in terms of ongoing management) for the healthcare provider (diZerega and Rodgers, 1992).

Postoperatively/postinfection, there may well be a degree of viscotrophic change to the peritoneal fluid, in that inflammatory products make it more thick/viscous and therefore slower to circulate, these factors contributing to adhesion formation. In general, the distance travelled by peritoneal fluid and the material within it (which is a measure of the effectiveness of peritoneal fluid flow) depends upon its volume, viscosity and the specific gravity of the material (diZerega and Rodgers, 1992). Peritoneal fluid is a serous fluid and, in a similar way to the reduced movement in joints affecting synovial fluid viscosity and hence function (Chapter 5), poor movement/mobilization of peritoneal fluid may affect its viscotrophic qualities. Poor cavity dynamics and reduced organ mobility may therefore affect the state of the peritoneal fluid in the region of reduced mobility and lead to a tendency to adhesion formation. Reduced organ movement and reduced cavity dynamics are associated with organ disease and surgical intervention and their healing consequences. However, if the organ mobility is not re-established, then the peritoneal fluid may remain in too adapted a state (viscous) and so promote adhesion formation rather than reducing the likelihood of it.

On that note, an understanding of the 'articulations' and 'sliding surfaces' within the abdomen and pelvis may help illustrate how body movement and therapeutic manipulation of the organs may be of benefit in improving, maintaining or even restoring fluid dynamics in the peritoneal space and in maintaining good abdominopelvic organ function. This will be reviewed below, and later.

Pleural drainage

The mechanics of the pleural space have long been controversial. There is some dispute as to the relevance of respiratory mechanics on pleural fluid transport (Allum *et al.*, 1995) but some authors do believe this factor to be an important part of a framework of factors influencing pleural fluid dynamics (Lai-Fook and Rodarte, 1991). This framework is as follows:

Pleural pressure, the force acting to inflate the lung within the thorax, is generated by the opposing elastic recoils of the lung and chest wall and the forces generated by the respiratory muscles. The spatial variation of pleural pressure is a result of complex force interactions among the lung and other structures that make up the thorax. Gravity contributes one of the forces that act on these structures, and regional lung expansion and pleural pressure distribution change with changes in body orientation. Forces are transmitted directly between the chest wall and the lung through a very thin but continuous pleural liquid space. The pressure in the pleural liquid equals the pressure acting to expand the lung. Pleural liquid is not in hydrostatic equilibrium, and viscous flow of pleural liquid is driven by the combined effect of the gravitational force acting on the liquid and the pressure distribution imposed by the surrounding structures. The dynamics of pleural liquid are considered an integral part of a continuous microvascular filtration into the pleural space. Similar concepts apply to the pulmonary interstitium. Regional differences in lung volume expansion also result in regional differences in interstitial pressure within the lung parenchyma and thus affect regional lung fluid filtration.

The essential part of this statement is that the elasticity and mechanics of the chest wall are important to pleural fluid flow. This indicates that poor biomechanics of the thoracic cage may have a degree of influence on pleural fluid transport, and with this in mind some researchers are looking into the clinical relevance of using respiration (for example) to increase pleural fluid drainage in cases of pleural effusion (Dechman *et al.*, 1993) although, so far, any positive clinical effects are short lived.

Clinical application

The maintenance of a sufficient pleural fluid distribution to all parts of the lung and pleural cavities is thought by osteopaths to be essential for the healthy and optimum function of the lungs and their ability to resist infection/other disease processes. Also, when there is dysfunction/ disease within the lung/pleural cavity it may be useful to ensure movement of the thoracic cage, so that lymph and pleural fluid movement are maintained at as optimal a level as possible. There are many situations in which pleural effusion occurs, the mechanisms of which can be complex (Sahn, 1990; Alberts *et al.*, 1991), and it may be that respiration or manipulation of the thorax is clinically useful in these cases.

This may not be therapeutically advisable in all cases, though, as certainly in acute bacterial infection of the lung, mobility of the thorax is naturally reduced to help combat and contain the infection, so externally overcoming this mechanism by physically manipulating the thorax might be counterproductive. However, in chronic inflammatory and infection states, this immobility may in fact be a maintaining factor for the chronicity of the disease state, as it further inhibits fluid drainage. Chronic respiratory diseases such as bronchitis and asthma are both associated with increased fluid in the lung tissues, which compounds the decreased lung function. In these long-standing situations, increasing the mobility of the thoracic cage may prove beneficial in that it aids the immune response and the local health of the tissues of the lung by improving interstitial drainage and fluid movement. (The osteopathic management of a case of asthma will be reviewed later.)

Although mobilizing diseased tissue remains rightly controversial, with any vigorous manipulations being strongly contraindicated, readers should note that there are a whole variety of gentle and indirect mobilizations that might be safely clinically employed by an experienced practitioner, with a view to improving the underlying pathological condition.

Pericardial fluid movement

With respect to pericardial fluid circulation, it can be seen that this fluid helps to permit relatively unobstructed cardiac movement within the mediastinum.

Pericardial sac mobility and elasticity are thought to be related to cardiac efficiency, and, if anything were to constrain the pericardium or limit its viscoelastic properties (which can normally accommodate a degree of change in the size of the heart itself; Freeman, 1990), this might affect cardiac efficiency or pericardial lymph flow/fluid mechanics.

The fibrous pericardium is attached via the sternopericardial ligament to the sternum and one osteopathic hypothesis is that injury and restriction within the sternal articulations and hence the sternopericardial ligament may influence the viscoelasticity of the pericardium and thus cardiac physiology. The sternopericardial ligament is shown in Figure 9.9.

As an aetiological factor in cardiac pathology it is probably very minor, but in situations of postmyocardial infarction or open chest surgery for cardiac pathology or other organ dysfunction, it may be relevant for posthealing fluid dynamics and consequent function of the cardiac/pericardial relationship. Osteopaths therefore have various ideas concerning supportive care for this type of patient, which at the very least may help with postoperative pain and discomfort and may have other beneficial effects in cardiac function.

All sorts of conditions and traumas may affect the mobility of the anterior rib cage and the mobility of the sternum in particular, which may in some way interfere with pericardial sac mechanics. These include blows to the anterior chest, whiplash/seat-belt injuries to the anterior chest, rib fractures and so on, all of which can be treated with osteopathic manipulations.

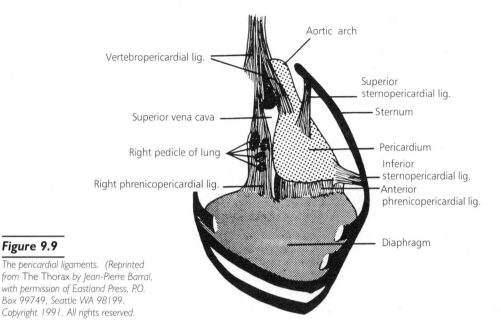

Aortic arch

Vertebropericardial lig.

Superior
sternopericardial lig.

Sternum

Superior vena cava

Right pedicle of lung

Pericardium

Inferior
sternopericardial lig.

Right phrenicopericardial lig.

Anterior
phrenicopericardial lig.

Diaphragm

Figure 9.9

The pericardial ligaments. (Reprinted from The Thorax *by Jean-Pierre Barral, with permission of Eastland Press, P.O. Box 99749, Seattle WA 98199. Copyright 1991. All rights reserved.*

Note: The above perspectives are not clinical fact and are only borne out empirically by various reports of osteopaths helping these types of patient. Unfortunately, there is currently insufficient clinical investigation of this approach to be able to comment further, although the approach is logical enough to warrant consideration.

VISCERAL BIOMECHANICS WITHIN OSTEOPATHY

The concept that organ mobility is important to fluid dynamics has now been mentioned several times. It is an interesting concept, and forms part of the osteopathic considerations of organ mobility and the effect this can have on both visceral function and musculoskeletal function. The author has a special interest in visceral biomechanics and function within osteopathy (Stone, 1992, 1995, 1996a, b) and what follows is a brief introduction to this very large subject.

Osteopathic techniques applied to the organs have a long history within the profession and are used not only in relation to fluid dynamics but also to aid smooth muscle function and influence

somatic biomechanics. A few decades ago, though, very few osteopaths were regularly using these types of technique, and much of value to the profession and its patients was being lost. However, over the last 5–10 years there has been a renewed interest in visceral techniques and the profession is at last re-grasping the significance of such concepts. Several European osteopaths have also been instrumental in re-establishing an interest in visceral biomechanics. J. P. Barral and P. Mercier have been two of the most ardent in this endeavour (Barral and Mercier, 1988).

Visceral biomechanics relate to the movements that the organs make against each other and against the walls of the body cavities that contain them. The viscera 'articulate' by utilizing sliding surfaces formed by the peritoneal (and pleural or pericardial) membranes that surround the organs and line the body cavities. The 'ligaments' that support the organs and guide their 'axes of movement' are formed by the peritoneal attachments of the organs to the body cavities (and pleural or pericardial attachments to the mediastinal fascia and thoracic cavity, for example).

Movement passes through the visceral structures as a consequence of normal locomotion, and other general body movements such as bending, and consequent to processes such as defecation, micturition and respiration. As the body cavities distort and change their shape, so the individual organs must adapt to these changes, and they do so by slightly sliding over each other, given the constraints of their attachments and surrounds.

Organ movement can help promote fluid flow within the cavities, as already suggested, and organ movement, in the sense of an external massaging of the organs by movement, seems to be beneficial to visceral function (as with the effect of respiratory motion on gut peristalsis). Restriction and tension in the body cavities can limit visceral motion possibilities and so compromise function and fluid flow. Conversely, restriction (tension, scarring and adhesion formation) within and between the organs and their sliding surfaces can create adverse tension within the suspensory ligaments of the organs and so create tension in those parts of the musculoskeletal system to which the organs are attached.

Thus there can be mechanical links between the viscera and the musculoskeletal system, and restrictions within the visceral field may be very relevant to the efficient functioning of the bio-mechanical arrangement of the musculoskeletal system. These links are in addition to the neural links (mediated by the autonomic nervous system) that were discussed in earlier chapters.

Outlined in Figures 9.10–9.13 are some examples of organ articulations, and some indication of which viscera may contribute tension (through their mechanical inter-relations) with the musculoskeletal system.

Considering organ biomechanics also includes looking at the state of the smooth muscle walls of the organs and the connective tissues within the organs. Many organ dysfunctions and disease express themselves as or are complicated by problems of visceromotion and elasticity within the soft tissues of the organ (adverse peristalsis, bladder contractility and respiratory system compliance, for example). Improving the tone of the smooth muscle walls of the hollow organs and improving the elasticity of the connective tissue

components can be beneficial for visceromotion and the internal circulation of the organ tissues. These concepts are also relevant for solid organs such as the kidneys and liver, and relate to their capsules and to their internal architecture and connective tissue components.

Tension and contracture can be induced in these tissues following inflammation and infection, but also by poor general movement through and within the tissues. All the discussion in previous chapters on movement and connective tissue function is relevant here. Altered movement, elasticity and compliance will, through the inter-relationship between extracellular matrix and fluid interactions and cell membrane function, influence cellular communication, health, immunity and therefore function. Many visceral disorders can be improved by releasing tensions within and around the organs, although this has to be done carefully, as visceral structures are delicate and there can be relative contraindications to manipulating tissues that are diseased, as has already been pointed out.

Visceral manipulation is a complicated subject and cannot be discussed in great detail here, although, as stated, it may have relevance to the osteopathic management of a variety of visceral diseases and dysfunctions, and musculoskeletal biomechanical problems. Several of the case studies will highlight these points, however.

OTHER LINKS BETWEEN BODY MOVEMENT AND FLUID DYNAMICS

Cerebrospinal fluid circulation

Fluid dynamics within the cranium and spinal column and the intervertebral foramina

The circulation of the cerebrospinal fluid is very important for the healthy and effective function of the central nervous system. The cerebrospinal fluid spaces, and direction of circulation are shown in Figure 9.14.

It is always surprising to realize that the brain is 80% water and that 20% of that water is extracellular (Kandel *et al.*, 1991). Cerebrospinal fluid

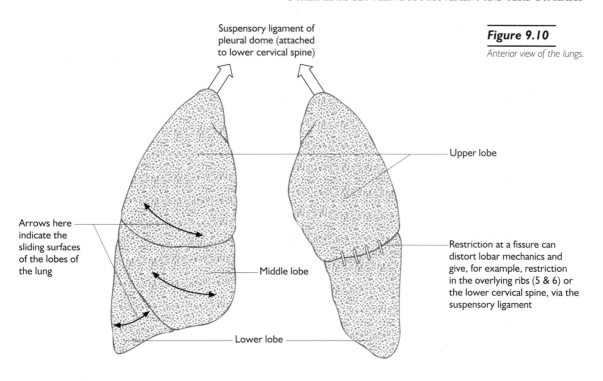

Figure 9.10

Anterior view of the lungs.

Suspensory ligament of pleural dome (attached to lower cervical spine)

Upper lobe

Arrows here indicate the sliding surfaces of the lobes of the lung

Restriction at a fissure can distort lobar mechanics and give, for example, restriction in the overlying ribs (5 & 6) or the lower cervical spine, via the suspensory ligament

Middle lobe

Lower lobe

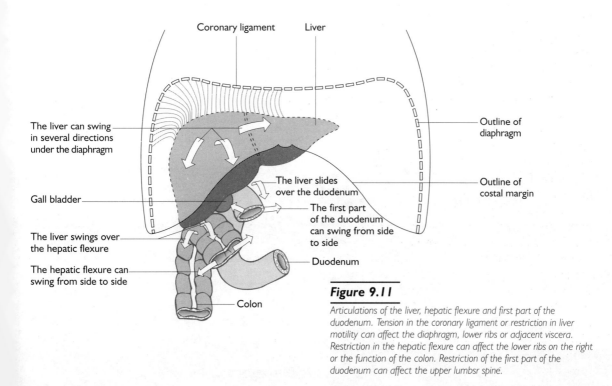

Coronary ligament

Liver

The liver can swing in several directions under the diaphragm

Outline of diaphragm

The liver slides over the duodenum

Outline of costal margin

Gall bladder

The first part of the duodenum can swing from side to side

The liver swings over the hepatic flexure

Duodenum

The hepatic flexure can swing from side to side

Colon

Figure 9.11

Articulations of the liver, hepatic flexure and first part of the duodenum. Tension in the coronary ligament or restriction in liver motility can affect the diaphragm, lower ribs or adjacent viscera. Restriction in the hepatic flexure can affect the lower ribs on the right or the function of the colon. Restriction of the first part of the duodenum can affect the upper lumbsr spine.

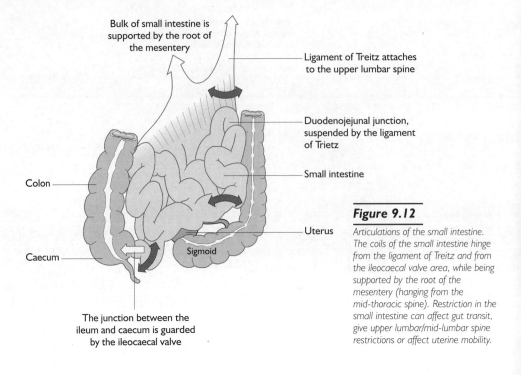

Bulk of small intestine is supported by the root of the mesentery

Ligament of Treitz attaches to the upper lumbar spine

Duodenojejunal junction, suspended by the ligament of Treitz

Small intestine

Colon

Uterus

Caecum

Sigmoid

The junction between the ileum and caecum is guarded by the ileocaecal valve

Figure 9.12

Articulations of the small intestine. The coils of the small intestine hinge from the ligament of Treitz and from the ileocaecal valve area, while being supported by the root of the mesentery (hanging from the mid-thoracic spine). Restriction in the small intestine can affect gut transit, give upper lumbar/mid-lumbar spine restrictions or affect uterine mobility.

Figure 9.13

The articulations of the uterus. Tension in the ligaments of the uterus can give a variety of problems – affecting the bladder, rectum, sacrum, piriformis and vaginal mechanics, for example.

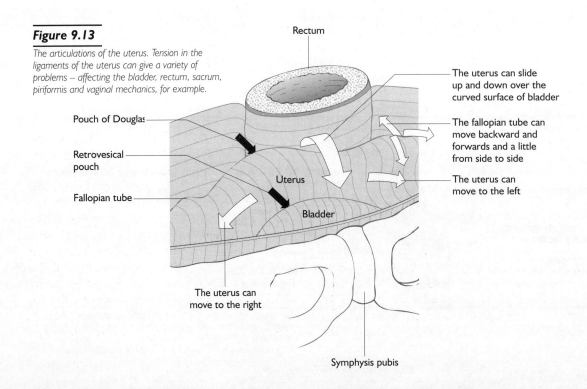

Rectum

Pouch of Douglas

Retrovesical pouch

Fallopian tube

Uterus

The uterus can move to the right

Bladder

Symphysis pubis

The uterus can slide up and down over the curved surface of bladder

The fallopian tube can move backward and forwards and a little from side to side

The uterus can move to the left

Figure 9.14

The distribution of the cerebrospinal fluid. (Reproduced with the permission of Appleton & Lange from Principles of Neural Science, 3rd edn, Kandel et al., 1991.)

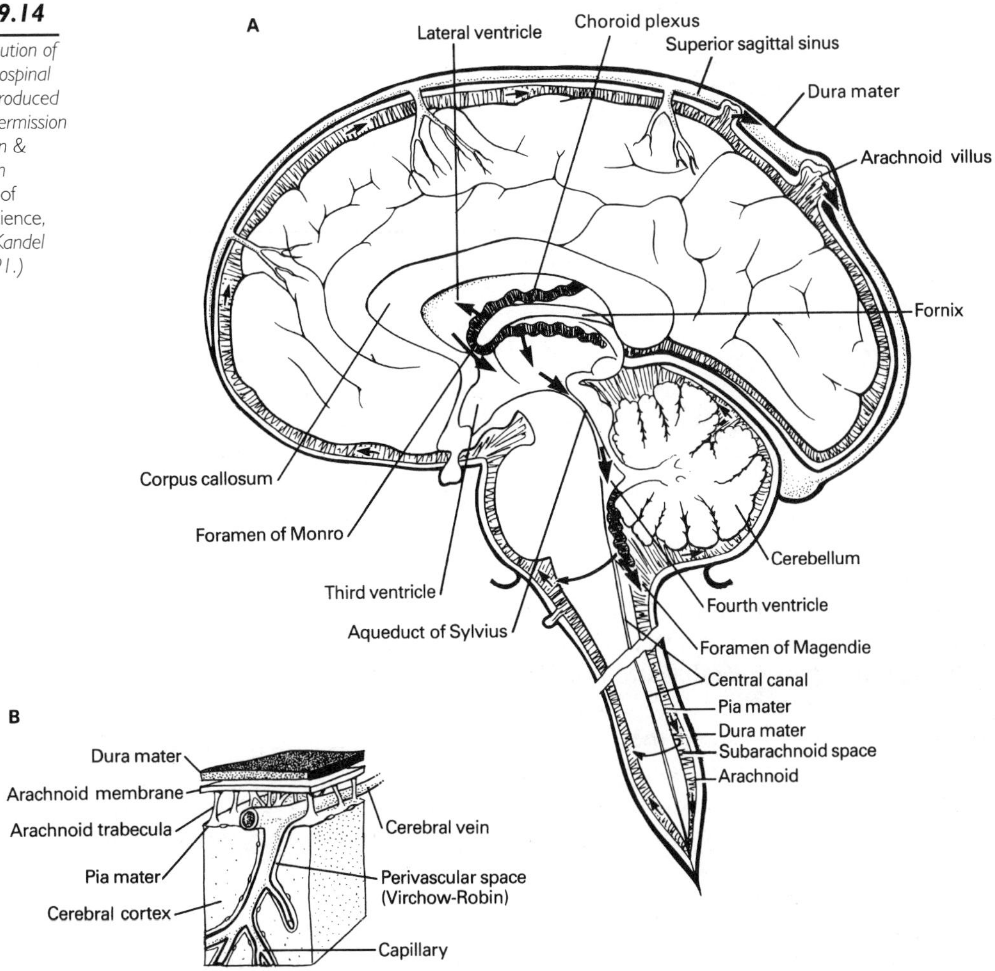

is an important determinant of the extracellular fluid that bathes neurones and glia in the central nervous system.

Most of the cerebrospinal fluid (CSF) is found in the four ventricles and it is secreted by the choroid plexus in the lateral ventricles. CSF flows from the lateral ventricles through the interventricular foramen (of Monro) into the third ventricle. From here it flows into the fourth ventricle through the cerebral aqueduct (of Sylvius) and then through the foramina of Magendie and Luschka into the subarachnoid space. The subarachnoid space lies between the arachnoid mater and the pia mater, which together with the dura mater form the three meningeal layers that cover the brain. Within the subarachnoid space, fluid flows down the spinal canal and also upwards over the convexity of the brain.

The CSF flowing over the brain extends into the sulci and the depths of the cerebral cortex in extensions of the subarachnoid space (called 'Virchow–Robin', or 'perivascular' spaces) along blood vessels. Small solutes diffuse freely between the extracellular fluid and the CSF in these perivascular spaces and across the ependymal lining of the ventricular system, facilitating the movement of solutes from deep within the cerebral hemispheres out to cortical subarachnoid spaces and the ventricular system. The CSF drains into the ventricular system through special

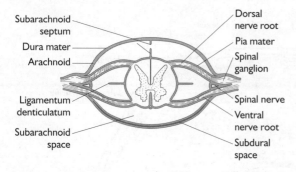

Subarachnoid
septum

Dura mater

Arachnoid

Ligamentum
denticulatum

Subarachnoid
space

Dorsal
nerve root

Pia mater

Spinal
ganglion

Spinal nerve

Ventral
nerve root

Subdural
space

Figure 9.15

*Transverse section through the spinal cord and its membranes.
(Redrawn from Gray's Anatomy, 36th edn, Williams and Warwick,
1980.)*

structures called arachnoid villi. It is generally held that there is less active flow within the vertebral canal but diffusion and body movement may aid fluid concentration throughout the whole extent of the subarachnoid space. The CSF is also thought to drain back locally into the venous system through the vertebral venous plexi, the intervertebral veins and the posterior intercostal and upper lumbar veins into the azygos and hemiazygos veins (Williams and Warwick, 1980). A transverse section through the spinal cord and its membranes, in Figure 9.15, shows the subarachnoid space.

In his book *The Philosophy and Mechanical Principles of Osteopathy*, A. T. Still said: 'A thought strikes him that the cerebrospinal fluid is one of the highest known elements that are contained within the body, and unless the brain furnishes this fluid in abundance, a disabled condition of the body will remain.' By this he understands the physiological importance of the CSF to nerve tissue function; something that is not in doubt.

Body movement and cerebrospinal fluid circulation

Although the production of CSF is a physiological event, giving a cyclical/wave-like production of fluid, body movement is thought to be influential to the flow of CSF through the spaces mentioned above (Flanagan, 1988).

The cranium and (to a lesser extent) the spinal column may seem like areas of the body whose internal shape and size are not very changeable (unlike the thoracic and abdominal cavities, in contrast). However, fluid circulation must also be maintained, and through the arrangement of the membranes, meninges and dura, there is a complex shifting web of subtle mechanical influence that can aid the circulation of the cerebrospinal fluid from deep within the cerebral hemispheres, around the brain and along the length of the spinal cord to the peripheral nerve roots of the spinal nerves and cranial nerves.

As we shall see, movement within the spinal column may affect the dural mechanics and so potentially influence cerebrospinal fluid flow, and may also affect neural mechanics. However, there is another idea within osteopathy, that movement of the bones of the skull, even in adults, may contribute to CSF flow. This is discussed below.

MOTION WITHIN THE HEAD

The idea that the different bones of the head actually articulate against each other and form an integrated part of the biomechanical arrangement of the body is one that is quite perplexing to the orthodox medical profession. However, it has a unique place within osteopathic thought processes, and has much clinical relevance for a very wide range of problems and disorders.

Figure 9.16 shows a drawing of a disarticulated skull. This picture of the component parts of an adult skull shows that, far from being one solid bony structure, the human skull has a very intricate design, with the bones of the skull interlocking into a three-dimensional cavity containing the central nervous system and other structures.

One fundamental osteopathic belief is that no part of the human form is designed 'by accident' – in other words, even given a darwinian approach to changes/variations in design between species, each part of that design has arisen to perform a given and important function.

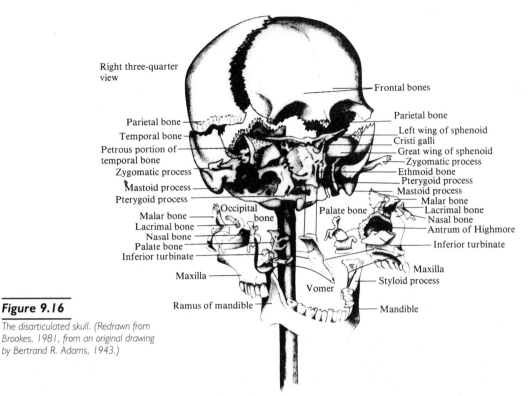

Right three-quarter view

Frontal bones
Parietal bone
Parietal bone
Temporal bone
Left wing of sphenoid
Petrous portion of temporal bone
Cristi galli
Great wing of sphenoid
Zygomatic process
Zygomatic process
Ethmoid bone
Mastoid process
Pterygoid process
Pterygoid process
Mastoid process
Malar bone
Occipital bone
Palate bone
Lacrimal bone
Malar bone
Nasal bone
Lacrimal bone
Antrum of Highmore
Nasal bone
Inferior turbinate
Palate bone
Inferior turbinate
Maxilla
Maxilla
Styloid process
Vomer
Ramus of mandible
Mandible

Figure 9.16

The disarticulated skull. (Redrawn from Brookes, 1981, from an original drawing by Bertrand R. Adams, 1943.)

Note: This concept of darwinian development in relation to improved function has been beautifully argued in a book by Richard Dawkins, *Climbing Mount Improbable* (1997).

The mere fact that there are these articulations, persisting through life, leads osteopaths to believe that their design serves some purpose. Quite what unique function the different articulations of the skull are designed to meet is open to much question and debate, but discussed below are some osteopathic contributions to this dialogue.

The changing form of the skull

The skull undergoes considerable change from the fetus to the newborn, through childhood and into adulthood. Some of the differences in suture arrangement are shown in Figure 9.17.

Movement between cranial bones is recognized during the birth process, where the skull undergoes a process of moulding. This arrangement of the skull allows some of its parts to fold over each other to allow the head to pass more easily along the birth canal. This is shown in Figure 9.18.

From there onwards, the orthodox profession subscribes to the opinion that the component parts of the skull gradually either fuse or come to interlock so completely that no movement and therefore no function can be ascribed to them: the sutures of the skull are thought to be unimportant.

For many osteopaths this is an alien opinion, as motion within the skull is considered fundamental to the function of the central nervous system, the hypothalamus and pituitary glands, the ears, eyes, sinuses and many other structures (Magoun, 1976).

In osteopathic texts motion within the skull is most frequently linked to the flow dynamics of the cerebrospinal fluid, and general fluid dynamics deep within the cranium where effective tissue circulation is vital. But other ideas have been considered, including the opinion that skull joints are necessary to provide a shock-absorbing arrangement to offset forces induced in mastication: a

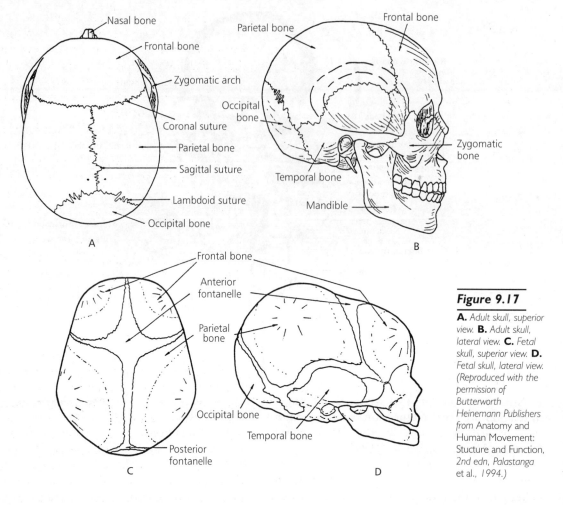

Figure 9.17

A. *Adult skull, superior view.* **B.** *Adult skull, lateral view.* **C.** *Fetal skull, superior view.* **D.** *Fetal skull, lateral view. (Reproduced with the permission of Butterworth Heinemann Publishers from Anatomy and Human Movement: Stucture and Function, 2nd edn, Palastanga et al., 1994.)*

mobile/absorptive face and cranium will help to offset shear forces acting upon the teeth, thus reducing wear (Upledger and Vredevoogd, 1983).

Another group of structures within the skull also have an unclear function: the sinuses. Whatever function they do actually have, there seems to be a bit of a design fault somewhere, as they are often prone to problems of poor drainage. Osteopaths would consider that the slightly shifting arrangement provided by the articulations of the skull helps to maintain tissue drainage within the sinuses and prevent congestion.

As stated, whatever the function of the articulations, it does seem that the sutures are each arranged differently to permit various permuta-tions of skull 'shift' (as opposed to gross move-ment). To appreciate the relevance of such shifts, one must remember that living bone is quite unlike most people's conception of it, which is based upon preserved cadaveric specimens. Living bone is malleable, springy and, especially when arranged into plates or thinner sections, able to sustain quite a degree of torque before re-coiling elastically back into its original orientation.

There are very many tissues – muscular, liga-mentous and fascial – that attach to the various skull bones, and the shifting tensions within these tissues during locomotion, general activity, eating, talking and so on will all pull upon the skull. This may be another reason why there are joints and sections within the skull – to allow

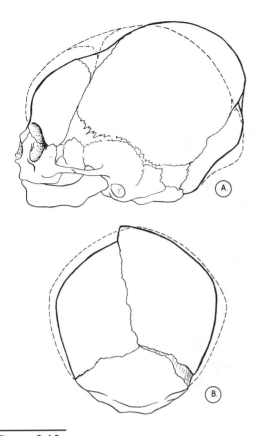

Figure 9.18

Moulding of the fetal skull. The dotted lines show the shape before moulding. (Reproduced with permission from Llewellyn Jones, 1986.)

these conflicting forces to be accommodated more readily without causing stress within those tissues or upon the bone of the skull itself. Some of the muscular attachments on to the inferior aspect of the skull are shown in Figure 9.19.

Given that there may be quite a bit of subtle shifting of shape within the living skull from the influence of soft tissues on the outside of the skull, it follows that the tissues on the inside of the skull might be subjected to a degree of torque or tension – especially in infants and children where the sutures are less well formed and permit much more motion anyway.

The shifting movements that take place within the cranium may have a role to play in flow dynamics of the cerebrospinal fluid in particular

but may also influence venous drainage (especially around the cranial nerves that pass through various holes and spaces (foramina) within the skull). For now, the concept of motion within the skull itself needs greater discussion, as it is fundamental to an osteopathic model of motion that has not yet been explored.

Within the skull (and indeed other body areas) osteopaths consider that there are two movements: 'voluntary motion' and 'involuntary motion'. Neither of these terms may be the most appropriate. 'Voluntary motion' relates to the discussions above of a passive shifting of skull sutures to accommodate the various pulls and tensions within the soft tissues that attach to the skull. In this sense it is not a 'voluntary' motion but where motion in the skull follows passively from the influence of a variety of voluntary movements.

'Involuntary motion' is something else.

'Involuntary motion'

Within orthodox science many motions within the body could be thought of as involuntary – for example, respiration, peristalsis, pulsation in the blood vessels and so on. Osteopaths recognize another category of motion within the human form. This idea remains controversial even within the profession and certainly is one that orthodox science does not recognize or validate. However, the concept has given rise to a model of osteopathic practice that has developed into a highly valuable and profoundly beneficial form of treatment (Sutherland, 1990).

Osteopaths who work with involuntary motion, or the involuntary mechanism (a phrase that will be expanded upon in a moment), can apply the concept throughout the body. But, as the phenomenon was first recognized within the cranium and much of the treatment given to help restore involuntary motion to the body centres on releasing tensions in and around the head, such osteopaths have been saddled with the term 'cranial osteopaths'. Unfortunately, this misnomer is one that will be virtually impossible to change as it is now part of lay terminology, with many patients enquiring after 'cranial osteopaths' as opposed to 'non-cranial osteopaths' (who are

259

Figure 9.19

Muscle origins and other structures on the base of the skull. (Redrawn from Clemente, 1987.)

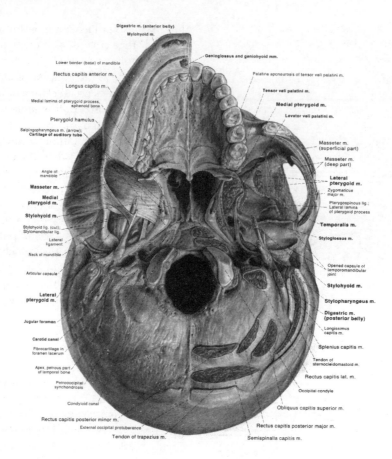

ones that do not utilize the concept of involuntary motion in their work).

Involuntary motion is a motion that passes through all the tissues of the body and, like respiration, should occur no matter what else is going on. It is a primary motion in the body and should not be compared to locomotion, which can be considered a voluntary act. In fact involuntary motion has been described by the man who first recognized it as associated with the **primary respiratory mechanism**. Involuntary motion is primary in the sense that it represents not mere thoracic respiration but the motion of life itself.

Several parts of the osteopathic profession are unhappy with this concept, but many feel it is correct. Whatever the extent of one's personal views, there is the assumption that there is some

sort of involuntary motive force behind this movement: something beyond our conscious control that initiates this motion and determines how it is expressed. The existence of such a mechanism has led to the concept of working with the primary respiratory mechanism – the motive force behind involuntary motion.

The origins of this motion are unclear but several ideas as to the nature of the involuntary/primary respiratory mechanism have been put forwards. These include:

• motion consequent to the cyclical production of cerebrospinal fluid (creating a hydraulic system that induces a wave-like motion that then permeates through the body);

• a combination of respiration, arterial pulsation, motility within the hollow organs (peristalsis) and general rhythmic skeletal muscle activity that is ongoing even when the body is comparatively at rest, such as when the person is asleep;

- 'energetic' considerations – electrical activity in and around the brain is thought to give it an active 'motricity' (contractility), which then radiates throughout the body;
- a remnant of the motive force that guided embryological formation, migration, folding and development of tissue within the fetus, infant and child, which continues right up to when we stop growing and developing.

The first, third and fourth suggestions were the original ones given by the osteopath who first recognized, described and worked with this model of motion, William Sutherland, an American osteopath who trained under Still, developed a treatment rationale based upon 'balanced ligamentous tension' (which we will refer to later) and coined the phrase 'primary respiratory mechanism' used above (Sutherland, 1990).

Considerations 1: Circulation of the cerebrospinal fluid

To many people, the idea that the force generated by the cyclical production of the cerebrospinal fluid is sufficiently strong to induce motion within the bones of the skull and through the rest of the body is not to be seriously entertained.

Considerations 2: Combined motion

This lack of belief in the motive force of cerebrospinal fluid flow led to the second supposition: that there was a combination of recognized movements in the body that would summate to provide a motion that would, among other things, aid the flow of cerebrospinal fluid within the cranium and spinal column. This latter opinion seems to be gaining support in some quarters, although many still subscribe to the first opinion. This combined action of 'ordinary' motion, which is recognized within the orthodox sense, was thought to be a more reasonable explanation of any involuntary motion that might be present. It also allowed many practitioners to put aside

the idea of a primary respiratory mechanism (with all its associated spiritual and energetic correlation), which they were uncomfortable with, but still work with a system of involuntary motion that passed through the head and rest of the body, which was physiologically useful and of therapeutic importance.

As stated above, though, the use of the involuntary mechanism within osteopathy is extremely popular and many practitioners work only from that perspective. These practitioners have made many valuable contributions to healthcare in general and, whatever lies behind their practice, one needs to recognize its empirical benefit and validity. Involuntary motion is now discussed in more detail.

What direction(s) does involuntary motion occur in?

Putting the matter of production of involuntary motion aside, followers of this model (of involuntary motion) will describe how the movement passes through the body (in terms of direction) and say that it is a cyclical motion, which is bilaterally symmetrical throughout the body and which should be focused or centred on a particular point or fulcrum (which is sited within the skull; Magoun, 1976). This is shown in Figure 9.20.

The motion passes throughout all the tissues of the body and if these latter are all even, balanced and not suffering contracture, spasm or scarring, for example, will permit the motion to be expressed in the above manner. However, should there be any tension or torsion within the tissues, then any involuntary motion that must pass through those tissues will be somewhat deflected from its original pattern, creating a shift in the fulcrum and a different pattern of expression from the one above.

The amount of deviation from the ideal motion pattern and the extent of change in position of the fulcrum about which the motion is performed are considered to be a measure of the gravity and nature of dysfunction within that person.

Such a system of membranes acting around a fulcrum, with tension in one part of the structure influencing the rest, should be considered as a

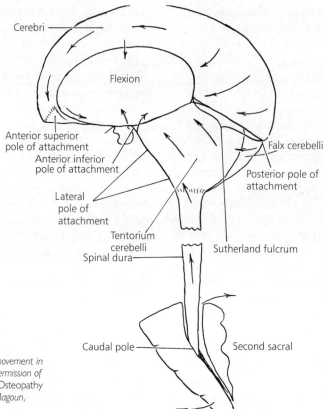

Cerebri

Flexion

Anterior superior
pole of attachment

Anterior inferior
pole of attachment

Lateral
pole of
attachment

Falx cerebelli

Posterior pole of
attachment

Tentorium
cerebelli

Spinal dura

Sutherland fulcrum

Caudal pole

Second sacral

Figure 9.20

Reciprocal tension membrane movement in flexion. (Reproduced with the permission of Journal Printing Company from Osteopathy in the Cranial Field, *3rd edn, Magoun, 1976.)*

'reciprocal tension membrane', with one of the most important aspects of the reciprocal tension membrane being the system of dural, meningeal and other fascial supports of the central nervous system contained within the cranium and spinal column. Reciprocal tension will be discussed below, but its presence is thought to influence fluid flow in and around the central nervous system and through to the peripheral nervous system, and it is this fluid flow that forms the next part of our discussion.

Tides, eddies and waves

One should emerge with the picture that involuntary motion permeates through the body in a cyclical rhythmic way, like a series of tides, eddies and waves, which are subtly expressed in all body tissues by engaging the system of reciprocal tension membranes, starting within the cranium and then spreading throughout the rest of the

body. These terms are particularly relevant, as the shifting tension within the reciprocal tension membrane is thought to influence the flow dynamics of the cerebrospinal fluid (CSF) both within the dural sleeve of the brain and spinal cord and also out into the connective tissues of the body (Erlingheuser, 1959). To palpate these motions and tides, one uses a light palpation and waits to passively pick up the underlying motion, as opposed to active motion testing of gross joint motion, which is the procedure in a lot of other osteopathic examination procedures.

Clearly, if one goes along with the association between involuntary motion and cerebrospinal fluid flow one can see how the watery terms used above can be relevant. However, they can also be relevant to those who postulate an energetic origin for involuntary motion, as described above. This third supposition in the list indicated that this involuntary motion has as much to do with energy and physics as it does with either fluid flow or respiration, peristalsis and so on. Physical laws illustrate that there are many motions akin to waves, tides and eddies, which may be related to the phenomenon of involuntary motion.

The Tide

Sutherland was, it is fair to say, profoundly interested in the CSF, and in the nature of its circulation. He called the fluctuation of the CSF 'the Tide', and felt that within the CSF was an 'invisible element' that he referred to as 'the breath of life', which imbued the CSF with a certain potency.

He felt that the flow dynamics of the CSF should be like a gentle fluctuation, like the ebb and flow of a tide. Articular restrictions within the cranium and spinal column were considered to disrupt this flow, which would then interfere with normal brain/nervous tissue function through inadequate tissue perfusion or drainage. He felt that one could palpate the ebbs and flows within the CSF and determine whether its flow and distribution were appropriate. He had the following to say about the Tide:

> If you were to take a glass of water, place it on the table, and shake the table, the water would spill therefrom. However, if I took my hand and gave a transmitted vibration from my shoulder to the table, you would see that water come up to the centre of the glass in a little quiver. This is what I want you to see in the potency of the Tide in the cerebrospinal fluid. Not this up and down fluctuation during inhalation and exhalation, but the condition where you get the movement down to a balance point between inhalation and exhalation, a midway point. This midway point is where you get a brief period where you observe that the diaphragm is moving gently at a fulcrum point. Then you get this vibration to the centre of the Tide, the point where you might say that you have come to what is known in a hymn as 'The Still Small Voice'. You have heard the hymn, 'Be Still and Know that I Am'. Do you get the point? It is the

stillness of the Tide, not the stormy waves that bounce upon the shore, that is the potency, the power. As a mechanic of the human body you can bring the fluctuation down to that short rhythmic period, that stillness, if you understand the mechanical principle of this fluctuation of the Tide.

Sutherland, 1990

This imagery led to the development of various techniques that could be applied (principally to the cranium and pelvis) throughout the body, which would gently encourage this type of fluctuation within the CSF and so promote healthy neural function. These techniques are extremely subtle, and discussing them in any detail is beyond the scope of the book.

However, one of them is worthy of a (very) brief note.

Compression of the fourth ventricle
Sutherland said:

> Beneath the tentorium cerebelli is a column of fluid that surrounds the brain stem and cerebellum as well as being within the brain stem (the fourth ventricle). Within this body of fluid is that 'highest known element' to which Dr Still pointed; and within the brain stem, within the medulla oblongata, are the primary centres controlling the physiology of the body, especially the centre for respiration.... 'When you do not know what else to do, compress the fourth ventricle.'

Sutherland, 1990

The fourth ventricle can be seen in Figure 9.14. As stated, how this is done in its entirety is beyond the scope of this book but it represents one of the most universally applicable techniques used by practitioners who follow Sutherland's approach.

Reciprocal tension

One way of approaching the mechanisms of involuntary motion is to use the concept of reciprocal tension as an examination and treatment tool.

The way that reciprocal tension permeates through all the membranes and connective tissue/fascial structures of the body is of great interest to osteopaths, even those who do not subscribe to the concept of involuntary motion. The tensegrity model discussed in earlier chapters is useful to recall here as it illustrates how tension in one part is immediately transferred to another area. This is very much the situation in the reciprocal tension system of membranes within the human body.

It is through the system of reciprocal tension that the osteopath working with the involuntary motion mechanism can take a contact point on any part of the person's body and influence the overall pattern of motion.

This is another reason why the term 'cranial osteopath' is a misnomer, and confusing to many patients and external observers.

Note: If one is not using the concept of involuntary motion, one can use general articulation, mobilization and other techniques such as the functional technique to influence this pattern of reciprocal tension.

Balanced membranous/ligamentous tension

The reciprocal tension system of membranes by its very name reveals that it is made up of several component parts. These consist of the dural membranes within the skull and spinal column, the ligaments in the spinal column and the ligaments and fascial sheaths in the limbs and cervical region that we have previously discussed, and all other fascia structures that run within the cavities of the body. Figure 9.20 shows the membranes in the skull, which together form the reciprocal tension membrane (as well as indicating the directions of shifts in tension during involuntary motion).

Being 'in reciprocal tension' is a very orthodox biomechanical principle, which can be appreciated from all the discussions in this chapter concerning the inter-relatedness of parts and the need for stability, flexibility and communication within the tissues of the body. Therefore one can either put the idea of balanced membranous/ligamentous tension alongside involuntary motion or consider it on its own.

Developing a system of balanced ligamentous tension begins within the embryological formation of the fetus and carries on through infancy to adulthood, as all the neurological reflexes and systems of control of muscle action develop in response to proprioceptive information arising from the ligamentous and fascial systems of the body as they are engaged during motion (triggered by muscular action).

Because of this association with embryology this discussion on balanced membranous/ligamentous tension will be continued under the section on embryology below.

A further point of clarification: to some people the motive forces behind embryological development are not completely removed from the energetic principles alluded to above; whereas many others can appreciate the physical and anatomical relationships within embryology and ongoing development within the human form without a single reference to energetic principles at all, nor indeed to any form of involuntary motion.

It is a great shame that the following concepts, which are very powerful and of particular therapeutic value, should be lost to a number of osteopaths because they cannot subscribe to the idea of involuntary motion. It is wrongly assumed that one needs to accept involuntary motion in order to work with embryological principles.

However, to exponents of the concept of the primary respiratory mechanism, the association of involuntary motion and the reciprocal tension membrane is something vital and special, which should not be forgotten.

Embryology

Recapitulation

In Chapter 5 the developmental process within the embryo was discussed, along with the concept of continued growth throughout life and factors that could influence this process. The idea that one never stops developing is fundamental to the concept of osteopathy.

The tissues of the embryo, and the person after birth, go through a functional differentiation process which takes the embryo from an undifferentiated primordium to a collection of cell aggregations (tissues) and tissue aggregations (organs) that is recognizable as a human infant, into the adult form (where aggregations of cells or tissues no longer dramatically change in relation to each other but still undergo a process of renewal and regeneration – the cell cycle). This means that the human form never stops developing in some way.

All this development is determined by forces external to the genetic material of the cell, which means that the way the body can either 'develop' or 'turn over its cells' is an adaptable process that can be influenced. As previously discussed, one of the greatest influencing factors is physical force.

For osteopaths who reflect upon these ideas of continued growth as directed/influenced by tissue tensions and torsions (which provide influential physical force upon the developing tissues), they lead to consideration of clinical relevance.

The importance of an intact and functioning central nervous system to life is beyond question. If one looks at the development of the nervous system and its bony protection – the skull (in particular) and the spinal column – one can see that much growth and development occurs after birth.

The relevance of this is that, if there are any limitations to growth of the central nervous system, perhaps caused by an uneven or incomplete expansion of the soft skull postnatally, through infancy and childhood, then the development of neural function may be impaired.

This is a profoundly logical conclusion for osteopaths but seems more elusive to the orthodox profession, except in extreme cases of fetal malformation or gross compression of the cranium during birth such that neural damage occurs (as opposed to having ongoing development interfered with by subtle physical tensions in the tissues of the head and neck).

The bony and membranous structures within the skull must accommodate the changing shape of the brain and, if the skull is unable to expand fully, for example because of unresolved physical stress during birth or as a result of tissue tension that arises after birth (as posture develops and the child starts to move) then the different lobes of the brain may come under different pressures

(Arbuckle, 1960). An indication of the changing shape of the brain during development is shown in Figure 9.21.

For example, if one looks at Figure 9.21, one can see that the direction of expansion of the cerebral hemispheres means that the temporal lobe is continually expanding into the temporal fossa of the cranial base, requiring the falx cerebri and the tentorium cerebelli to stretch out to accommodate this. The impetus for the development for the fossa within the cranial base itself comes from the ever-expanding brain tissue. Thus the brain is literally moulding the skull. Any tension within the developing bony cranium may lead to tension in the skull that is greater than the brain can overcome, meaning that it is always somewhat behind in fulfilling its developmental impetus (Korth, 1982).

Removing the tissue tension that is constricting skull growth and expansion will then reduce the limiting influence this has upon brain expansion and allow the nervous system to fulfil its developmental process and therefore function effectively.

Paediatric osteopathy

From this type of background and approach, paediatric osteopaths (osteopaths who work with infants and children) feel that they can help central nervous system development and ongoing function, which could be extremely relevant in many infants, as well as providing a unique and novel approach to the management of developmental or nervous system disorders such as cerebral palsy and autism, and Down's syndrome (Handoll, 1998).

The developmental forces acting upon and within the developing skull are concerned with the three-dimensional growth and expansion of tissues around a core 'blueprint' as well as the differentiation of early tissue types into their (eventual) adult form. Developmental strains within the cranium are related to the phenomenon of intraosseous strain (which has been introduced before).

These embryological bony developmental forces are also allied to the concept of reciprocal tension and so will be reviewed below.

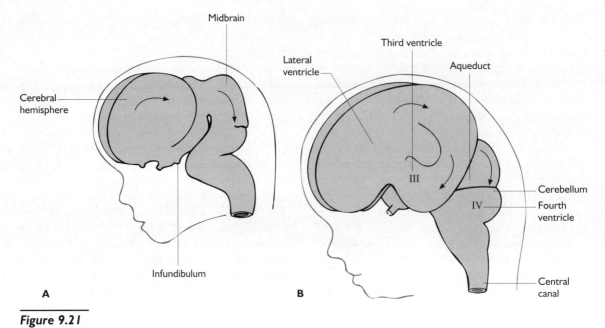

Figure 9.21

*The central nervous system at (**A**) 8 weeks and (**B**) 3 months. (Redrawn with permission from Sutherland Society Notes.)*

Developmental considerations within the cranium and spine

One of the first things to realize is that muscles form from different embryonic tissue from bones, ligaments and connective tissues. These latter all form from the same tissue type. This implies that bones, ligaments and connective tissue sheaths are functionally connected, and muscles, although they may attach to these structures, are part of a different functional system.

The second thing to realize is that there is a core 'blueprint' laid down within the developing embryo that determines the ideal position and orientation of all parts of the body, including the head, spine and limbs, through birth and beyond. (Much study has been done that indicates that there is a molecular basis for pattern formation in the limbs, which probably works throughout the whole embryo.)

A three-dimensional blueprint

As the embryo grows, it does so on three different axes, and any developing cell must know where it is in relation to these three axes, so that it can 'know' where to migrate, where to divide and so on (Blechschmidt and Gasser, 1978). Having a positional sense is vital if any cell is to differentiate into the correct tissue in the correct position relative to other cells within the exceptionally complex and irregular structure that is the developing fetus.

We will be concerned with development of the spine and limbs, and of the cranium.

The developing spine and limbs

As far as the spine and the limbs are concerned, these 'blueprints' are laid down by particular structures called the sclerotomes (developing in association with the notochord) and the axial mesenchymal condensations of the limb buds, respectively (Larsen, 1993). This is illustrated in Figures 9.22 and 9.23, as well as in Figure 5.4.

All these figures indicate that there is a core of embryonic tissue that essentially remains throughout life, around which the other tissues of the area are oriented. The spine and limb articulations condense from these cellular collections and form pretty much along the lines discussed during the introduction to tensegrity

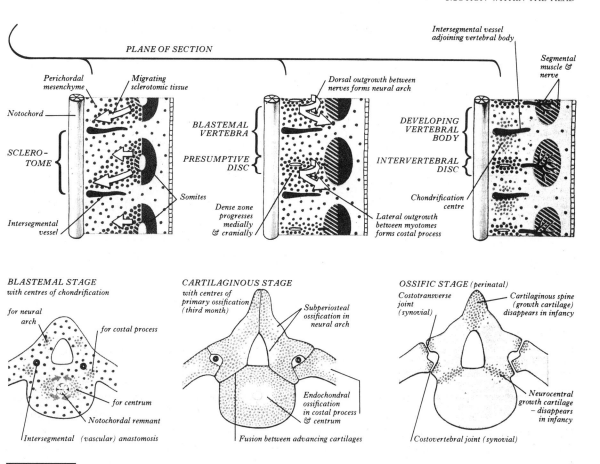

Figure 9.22

Sequential diagrams of development from somites to prenatal ossificatory stages. (Reproduced with the permission of Churchill Livingstone from Gray's Anatomy, 36th edn, Williams and Warwick, 1980.)

in Chapter 5. In essence, the bones of the limbs and the spine first form as whole (continuous) structures, forming struts/rods that support the tissue of the embryo like the poles holding out the spine of the tent-man (the analogy that was used to introduce tensegrity). As development continues, changes appear within these columns/cores of tissues (precursors to bones) and they segment themselves into a number of different sections.

Each section of the rod is still linked by a thin tissue sheet from the original core structure. These linkages form the ligaments and joint capsules/intervertebral discs between the bones

of the limbs and spine. Thus the spine has a ligamentous sleeve formed by its anterior and longitudinal ligaments, annular fibres and intervertebral discus, and the limbs have a sleeve at the level of each joint formed by the joint ligaments and capsule. These sleeves are continuous with the periosteum of the bone and therefore indirectly to the internal structure of the bone.

The development of the single bony column into a multisectional column held together by ligaments/connective tissue provides for greater flexibility of the limb or spine (a multisectional rod clearly has more movement possibilities than a single rod). Multisectional rods therefore

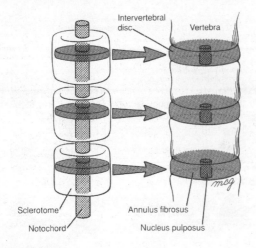

Figure 9.23

Contribution of the sclerotome and notochord to the intervertebral disc. When the sclerotome splits, cells remaining in the plane of splitting coalesce to form the annulus fibrosus of the disc and the notochordal cells enclosed by this structure differentiate to form the nucleus pulposus of the disc. The regions of the notochord enclosed by the developing vertebral bodies degenerate and disappear.
(Reproduced with the permission of Churchill Livingstone from Human Embryology, *Larsen, 1993.)*

require a stabilizing system to prevent them from becoming unstable.

Hence the muscles (which migrate in from another type of embryonic tissue) move into place around the limb sections or spine segments and provide both a stabilizing system and a motive system.

In this type of developmental pattern, the limb bones with their linking ligaments and connective tissue structures have developed from and are therefore oriented around the 'blueprint' of the core structure (the notochord for the spine and the axial mesenchyme core for the limbs). In concurrence with tissue memory and pattern recognition concepts, the limbs and spine will always try to be aligned around these core structures throughout life, if permitted.

The tension in the ligaments of the limbs and spinal column should be evenly balanced, such that the bony elements are evenly oriented around the core axis. If all tissue tensions are equally balanced, then the area/limb is said to be held in balanced ligamentous tension.

One of the things that might compromise this is the pull exerted by the muscular structures acting upon the area, which may well pull the limb or spinal bony component 'out of alignment' with its central axis.

Using balanced ligamentous principles in treatment

Therapeutically, this alignment or distortion can be palpated, using a technique where one feels how the limb is twisted and orientated in space and whether the axis around which it is longitudinally orientated actually corresponds to where one might expect the spinal or limb core axis to be (in the adult form). If one holds the limb/spinal area into a position that in some way corresponds to the hypothetical core axis, then the reciprocal tension within the ligamentous structures will realign the limb/spine around this original core axis, resulting in a more harmonious relationship between all component parts.

Balanced ligamentous tension concepts can be used throughout the entire body and in all tissue systems. It represents a fundamental and unique opportunity to work with the formative processes of life, throughout life. This type of system has an enormous and as yet largely untapped therapeutic potential.

Intraosseous strain

These discussions of tension acting in and around bones should remind readers of the previous discussion we had concerning bony development and growth throughout life.

Intraosseous strain within the skull, and the cranial base in particular, could be profoundly influential to nervous function as discussed above, and is a phenomenon that means that the bone will literally grow differently (or more correctly, will expand inefficiently or unevenly). This means that, unless one resolves these types of problems of conflicting forces acting upon the bones, as ossification proceeds then the bones will become permanently moulded into that slightly torsioned shape. This could have permanent repercussions for articular function, and physiological function of the brain and nervous system.

In order to appreciate the shifting dynamics of reciprocal tension within the skull, and to appreciate how intraosseous strain within the cranium can arise, we need to review the embryological formation/development of the skull.

The developing cranium

Very early in fetal development the cranium begins as a collection of mesenchymal cells surrounding the developing brain (at the end of the first month). These mesenchymal structures expand and develop, wrapping themselves around the brain and the emerging peripheral (cranial) nerves as they grow. Some of these mesenchymal structures will differentiate into cartilaginous structures before ossifying, and some will differentiate into membranous structures before ossifying; and so some parts of the skull develop in diverse ways as a result of this differentiation (Williams and Warwick, 1980).

These cartilaginous and membranous structures will come under different mechanical influences as they try to develop around their 'core blueprint', the existence of which was introduced earlier. Cartilaginous structures often differentiate further under the influence of compressive forces and membranous ones do so under the influence of stretching or expansive forces. There is a clinical relevance to this, which we will discuss in a moment.

The bones of the skull that become cartilaginous are:

- the occiput (except its upper squamous part);
- the petrous portion of the temporal bone;
- the body, lesser wings and roots of the greater wings of the sphenoid;
- the ethmoid.

The bones of the skull that become membranous are:

- the frontal bones;
- the parietals;
- the squamous parts of the temporal bones;
- the upper (interparietal) part of the occiput.

The cartilaginous parts of the basicranium are particularly subject to compressive forces during childbirth, which may produce strain on the cartilaginous parts of the bone such that they subsequently ossify under a degree of torsion/altered shape. The membranous portions (the cranial vault) are particularly affected by tensions in the cranial base and the way in which the internal membranes (dural and so on) of the skull may limit their movement and expansion capacities as growth continues. They are also subject to strain during birth, as they may become stressed through the process of fetal moulding (Magoun, 1976).

Some of these forces can be appreciated if one looks at what happens to the fetal skull during birth (Figures 9.18, 9.24).

The rotatory forces are particularly interesting as they can determine the developing orientation of the condylar parts of the occiput and therefore the mechanical relationship between the head and the cervical column of the spine.

The whole arrangement and orientation of the cranial base is vitally important for the uninterrupted and uncompromised function of the cranial nerves, which have to exit the skull from foramina within and between the bones of the cranial base (Magoun, 1967, 1968a, b). Torsion in the cranium can affect these nerves, as we shall discuss later.

As the cartilaginous and membranous parts of the skull do not fully ossify until some years after birth, continuing to release mechanical strain and stresses may lead to a more optimal shape of the cranium that places less strain on the neural structures within.

The developmental strains discussed, if unresolved, lead to the formation of intraosseous strain, which we have discussed in a previous chapter.

Summary at this point

This section has given a very brief introduction to the concept of motion within the head, and to the subject of paediatric osteopathy. Much more could be (and is) said about such things, but that is left to other books to describe.

Figure 9.24

Birth stresses on the basicranium and atlas. **A.** *Rotatory forces (inferior view of cranium).* **B.** *Axial forces (cross-section of C1/C2). Shaded areas indicate cartilaginous portions of the basicranium and C1.*

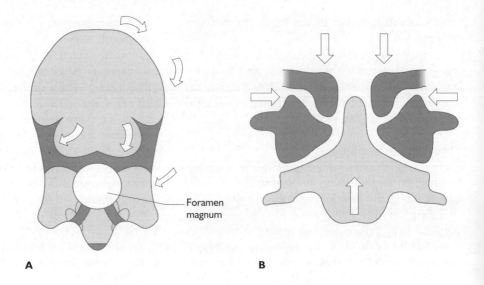

Foramen magnum

A   B

OTHER ASPECTS OF FLUID CIRCULATION AND THE HEALTH OF THE NERVOUS SYSTEM

Neural biomechanics

The brain, spinal cord and peripheral nerves can be considered as a unified structure, which has a degree of elasticity and a variety of movement possibilities. Neural biomechanics are important not only for neurosurgeons (McCormick and Stein, 1990) but for any manipulative practitioner.

Discussions of neural biomechanics do not depend upon the involuntary mechanisms of Sutherland, and management can be approached using a variety of 'standard' osteopathic procedures. Neural biomechanics is the study of the normal movement, sliding and articulation of neural structures within and against surrounding structures. The normal movements of the brain, spinal column and peripheral nerves depend on the elasticity, pliability and orientation of the dural (and other) membranes surrounding the neural structures. Because of the attachment of the dural membranes to various parts of the spinal column and cranium, biomechanical torsion in these parts could limit the normal movement dynamics of the neural tissues. Normal neural tissue is also elastic to a degree, and any tension in the dural sleeves and membranes of the nervous system may constrict this neural elasticity and possibly result in neural injury as the body continues to move (Butler, 1991).

Such tensions could lead to a variety of clinical syndromes (Breig, 1970; Breig and el-Nadi, 1966), the peripheral entrapment of the spinal nerve roots within the intervertebral foramen being one of the most commonly noted.

Indeed, irritation and compression of the spinal peripheral nerve roots within the intervertebral foramen is a condition that is perhaps the largest element of most osteopaths' practices. It constitutes one of the most frequently encountered 'neural pathologies' in practice.

Neural biomechanics also apply throughout the length of the peripheral nerves, and cases of peripheral entrapment are common at such sites as the sciatic nerve passing through or next to the piriformis muscle, the common peroneal nerve around the knee and the median nerve within the carpal tunnel. In these regions, the fascial surrounds of the nerve will normally ensure that it slides against surrounding structures and is permitted a degree of elasticity.

Peripheral nerves

The general arrangement of the nerves gives several mechanical possibilities and is designed to withstand compressive and tensile forces. The

270

peripheral nerves are composite structures consisting of fascicles, blood vessels and connective tissue supports and capsules.

Surrounding each fascicle of the nerve is a layer of connective tissue called the endoneurium. This plays an important role in maintenance of the endoneurial space and fluid pressure, and provides a resistance to tensile forces. Fascicles are often arranged in groups, and surrounding each of these is a layer of connective tissue called perineurium. This layer protects the endoneurial tubes, acts as a mechanical barrier to external forces and serves as a diffusion barrier, keeping certain substances out of the intrafascicular environment. The perineurium is also well designed to resist tensile forces. Numbers of perineurial bundles are grouped together and are bounded by another connective tissue layer called the external epineurium. This layer supports the perineurial bundles within a looser connective tissue web called the internal epineurium. This allows movement between the perineurial bundles, within the external epineurium. This arrangement will protect the nerve against compressive forces and it seems that nerves that have more fascicular and perineurial bundles can withstand compression more efficiently than those with just a few. Surrounding all of this is a final connective tissue layer called the mesoneurium. Blood vessels enter the nerve through this layer and it allows a degree of slide and lateral movement against surrounding muscular and bony structures (Butler, 1991). These layers are shown in Figure 9.25.

The fascicles, as they pass along the nerve, are arranged in an uneven manner – they branch and re-branch as they pass along the nerve, thus giving further protection from compressive and tensile forces. This is shown in Figure 9.26.

Fascial injury, inflammation and scarring/tethering of the neural tissue can disrupt these relationships and the normal pattern of mechanics within the nerve, and lead to neural irritation, giving a variety of consequent neuropathies (motor, sensory and/or autonomic). Manipulations can be given along the length of the nerve to release con-

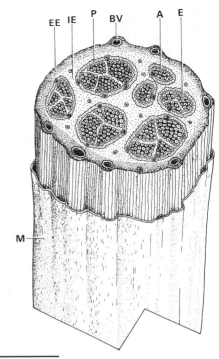

Figure 9.25

The connective tissue sheath of a multifascicular segment of peripheral nerve. A = axon; BV = blood vessel; E = endoneurium; EE = external epineurium; M = mesoneurium; P = perineurium. (Reproduced with the permission of Churchill Livingstone from Mobilisation of the Nervous System, Butler, 1991.)

straining tensions and allow a better mobility of the whole of the nerve. Tensions within muscular structures in between which the mesoneurium runs and which it is attached to can also limit neural mobility and should be explored in cases of unresolved peripheral neuropathy.

The nervous system does not consist of just peripheral nerves and, as we said before, should be thought of as a uniform structure when it comes to neural biomechanics. The membranes surrounding the whole of the nervous system attach both to it and to various parts of the spinal column, pelvis and cranium and contribute to its mechanical function.

To appreciate these ideas, we need to look at the attachments of these dural and other membranes to the musculoskeletal system and consider how peripheral neuropathy may come about as a result.

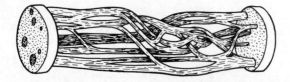

Figure 9.26

The fascicular branching in the musculocutaneous nerve. (Reproduced with the permission of Churchill Livingstone from Nerves and Nerve Injuries, 2nd edn, Sunderland, 1978.)

Dural attachments, spinal torsion and neural mobility

Three connective tissue layers (meninges) surround the spinal cord. The inner two, the arachnoid mater and pia mater, are known as the leptomeninges and are somewhat elastic. The outer layer is thicker and stronger and is called the dura mater. The dura mater is attached segmentally to each vertebra and will be moved by vertebral motion. This arrangement is shown in Figures 9.27 and 9.28.

Between the dura mater and the pia mater run a number of suspensory ligaments that help to keep the spinal cord oriented within the dural sleeve. These are called denticulate ligaments and allow a degree of freedom of motion of the cord within the dural sleeve. Within the cranium the dura is attached to various parts of the cranial base (as we shall see later) and, inferiorly, to the coccyx via the filum terminale.

Spinal torsion patterns are interesting not only because they induce more relative closure of one foramen compared to another but because of the way that they twist and pull the dural sleeves that the nerve roots are sitting in. This torsion of the dural sleeve arises because the sleeves are attached to the accompanying bony structures and move in accordance with bony vertebral movement, as indicated above. This makes them gently twist and tense and relax around the nerve root, depending on intervertebral movement. Clearly, this would aid fluid movement in the subarachnoid space and also allow the nerve root a little bit of 'slip and slide' within its dural sheath during grosser spinal column and limb

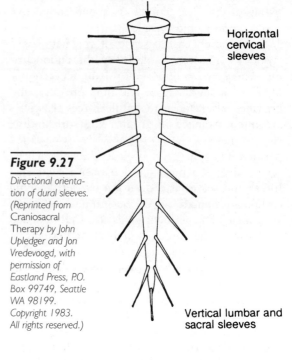

Figure 9.27

Directional orientation of dural sleeves. (Reprinted from Craniosacral Therapy by John Upledger and Jon Vredevoogd, with permission of Eastland Press, P.O. Box 99749, Seattle WA 98199. Copyright 1983. All rights reserved.)

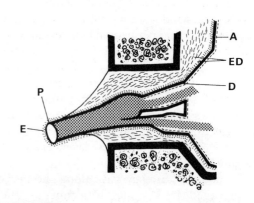

Figure 9.28

The junctional zone between the peripheral and central nervous systems. A = arachnoid; D = dura; ED = epidural tissue; P = perineurium; E = epineurium. Not to scale. (Reproduced with the permission of Churchill Livingstone from Mobilisation of the Nervous System, Butler, 1991.)

movements (which is necessary to avoid unnecessary stretch on the nerve root during such actions).

The superior and inferior attachments of the dural tube

As indicated, not only do the dural sleeves attach at a segmental level but the dural tube is attached at either end to the foramen magnum (and through on to the inner aspects of the cranium) and to the sacrum (Barbaix *et al.*, 1996) and coccyx. It is connected along its length to the posterior longitudinal ligament but this arrangement allows the dural tube to move up and down within the spinal column and does not fix it nearly as greatly as the superior and inferior attachments. Additionally, osteopaths believe that there are strong attachments of the dural tube to the upper cervical vertebrae (especially C1 and C2), although not all anatomists would agree that this is so. (The other superior and inferior and longitudinal attachments are not in doubt, however.)

The fact of these attachments to bony articulations means that the dural tube may become twisted along its length if either the upper cervical and occipital relations are disturbed or sacral and coccygeal torsion develops. In these circumstances the dural tube will still move but it may do so in a slightly altered way, with tension acting slightly differently along its length compared to before. This, coupled with any local torsion acting at a segmental spinal level, may lead to a variety of places where the dural tension compromises neural mechanics and leads to symptoms of entrapment/peripheral neuropathy.

Intervertebral neural entrapment/compression

The mechanics of the intervertebral foramen are therefore important, as any constraint or adaptation within spinal biomechanics can influence the size and movement patterns within this space. This can be appreciated by looking at the dural and meningeal attachments at the level of the intervertebral foramen (Figure 9.28).

Normal spinal movement

Normal, physiological movement within the apophyseal articulations should allow the nerve roots to slide within the foramen and also, through the subtle tensioning of the membranous 'anchorages' of the nerve root, promote the flow of fluid that passes within these spaces and in the perineural vasculature.

Altered spinal movement

Muscle spasm of the locally acting paravertebral muscles can compress the apophyseal facet joints and reduce the intervertebral foraminal space. This in itself is not enough to physically compress the nerve root. However, as muscular spasm normally results from injury to the spinal articulations, the ligaments, capsule and surrounding soft tissues are often inflamed and swollen. Consequent oedema within the foramen is capable of compressing the tissues around the nerve root and ultimately interfering with nerve root circulation, hence causing an 'entrapment' of the nerve root.

Any other space-occupying lesion within the spinal column, such as degenerative conditions of the bone giving spurs/osteophytes, or intervertebral disc herniations or prolapses, or tumours, can all induce direct tissue compression, lead to oedema or be the origin of substances that will irritate the neural tissue (such as the constituents of the disc when this becomes ruptured/prolapsed). Additionally, scar tissue and fibrosis that builds up consequent to injury and inflammation (perhaps as a result of the above type of situation) may lead to perineural adhesions, which limit nerve root motion and also cause irritation of that nerve (Garfin *et al.*, 1995).

Peripheral neuropathy

The neuropathies that result from all these types of compression can be motor (lower motor neurone) and/or sensory, and their severity depends on the amount of compression and neural irritation and so the amount of ischaemic radiculopathy (see below). The problems mostly come about because of the effects this compression has on the vasculature of the nerve root (Breig *et al.*, 1966).

Peripheral nerve root vasculature

The spinal cord is served by a number of vessels that ensure adequate blood supply and drainage. These are indicated in Figure 9.29.

Figure 9.29

Diagram of the intrinsic blood vessels of the spinal cord. The position of the veins is quite variable. (Reproduced with the permission of Churchill Livingstone from Gray's Anatomy, 36th edn, Williams and Warwick, 1980.)

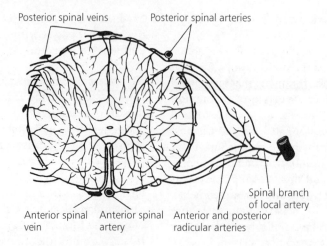

Posterior spinal veins

Posterior spinal arteries

Spinal branch of local artery

Anterior spinal vein

Anterior spinal artery

Anterior and posterior radicular arteries

There are a number of different anastomoses between capillaries within and around the spinal cord and nerve roots. However, despite this, it has been observed (as early as 1946) that the intraneural vasculature is only just sufficient for the tissue's needs: 'There exists a very close relationship between the metabolic requirements of the nervous tissue and the final distribution of intraneural vessels in the adult, a relationship which functions in such a way as to provide the nervous system with a blood supply just adequate for its needs.'

The neural and vascular structures within the spinal canal, together with the fatty tissue and integument, constitute an intricate anatomical complex in which variations of pressure produce varying results. The neural tissues are less vulnerable to changes in physical pressure because of the substantial positive pressure in the subarachnoid, fluid-filled space. The vascular structures are most vulnerable to any pressure changes because of the low intra-arteriolar and intracapillary pressure, and because of the low-pressure venous system.

However, if the blood supply or drainage is compromised, then the neural tissue will also suffer as a result.

The effects of ischaemia on spinal cord and peripheral nerve tissue have been well studied, and increasing interest in the pathophysiology of nerve compression has indicated that any rise in intrafascicular pressure – as a result of oedema, for example – can also be devastating to neural tissue (Gorio *et al.*, 1981).

So, however the compression arises, neural tissue can become damaged. The amount of compression needed is quite small and, especially if maintained over a period of time, can lead to substantial changes. These changes include such things as axonal swelling, myelin degeneration, myelin sheaths becoming detached from the axolemma, Schwann cell necrosis and wallerian degeneration.

Axonal transport

Additionally anterograde and retrograde axonal transport may be altered, which could have far reaching and long lasting effects.

Because the axon and the nerve cell body are components of the same cell, the neurone, there are extraordinary requirements on the system for intracellular communication between the cell body and its axon's proximal and distal parts. Most of the metabolic machinery of the neurones is concentrated in the cell body, where synthesis of materials necessary for the maintenance of structural and functional integrity of the axon and its terminal takes place. Materials synthesized in the cell body are transported distally via anterograde axonal transport.

There is also a constant retrograde transport of material from axon terminals toward the cell body. One function of retrograde transport is to recycle materials that were originally transported from the cell body to the axon. Various extracellular materials can also be taken up by the nerve terminals and transported in a retrograde direction. Some of the most important of these are the trophic factors, such as nerve growth factor, which may be taken up by special receptors at the nerve endings and then translocated by retrograde transport. It is believed that retrograde transport of trophic factors to the nerve cell body is of great importance for the survival and viability of the cell body.

Readers are reminded that this discussion represents a continuation of the information given in Chapter 4 and should serve to expand upon the potential ramifications of altered communication and information processing that were discussed in that chapter. It is yet one more component of how somatic dysfunction can lead to neural dysfunction and eventually contribute to distortion of the homeostatic and immune functions of the body.

Clinical management

Readers are reminded that, in order to maintain mobility at any of these sites or in any of these situations, one might have to look at wider biomechanical influences on spinal mechanics, as discussed within the preceding chapters.

Management centres on re-establishing normal (or as near normal as possible) spinal intervertebral mechanical relations and soft tissue tensions. Maintaining fluid flow around the nerve is of great importance, as this will reduce pressure within the foramen and lead to an increased possibility of nerve healing. Because of the attachment of the spinal nerve root to the vertebrae (via its dural sleeve) mobilization of the intervertebral segments and restoring normal flexible and dynamic motion to this region should have the effect of promoting fluid flow and hence reduce intrafascicular pressure and aid neural healing. Working along the whole length of the dural tube, from the cranium to the sacrum and coccyx, will also help to improve dural mechanics at a segmental level, by releasing longitudinal tension and allowing the dural membrane to act in reciprocal tension once more, thus giving more freedom of movement along any part of its length.

As stated, this can help the management of peripheral nerve root entrapment but may also be relevant in cases of cranial nerve entrapment.

Cranial nerve entrapment

The same principles of neural compression through soft tissue tension and tissue oedema apply to the cranial nerves. Constriction can occur within and around the foramina of the skull, which could interfere with the cranial nerves as they pass through them. Various peripheral neuropathies of the cranial nerves may result – giving trigeminal or vagal neuralgia, for example. However, working on such conditions through manipulative procedures is not a concept that is nearly so familiar to orthodox practitioners as it is to osteopaths. To understand it further, we must revise the dural attachments within the cranium, so that we can appreciate how motion in and around the head may compromise the movement of cranial nerves as they pass through the foramina of the skull and into the tissue of the face, orbits, neck and throat.

Dural attachments in the cranium

The cerebral dura mater is an extension of the spinal dura mater and lines the inside of the skull, where it serves the twofold purpose of providing an internal periosteum to the bones and a supportive membrane for the brain. It is composed of two layers, a meningeal one and an endosteal one, which are closely united, except where they separate to enclose the venous sinuses that drain the blood from the brain. Figures 9.30 and 9.31 illustrate these membranes.

The endosteal dura mater adheres to the inner surfaces of the cranial bones, with the strongest attachments being at the sutures (where it passes through the sutures to become continuous with the pericranium), the base of the skull and the foramen magnum. The meningeal layer provides tubular sheaths for the cranial nerves as they pass through the foramina at the base of the skull. Outside the skull these sheaths fuse with the epineurium of the nerves, and the sheath of the optic nerve is continuous with the sclera of the eyeball. The meningeal layer also extends

Figure 9.30

The cerebral dura mater and its reflexions, exposed by the removal of a part of the right half of the skull and brain. (Reproduced with the permission of Churchill Livingstone from Gray's Anatomy, 36th edn, Williams and Warwick, 1980.)

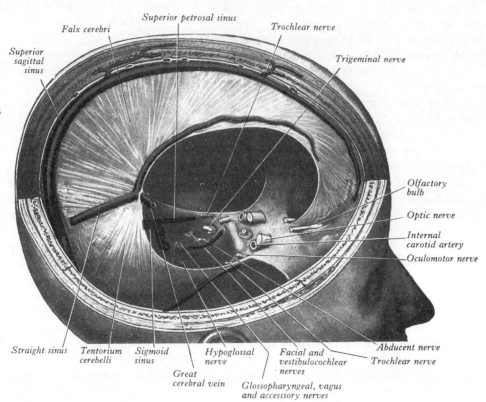

internally as four processes or septa, which partially divide the cranial cavity into a series of freely communicating spaces. These septi are the falx cerebri, the tentorium cerebelli, the falx cerebelli and the diaphragma sellae.

The falx cerebri is fixed to the ethmoid bone anteriorly and the tentorium cerebelli posteriorly. The tentorium cerebelli is attached to the occipital and parietal bones posteriorly, the petrous portion of the temporal bone laterally, where it also forms a pouch for the trigeminal nerve and attaches to the trigeminal ganglion, and to the clinoid processes of the sphenoid anteriorly. The falx cerebelli attaches to the tentorium cerebelli and the foramen magnum. The diaphragma sellae is a small pouch of meningeal dura that surrounds the infundibulum of the hypothalamus, where it attaches to the sphenoid portion of the cranial base as it blends with all the other membranes of the brain at this point.

All of these attachments allow tension to subtly shift from the periphery to the inner aspects of the cranium, where it can act reciprocally and lead to torsion at the level of the foramina.

One can watch tension accumulate around the cranial nerves from the inside of the skull outwards, or one can watch it from the external perspective, where soft tissues around the external aspects of the foramina pass tension through to the cranial nerves and dural sleeves as they pass internally into the skull.

Many of the motion concepts that relate to this area find a natural home in the concepts of the primary respiratory mechanisms and involuntary motion discussed above, and practitioners in this field have a great understanding of how tension in these membranes could eventually accumulate around the cranial nerves, leading to a cranial nerve neuropathy (Upledger, 1987).

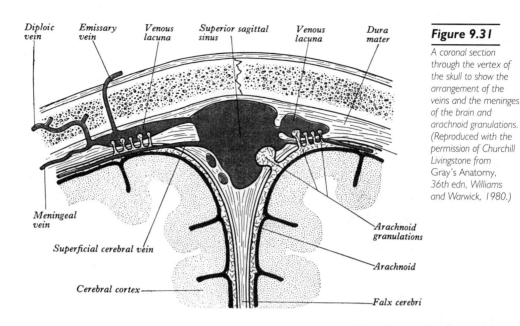

Diploic vein — Emissary vein — Venous lacuna — Superior sagittal sinus — Venous lacuna — Dura mater

Meningeal vein

Superficial cerebral vein

Cerebral cortex

Arachnoid granulations

Arachnoid

Falx cerebri

Figure 9.31

A coronal section through the vertex of the skull to show the arrangement of the veins and the meninges of the brain and arachnoid granulations. (Reproduced with the permission of Churchill Livingstone from Gray's Anatomy, 36th edn, Williams and Warwick, 1980.)

Clinical management

Treatment is along the same lines as for the spinal peripheral nerves, although resolution of irritation is more complex as the moveable parts are less moveable in the first place! For this reason, soft tissue perspectives are as useful as articular ones, and treatment can be orientated to these sites indirectly through working on surrounding soft tissues such as the suboccipital region, the anterior throat and the upper cervical articulations to reduce dural tension from that level. Thereafter, other parts of the spine, temporomandibular articulation and pelvis can be considered, as all will be influential to movement and torsion around the cranial nerves through the reciprocal tension relationships within the dural sleeve.

SUMMARY

This whole chapter has illustrated how fluid mechanics throughout the body can either be supported or confounded by movement and activity within the musculoskeletal system. Whether one is talking about the systemic circulation, the organs, the fascial compartments, the body cavities or the nervous system, fluid dynamics are always of vital importance and if disturbed can lead to a variety of clinical syndromes and contribute to poor tissue health and cellular function. It is hoped that the reader will have gained some insight into the statement by A. T. Still that 'the artery rules supreme' and have an appreciation of the wide considerations that osteopaths give to fluid dynamics within their work.

What is left now is to put all the preceding chapters together and look at an integrated picture of structure and function. Recipes for treatment and management can never be given, although they are always asked for by all students! The application of principles is individual for each case and for each practitioner. The reader must remember what has been said about the importance of movement and tissue quality, about neural, mechanical (fascial) and fluidic (chemical) links between the different parts of the body, and how altered movement is thought to interfere with communication, homeostasis, immunity and tissue health. It is only by working through each component for each individual patient that an appreciation of their problem according to osteopathic principles can be achieved.

That said, the last two chapters will look at the approach osteopaths take to evaluation and case analysis, and will look at a series of case studies.

This should give some insight as to how osteopaths evaluate and manage a variety of conditions.

REFERENCES

Ahrenholz, D. N. and Simmons, R. L. (1988) *Peritonitis and Other Intra-abdominal Infections*, 2nd edn, Appleton & Lange, Norwalk, CT.

Alberts, W. M., Salem, A. J., Solomon, D. A. and Boyce, G. (1991) Hepatic hydrothorax. Cause and management. *Archives of Internal Medicine*, **151**, 2383–2388.

Allum, J. H., Honegger, F. and Acuna, H. (1995) Differential control of leg and trunk muscle activity by vestibulo-spinal and proprioceptive signals during human balance corrections. *Acta Oto-Laryngologica*, **115**, 124–129.

Arbuckle, B. E. (1960) *The Selected Writings of Beryl E. Arbuckle, D.O., F.A.C.O.P*, Privately published.

Aukland, K. and Reed, R. K. (1993) Interstitial–lymphatic mechanisms in the control of extracellular fluid volume. *Physiological Reviews*, **73**, 1–78.

Barbaix, E., Girardin, M. D., Hoppner, J. P. *et al.* (1996) Anterior sacrodural ligaments – Trolard's ligaments revisited. *Manual Therapy*, **2**, 88–91.

Barral, J.-P. (1991) *The Thorax*, Eastland Press, Seattle, WA.

Barral, J.-P. and Mercier, P. (1988) *Visceral Manipulation*, Eastland Press, Seattle, WA.

Blanchard, B., Blanchard, G., Forcier, P. and Cloutier, L. G. (1992) [The thoracic outlet: true syndromes, disputed syndrome (TOS, thoracic outlet syndrome). Current status 1991]. *Revue Medicale de La Suisse Romande*, **112**, 253–266.

Blechschmidt, E. and Gasser, R. F. (1978) *Biokinetics and Biodynamics of Human Differentiation. Principles and Application*, Charles C. Thomas, Springfield, IL.

Breig, A. (1970) Overstretching of and circumscribed pathological tension in the spinal cord – a basic cause of symptoms in cord disorders. *Journal of Biomechanics*, **3**, 7–9.

Breig, A. and el-Nadi, A. F. (1966) Biomechanics of the cervical spinal cord. Relief of contact pressure on and overstretching of the spinal cord. *Acta Radiologica [Diagnostica] (Stockholm)*, **4**, 602–624.

Breig, A., Tumbull, I. and Hassler, O. (1966) Effects of mechanical stresses on the spinal cord in cervical spondylosis. A study on fresh cadaver material. *Journal of Neurosurgery*, **25**, 45–56.

Butler, D. S. (1991) *Mobilisation of the Nervous System*, Churchill Livingstone, Edinburgh.

Clemente, C. D. (1987) *Anatomy. A Regional Atlas of the Human Body*, 3rd edn, Urban & Schwartzenberg, Baltimore, MD.

Colbert, D. (1993) *Fundamentals of Clinical Physiology*, Prentice Hall, Englewood Cliffs, NJ.

Dawkins, R. (1997) *Climbing Mount Improbable*, Penguin Books, Harmondsworth, Middlesex.

Dechman, G., Sato, J. and Bates, J. H. (1993) Effect of pleural effusion on respiratory mechanics, and the influence of deep inflation, in dogs. *European Respiratory Journal*, **6**, 219–224.

DiZerega, G. S. and Rodgers, K. E. (1992) *The Peritoneum*, Springer-Verlag, New York.

Erlingheuser, R. F. (1959) The circulation of the cerebrospinal fluid through the connective tissue system. *Academy of Applied Osteopathy Year Book*, 77–86.

Flanagan, M. F. (1988) Relationship between CSF and fluid dynamics in the neural canal. *Journal of Manipulative and Physiological Therapeutics*, **11**, 489–492.

Freeman, G. L. (1990) The effects of the pericardium on function of normal and enlarged hearts. *Cardiology Clinics*, **8**, 579–586.

Garfin, M. D., Rydevik, B., Lind, B. and Massie, J. (1995) Spinal nerve root compression. *Spine*, **20**,1810–1820.

Gerow, G., Matthews, B., Jahn, W. and Gerow, R. (1993) Compartment syndrome and shin splints of the lower leg. *Journal of Manipulative and Physiological Therapeutics*, **16**, 245–252.

Gorio, A., Millesi, H. and Mingrino, S. (1981) *Post-traumatic Peripheral Nerve Regeneration. Experimental Basis and Clinical Implications*, Raven Press, New York.

Gupta, A. and McCarthy, S. (1994) Pelvic varices as a cause for pelvic pain: MRI appearance. *Magnetic Resonance Imaging*, **12**, 679–681.

Handoll, N. (1998) The osteopathic management of children with Down's syndrome. *British Osteopathic Journal*, **21**, 11–20.

Hill, L. L. (1990) Body composition, normal electrocyte concentrations, and the maintenance of normal volume, tonicity, and acid-base metabolism. *Pediatric Clinics of North America*, **37**, 241–256.

Jacob, S. W., Francone, C. A. and Lossow, W. J. (1982) *Structure and Function in Man*, 5th edn. W. B. Saunders, Philadelphia, PA.

Kandel, E. R., Schwartz, J. H. and Jessel, T. M. (1991) *Principles of Neural Science*, 3rd edn, Prentice Hall, Englewood Cliffs, NJ.

Korth, S. (1982) Primary respiration in relation to child development. *British Osteopathic Journal*, 14, 141–142.

Lai-Fook, S. J. and Rodarte, J. R. (1991) Pleural pressure distribution and its relationship to lung volume and interstitial pressure. *Journal of Applied Physiology*, 70, 967–978.

Larsen, W. J. (1993) *Human Embryology*, Churchill Livingstone, New York.

Liebenson, C. S. (1988) Thoracic outlet syndrome: diagnosis and conservative management. *Journal of Manipulative and Physiological Therapeutics*, 11, 493–499.

Llewellyn-Jones, D. (1986) *Fundamentals of Obstetrics and Gynaecology, vol. 1: Obstetrics*, 4th edn, Faber & Faber, London.

Mabee, J. R. and Bostwick, T. L. (1993) Pathophysiology and mechanisms of compartment syndrome. *Orthopaedic Review*, 22, 175–181.

McCormick, P. C. and Stein, B. M. (1990) Functional anatomy of the spinal cord and related structures. *Neurosurgical Clinics of North America*, 1, 469–489.

Magoun, H. I. (1967) Entrapment neuropathy of the central nervous system. *Journal of the American Osteopathic Association*, 643, 68–75.

Magoun, H. I. (1968a) Entrapment neuropathy of the central nervous system: Part II. Cranial nerves I–IV, VI–VII, XII. *Journal of the American Osteopathic Association*, 779.

Magoun, H. I. (1968b) Entrapment neuropathy of the central nervous system: Part Ill. Cranial nerves V, IX, X, Xl. *Journal of the American Osteopathic Association*, 889.

Magoun, H. I. (1976) *Osteopathy in the Cranial Field*, 3rd edn, Journal Printing Company, Kirksville, MO.

Negrini, D., Ballard, S. T. and Benoit, J. N. (1994) Contribution of lymphatic myogenic activity and respiratory movements to pleural lymph flow. *Journal of Applied Physiology*, 76, 2267–2274.

Palastanga, N., Field, D. and Soames, R. (1994) *Anatomy and Human Movement*, 2nd edn, Butterworth-Heinemann, Oxford.

Sahn, S. A. (1990) The pathophysiology of pleural effusions. *Annual Review of Medicine*, 41, 7–13.

Shields, J. W. (1992) Lymph, lymph glands, and homeostasis. *Lymphology*, 25, 147–153.

Stone, C. (1992) *Viscera Revisited*, Tigger Publishing, Maidstone.

Stone, C. (1995) Osteopathy and urinary incontinence. *British Osteopathic Journal*, 17, 6–8.

Stone, C. (1996a) Literature review of the potential relationship between pelvic biomechanics and lower urinary tract dysfunction. *Physiotherapy*, 82, 616–620.

Stone, C. (1996b) Extrinsic mechanisms of continence. *British Osteopathic Journal*, 18, 8–9.

Sunderland, S. (1978) *Nerves and Nerve Injuries*, 2nd edn, Churchill Livingstone, Edinburgh.

Sutherland, W. G. (1990) *Teachings in the Science of Osteopathy*, Rudra Press, Cambridge, MA.

Tortora, G. J. and Anagnostakos, N. P. (1981) *Principles of Anatomy and Physiology*, 3rd edn, London, Harper & Row.

Tretbar, L. L. (1995) Deep veins. *Dermatologic Surgery*, 21, 47–51.

Triedman, J. K. and Saul, J. P. (1994) Blood pressure modulation by central venous pressure and respiration. Buffering effects of the heart rate reflexes. *Circulation*, 89, 169–179.

Tucker, B. and Jenkins, S. (1996) The effect of breathing exercises with body positioning on regional lung ventilation. *Australian Physiotherapy*, 42, 219–227.

Upledger, J. E. (1987) *Craniosacral Therapy: II. Beyond the Dura*, Eastland Press, Seattle, WA.

Upledger, J. E. and Vredevoogd, J. D. (1983) *Craniosacral Therapy*, Eastland Press, Seattle, WA.

Wall, L. L. and DeLancey, J. O. (1991) The politics of prolapse: a revisionist approach to disorders of the pelvic floor in women. *Perspectives in Biology and Medicine*, 34, 486–496.

Wallace, K. (1994) Female pelvic floor functions, dysfunctions, and behavioral approaches to treatment. *Clinics in Sports Medicine*, 13, 459–481.

Williams, P. J. and Warwick, R. (1980) *Gray's Anatomy*, 36th edn, Churchill Livingstone, Edinburgh.

10 EVALUATION: ANALYSIS; REFLECTION; CRITICAL BEING

Evaluation within osteopathic practice is a complex thing. One way of understanding how osteopaths approach this is to first look at various philosophical concepts behind being a profession; to look at educational methods within osteopathy; and at paradigms of thought relating to research methods that would be applicable to the osteopathic model of healthcare. This cannot be a very extensive discussion but should help set the scene for the framework that osteopaths use to support their reflective practice and how they may develop and evaluate their thoughts and practice.

OSTEOPATHY IS A PROFESSION

The following passage from *Quality Clinical Supervision* is very interesting (this text has been used as the basis for much of the discussion in this section):

> *A profession is a body of practitioners who offer public service for the public good, rather than working with products for their own profit. This indicates clearly that there is a strong moral dimension to professionalism. To be a professional is to have expert know-how underpinned by theoretical knowledge at graduate or graduate-equivalent level. The 'goods' emanating from this knowledge and accruing to individual clients must be distributed fairly and disinterestedly. Becoming a member of a profession is achieved by being approved and accepted (given professional status) as a result of assessments in both practical and theoretical dimensions of knowledge by those who are already members of the body. That approval traditionally rests not on a demonstration of mastery as a result of training but on evidence of the ability to think critically and to exercise professional judgement as a result of education. Such a professional must maintain personal standards of theoretical and practical knowledge, discipline and ethical behaviour (although there is also usually an overseeing professional council which broadly ensures standards). Professional practitioners must*

operate effectively and conduct themselves appropriately according to the purposes and procedures that are traditional to the profession. Central to these traditions is the (currently unfashionable) concept of service. Professionals are thus autonomous operators, in that within professional parameters they must, during practice, make considerable numbers of their own decisions using personal judgement. There is a moral dimension to this decision-making precisely because the professional's goal is to offer public service for the public good.

Fish and Twinn, 1997, p. 35

There are two main models of professional practice, the technical–rational model and the professional artistry model, which we will briefly review, to see which best relates to the above concept of 'profession'.

The technical–rational model

The technical–rational model characterizes professional activities as essentially simple, describable and able to be broken down into their component parts (skills) and therefore mastered. In this model, the initial preparation of practitioners is seen as offering would-be professionals a set of clear-cut routines and behaviours and a prepackaged content that requires only an efficient means of delivery. This approach provides students with a clearly defined set of competencies in a specific area of practice. The idea that practitioners are accountable for a set of competencies within a defined area of practice, however, suggests that they are answerable only to the technical accuracy of their work within the bounds of achieving other people's goals.

This is a limited view of professionalism, and it could be said that the technical–rational view of professionalism, offering simple preset routines and procedures, skills and knowledge, does not meet the real needs of practice. In its document: *Competences Required for Osteopathic Practice (C.R.O.P.)* (Education Department, 1993) the General Council and

Register of Osteopaths (no longer in existence since the establishment of the statutory self-regulatory body, the General Osteopathic Council) seems to list a whole variety of competencies yet does not describe the framework that should be used behind such categories to turn their use into professional practice, rather than a practice based on technical efficiency and routine craft skills. This is a large omission, as in fact osteopathic thought processes during practice are much more than adherence to a list of competencies.

There is perhaps a confusion of terms here, which should be clarified.

'Competence' is a broad ability (undeniably part of professionalism) that is different from 'competencies' or 'competency', which are individual skills that can be identified by analysing professional practice down to its last subskill. Competence will be striven for by an educated practitioner who is free to make professional judgements in the practical context according to his or her own reading of that situation, whereas competencies can enslave the practitioner who has been trained to operate prelearned skills in the practical situation without a prior and detailed reading of that context and who has become not an autonomous professional but merely a puppet of others.

To be fair to the C.R.O.P. document, within its listing of competencies it does imply that other thought processes should be occurring, but it does not make them explicit enough. It is a widely valued document and contains much that is essential to good practice but should now be revised to make clear the extent of reflection within osteopathic analysis. This process is in fact well under way, as evidenced by the format of the professional profile and portfolio (PPP) being used by the General Osteopathic Council (GOsC) as part of the application procedure to join the register of the GOsC.

Osteopathic thought processes are in fact more closely allied to the second model of professional practice: the professional artistry model (which is demonstrated in the PPP mentioned above).

The professional artistry model

The professional artistry model views professional activity as being concerned with both means and ends. Here, professional activity is more akin to artistry and practitioners are broadly autonomous, making their own decisions about their actions and the moral basis of those actions. Practice is viewed as messy, unpredictable, unexpected and requiring the ability to improvise – an ability often diminished by training and routine. To improve practice is to treat it more holistically; to work to understand its complexities; to look carefully at one's actions and theories as one works and, subsequently, to challenge them with ideas from other perspectives; and to seek to improve and refine practice and its underlying theory. Here, the professional is working towards increased competence and should be seen as an eternal seeker rather than a 'knower'.

Inherent within the model of professional artistry are the concepts of critical thinking and reflection.

Reflective practice is a part of experiential learning, which recognizes four stages of learning: experience, observation and reflection, abstract reconceptualization, and experimentation. Experiential learning is illustrated by the following passage from *Reflective Practice for Educators*:

> *In this cyclical process, learning or the process of inquiry begins with what Dewey (1938) described as a problematic or an indeterminate situation: a troublesome event or experience, an unsettling situation that cannot be resolved using standard operating procedures. Prompted by a sense of uncertainty or unease, the reflective practitioner steps back to examine this experience: What was the nature of the problem? What were my intentions? What did I do? What happened? In the process of observing and analysing this experience, problems emerge. The problem – a discrepancy between the real and the ideal, between intention and action, or between*

> *action and effects – further stimulates the inquiry and motivates the learner to absorb new information as part of an active search for better answers and more effective strategies. The final stages of the process involve reconceptualization and experimentation. Having examined and analysed the experience, the learner moves again into the realm of theory. Now motivated by an awareness of a problem, the learner uses new information to develop alternative theories that are more useful in explaining the relationship between actions and outcomes and to begin the search for strategies that are more consistent with espoused theories and more effective in achieving intended outcomes. This changed perspective becomes a stimulus for experimentation: New theories suggest different strategies that can be tested through action. In short raising questions about practice begins a learning process that leads to behavioural change.*
>
> Osterman and Kottkamp, 1993, p. 21

In order to participate in experiential learning, one must be a critical person. Critical persons are more than just critical thinkers. They are able critically to engage with the world and with themselves as well as with knowledge. Within this process there is a concept of critical being, which embraces critical thinking, critical action and critical self-reflection (Barnett, 1997). This can ultimately lead to someone being an intellectual (where one looks outwards to the wider society) rather than an academic (who looks inwards, to the peer community, to the internal norms and values of the academic subculture).

As we shall see later, the models used by osteopaths within their analytical thought processes include the concepts of reflection, critical thinking and experiential learning. But, before going on to these thought processes, it is useful to remember that there is another important difference between the two models of professional practice. The technical–rational model is related to a different scientific paradigm to the professional artistry model.

Paradigms

The technical–rational model relates to the scientific paradigm that has been predominant since the age of Descartes but which is now faltering. This was based upon universal truths and the existence of a fundamental particle, of linear cause and effect (one aetiology for each condition). However, it is now well demonstrated that there is no such thing as a fundamental particle: at the basis of all matter is energy, which changes as it is observed and changes according to events and environments in its domain. Therefore, the fundamental aspects of nature are unproven. There is therefore no such thing as scientific fact, and objective findings are not absolute. Looking for universal truths (the current scientific model) is flawed, as it is now being appreciated that individual variation and networking of diverse events lead to non-universal outcomes.

Additionally, to be objective (separate from what is being observed) is not possible.

There are two worlds in which we all live: a real world outside us and the world within. We are separated from the outside world by our sensory organs, which buffer us from experiencing something without reference to what is occurring within our internal world (as the neural networks interpreting these events are doing so with reference to internal preconceptions and events, biological and emotional, that are individual for each person). Therefore any judgements, ideas and concepts we form about the outside cannot be strictly objective. We cannot therefore separate ourselves from what we are observing, and so cannot research into ideas using a linear cause-and-effect analysis, which does not take into account how many variables may individually summate to give an outcome. Linear cause-and-effect research looks to separate out variables, to isolate them and therefore to remove any chance of observing real-life situations. Cooperative inquiry, where the researcher and subject work together to investigate inter-relations, seems to be the way forwards (Reason, 1994).

The professional artistry model, using much wider reflection, recognition of integrative interaction between parts and a broader base of critical analysis, seems to fit much more into a cooperative model of inquiry. This can be allied to this new paradigm: a move away from the narrow, positivistic and materialistic world view that relies on universal truths and the technical–rational model.

The professional artistry model is better placed to analyse and understand the healthcare conundrums relating to such things as degenerative, functional and malignant disorders, which are multifactorial and do not follow linear cause-and-effect analyses. These need to be evaluated in a global, integrative way, in order to appreciate the individual nature of how events accumulate to eventually lead to various pathological states. The professional artistry model then best fits the description of professionalism that was given at the beginning of this section.

One interesting thing about the outdated paradigms of research is that they attempt to exclude the placebo effect and find out what is 'really' helping the patient. This makes no sense when you think about it. Whenever we are 'treated successfully' it is in fact our inherent healing mechanisms that are being activated/engaged, thereby leading to the resolution of dysfunction and disease. Even the most powerful drug or surgical procedure in the world will not work in isolation from this phenomenon.

The placebo effect is not understood and is used as a damning term when orthodox professionals try to discount any supposed benefit from an intervention that does not follow their own approaches. They consider that the 'alternative' treatment was in fact useless, and the patient only got better because of the placebo effect. In reality, it could be considered that the alternative treatment was triggering a better inherent function of the patient, engaging their own mechanisms and thus more effectively ensuring that the 'placebo effect' should come into being.

Research would be more realistically directed at discovering why the placebo effect doesn't work in every case, rather than trying to diminish its importance. Investigating the placebo effect does not negate the therapeutic models within the alternative management model. In fact, it should help everyone realize how the various components within those models interfere with normal and effective body systems and responses and so lead to a diminution of the placebo effect. Understanding such things will help everyone to appreciate how patients can be individually helped rather than being written off because the universal approach has failed them.

This is new paradigm research at its best.

Having introduced the idea that osteopathic practice is allied to the professional artistry model and the paradigm of inter-relatedness that goes with it, it is now time to look in detail at the thought processes that osteopaths use.

THOUGHT PROCESSES DURING CASE ANALYSIS

Throughout the consultation period and treatment of a case, there should be an ongoing analysis of information within a framework that allows sound clinical practice and a growth of knowledge and experience.

Each time a patient is seen a cycle of events are followed, which are the same no matter what stage of management the patient is at.

The first consultation

This consists of case history taking, examination and formulation of a management plan, which may or may not include treatment.

The aim of the case history and examination is to come to a considered opinion as to the nature of the patient's problem and what that means within the context of the patient's life. Having come to a considered opinion, one then formulates a working hypothesis, to which a management plan can be applied. Often, several ways of managing the identified problem can be suggested, each one having an individual bearing upon the overall prognosis of the case. With the informed consent of the patient, a particular management is agreed upon, and the osteopath and the patient enter into a contract of care. This is then carried through, with constant reflection

on the ongoing validity of the hypothesis, and in consideration of any changing factors. Diagnosis is often 'most valid' retrospectively, as, when the patient is discharged, all details of the case can again be reflected upon and their relevance and meaning re-analysed and learned from.

Note: The term 'working hypothesis' is used on the basis that it reflects the strongest consideration possible of the nature of the case details and their meaning. However, it also 'allows' within it the possibility of growth and expansion of the original idea, or even its adaptation if it proves incorrect. The word 'diagnosis' is somehow more final and perhaps subconsciously may not engender the same reflection as 'working hypothesis'.

The basic stages

These are as follows (key words are highlighted):

1 **Exploration** – case history taking.
2 **Formulation of working hypotheses** that suggest themselves from the case history, and an acknowledgement of whether these are immediately concerned with the presenting symptoms or arise as part of a general screening process that is the concern of any primary healthcare practitioner.
3 **Identification of an examination plan** that should explore and aim to confirm or deny the working hypotheses identified so far.
4 At this stage there should be recognition of the aspects of the examination that are **routine screening**, and those that specifically **confirm or deny hypotheses** concerning the patient's presenting symptoms. This allows a possibility of choice of examination being employed if there are constraints of time within the initial consultation. The examination also allows an analysis of the **inter-relatedness** of parts, which is vital to the practice of osteopathy.
5 **Execution of the examination** and reflection upon whether the patient's symptoms can be explained by the preceding hypotheses or not. If not, an adaptation of

the hypotheses is necessary and some aspects of the case details may need to be re-visited or explored, and an adapted examination re-performed. Within the examination it is always possible to discover factors that were not expected and the practitioner should always try to fit the hypothesis to the findings, not the other way around. The practitioner should always be on guard against 'only seeing what they want to see'. If any non-vital part of the examination is to be left undone at this stage it must be recorded as such and performed at the next consultation, so that the formulation of the overall hypothesis can be completed. Throughout the examination the osteopath is continuously exploring the tissues of the patient, and should strive to be open to any subtleties within those tissues.

6 **Formulation of a management plan.** At the end of this process all possible lines of enquiry that are appropriate and possible (in the confines of an osteopathic consultation room) should have been explored (by questioning and examination) and a final working hypothesis should have emerged. This hypothesis guides the formulation of a management plan, which, as stated earlier, may or may not involve treatment by the osteopath.

If a final hypothesis is arrived at that is within the scope of care for that osteopathic practitioner, then a management plan is discussed and a variety of options are placed before the patient. The practitioner and the patient must come to an agreed approach that should compromise neither party and effect an alleviation of symptoms or be supportive to another regime of care and treatment, perhaps by a general practitioner (doctor) or other specialist.

If a final hypothesis has not been arrived at, and the patient's symptoms cannot be fully explained, then the management plan is concerned with finding the best avenue for the further exploration of the patient's symptoms. If the symptoms cannot be explained, an interesting point is introduced: does this mean that no treatment can be applied by the osteopath until an explanation is clear? Perhaps not: it may be that the symptoms indicate that an immediate or sudden life-threatening clinical situation is not imminent and that, while the patient is being directed for further evaluation, the osteopath could undertake to give a treatment that the symptoms and general state of the patient suggest should not be harmful in any way. In other words, conservative care may be given, which does not interfere with the continued exploration of the patient but lends support, both physical and emotional, to the patient. This latter approach always needs careful ethical consideration as, in general, treatment initiated without a diagnosis/hypothesis is unsound and potentially damaging in many ways.

7 **Sharing and mutual education.** Throughout this whole process there is an ethos that the practitioner and patient can each learn from each other.

Subsequent consultations

The pattern is similar:

1 There is a brief 'case history' when the progress of the patient is elicited and contrasted with what was expected. Any additional information that comes to light or any changing symptoms must be considered at this point before proceeding to the examination.

2 The examination should first consider those areas that were addressed within the previous consultation, to see if the objectives of that treatment have been maintained. If not, this may be because the areas require more work, because other areas have to be addressed before they will release; or perhaps the original hypothesis regarding management needs to be updated;

or there may be other factors for lack of change or differences to expected findings, e.g. work or activities the patient has undergone or perhaps some degree of stress that has interfered with the healing process.

An important point not to be overlooked is that any outstanding examination from the previous consultation (which may be necessary to complete the hypothesis and therefore the overall management plan) must be performed and analysed at this point before proceeding into treatment.

3 Once the current state of the patient has been assessed and reflected upon with respect to the expected prognosis, then further treatment can be carried out.

4 At the end of each consultation, some attention should be paid to the condition of the soft tissue and other structures worked upon once treatment has been concluded. This gives a point of reference for the next consultation. Any advice or comments to the patient should be given and their continued compliance with the management plan elicited.

Synopsis of important terms/stages related to the consultation process

Case history
This centres on **enquiry** (information retrieval) and **broadness** (of information sought). Case histories should be **directed**, and should not be done by routine/non-specific questioning.

Discussion/analysis of initial working hypotheses (prior to the examination)
This centres on **summation** (of the case, when presented to the tutor in an undergraduate situation or to one's self in practice), **prioritization** (of information discussed) and **recognition** (of the meaning of information retrieved).

This leads to **identification** of working hypotheses, which should be able to be **justified** by **cross-referencing** to information within the case history.

Formulation of the examination plan
This centres on the **confirmation** or **denial** of hypotheses and requires **observation**, and **breadth** of evaluation.

Examination
This centres on **consistency** (between examination actually performed and the previously identified hypotheses) and **accuracy** of testing and palpation.

Formulation of the final working hypothesis
This centres on **reflection** (of information within the examination and the case history) and **consistency** (between initial hypotheses and the final outcome). **Justification** of the hypothesis should be possible between many and varied details of the case history and examination.

Formulation of a management plan
This should encompass all aspects of the case (**broadness**), and should show **recognition** of the importance of, and implications of, the hypothesis. It should involve an **acknowledgement** of the normal bounds of osteopathic practice and the most **appropriate care**, determined by a dynamic balance between osteopathic approaches and standard (allopathic) medical practice for the hypothesis made. It should incorporate an identification of **prognosis**, which could be varied depending upon what (or even if any) **intervention** is given. Finally a **contract** for care should be reached that is **satisfactory** and **ethical** for all parties.

It is necessary, though, to appreciate that case analysis and reflection between an individual practitioner and patient goes on against the individual background of knowledge and experience within that practitioner. This means that individual choices developed within the management plan may vary between practitioners, based on their skill repertoire and experiences to date. However, the thought processes outlined above mean that the practitioner is continuously involved in experiential learning and brings continued reflection to his/her appreciation of

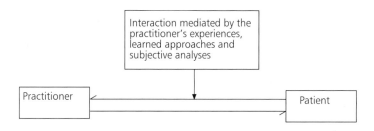

each case. As s/he develops one protocol for the patient, tests it out, and observes the outcomes, both s/he and the patient are involved in a co-operative learning experience that means that ongoing care strategies are continuously being revised and refined. This dynamic is shown in Figure 10.1.

INTER-RELATIONS BETWEEN PARTS

The aim of this whole process is to explore the nature of the patient's problem, to place it in the context of their lives and personal histories and to discover ways of helping them that come forward through the application of osteopathic principles to the person in question. Thus case analysis not only involves recognizing the pathological state of the patient's tissues but allows reflection and interpretation of the inter-relations between all aspects and areas of the patient's problem, to bring about increasingly refined and relevant ways of helping the person return towards health and good function and to become re-adapted to meet the needs of their life. It also allows a deepening appreciation of the integrated activities of the physiological and structural components of the body, leading to a more full understanding of health, disease and dysfunction.

Case analysis therefore involves a continuous development and reflection, and critical analysis of what osteopathy is and how one carries it out in practice.

This then is the abstract theory in broad outline. Understanding a little more of the specifics allows the theory to be more easily appreciated in practice.

BREAKDOWN OF THE STAGES, IN DETAIL

The case history

The case history is a very fluid information retrieval system and depends on the varied skills of the practitioner and the level of his/her base knowledge. Its purpose is not just to enable the differential diagnosis of the symptom(s), but to gain an understanding of the person who comes seeking help and to appreciate what is being asked for (on whatever level). The practitioner must seek to gain a holistic perspective of the patient, so that their problem can be placed in as broad a context as possible. This has relevance later, for prognosis and management.

Information retrieval should always be directed – a skilled practitioner does not ask questions by rote but develops a dialogue and employs lines of enquiry that are structured to explore certain relevant avenues as they become evident and to ensure that confusion of detail is eliminated as far as possible.

Skills

Note: Many of these skills are used throughout the consultation (not just at the case history stage) but are introduced here as it is timely to do so.

Common sense and maturity (of mind, not necessarily of years!) are great assets. The practitioner must make every effort to establish the reasons for presentation, which in themselves may or may not be related to the presenting symptoms. The person must be explored with respect to their symptoms and for any other factors that they may not have recognized or considered relevant but that may be vital, as they may be indicators for some perhaps unrelated disorder or problem. A good history should enable the practitioner to 'put themselves in the patient's shoes' so that a good impression of the context of the patient's problem is gained.

Interpersonal skills are required so that the patient is put at their ease and the delivery of information is not hindered by any sense of the practitioner not appreciating what is being said, or not being sensible to the emotions allied to it and to the needs of the patient. A sense of professional boundaries is essential, both to avoid becoming emotionally 'overpowered' by the patient's need for help or expectations of relief and to prevent the patient having an inappropriate idea as to the nature of the consultation, and it is vital to remain steadfast in the desire to help and not to harm the patient in any way (including psychologically).

One's base knowledge must be sound, and it is important to be able to use it/refer to it in a very flexible way. Rarely do things present as in the text book and, although common things do present commonly, one must always be 'on guard' for a slightly different presentation, whether of something frequently occurring or of something more unusual or out of the normal scope of the practitioner. Therefore the efficient use of reflection and the ability to think laterally are very important.

It is useful to be able to consider the information in such a way as makes the appreciation of what may be accounting for the symptoms more simple, and to allow the information retrieval to be adapted in the light of the response received. One structure that can be used for this purpose is 'the osteopathic sieve'.

The osteopathic sieve

This concept is based on the fact that there are several basic pathological processes and there are several 'families' of tissues to which these processes can occur. This combination of tissues and pathological process leads to a variety of syndromes/conditions, which have recognizable patterns of presentation. Therefore, when one starts to receive certain information about the symptoms, these can be cross-referenced to the syndromes known and an appreciation of what processes are involved with what tissues emerges.

As the information is being gathered, several ideas will present themselves, and the practitioner must direct the interview to explore these avenues until a more clearly defined picture is presented and an identification of what is most likely to be occurring is made. At the end of the case history it is likely that there will be one or two current working hypotheses that need to be explored within the examination, but it is rare that there is no hypothesis possible at all. The practitioner does not aim to diagnose the problem before s/he puts his/her hands upon the patient but it is important to have direction for the examination, and more importantly to recognize whether an examination is appropriate at all.

The osteopathic sieve was first described by Audrey Smith (an osteopath) and started out as a two-dimensional framework, but has now developed into at least five dimensions, which can enable the practitioner to move between information retrieval, examination, reflection and analysis. (Ms Smith wrote six papers on this subject, published in the *British Osteopathic Journal* from 1968–1973, and these were republished collectively by the British School of osteopathy in 1984).

The sieve in two dimensions is illustrated in Figure 10.2.

When certain processes occur in certain tissues, they give rise to certain syndromes/conditions. They can be recognized by their associated epidemiological factors and common presenting symptoms. This is the basic knowledge foundation upon which differential diagnosis is based. When patients present, they have various symptoms, in various sites, with various aggravating and relieving factors associated with them. When working with the osteopathic sieve above, a third dimension of body area (i.e. site of the symptoms) is added. Knowing where a symptom is sets off a whole chain of questioning based upon what tissues are at that site, what pathological conditions can affect the tissues in that area, and how that relates to the age, sex and

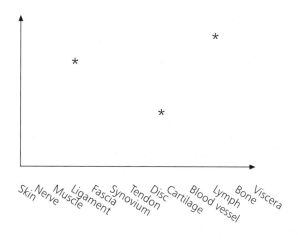

Pathological
processes

Figure 10.2

Basic classifications of pathological
processes are listed on the vertical
axis and the various tissue types of
the body are listed on the
horizontal axis. A patient could
present with a whole variety of
conditions, such as a degenerative
condition of the ligaments (post-
traumatic, for instance), a congenital disorder of the organs (such as
polycystic kidneys) and an inflammatory condition of the blood vessels (such as temporal arteritis).
This is indicated by the starred
boxes in the graph.

Tissue
types

family history (for example) of the patient concerned.

This third dimension is very important, as there can be several things that present with, for example, pain and swelling in the knee, each one having a partially or wholly different set of identifying categories/factors such as age, sex, nature of the pain, aggravating and relieving factors, progression and associated symptoms. Through reflecting upon these different possibilities, the practitioner must ask further questions to direct the flow of information to attempt to confirm or deny the possibilities. One therefore works 'backwards' from the number of things that can give rise to pain in the knee in young males (for example) to arrive at a potential hypothesis. Examples of these different identifying categories are listed in the box below, for reference. The third dimension is illustrated in Figure 10.3.

This type of analytical questioning requires a good memory and an agile mind that can hold several possibilities at once, explore them (by following various lines of enquiry) and so tick things off mentally when the door seems to be closing on one idea more than on another. The person taking the history should also try not to be

deflected from his/her lines of enquiry by a patient who reveals only part of the story, by mentioning only what they feel is relevant or by diverging from the question asked (or ignoring it completely).

As the case history develops, one forms links and patterns or relationships between all the various different categories of information, from the details provided by the patient. This whole process leads to an identification of a number of working hypotheses, such as a traumatic condition of the ligaments, a congenital condition of the bones or an infective disorder of an organ, for example. This is indicated in Figure 10.3.

Clearly, one can gather a great deal of information about the patient in this way, and one needs to analyse what is **relevant** for the presenting symptoms of the patient. 'Relevance' is a very intriguing concept. Have the new symptoms come 'out of the blue' or are they in some way related to the summation of effects caused by the presence of the other (preceding) problems and processes that the patient has experienced?

In order to appreciate 'relevance', the osteopath considers a fourth dimension – that of the number of body areas and systems that are involved and the timing of the events/conditions within these areas. This is done before the

Identifying categories

General information
- Sex, age and weight of the patient
- Observation of their general demeanour and appearance

Details of
- The symptom, e.g. pain
- The site
- Nature/quality
- Radiations
- Associated factors
- Onset
- Aetiology
- Progression since onset
- Daily pattern
- Aggravating factors, relieving factors and things that make no difference
- Previous history, of the presenting symptom(s) or of other symptoms

Other general information
Within the case history taking as a whole, other categories of information are also important:
- Other presenting symptoms (and their site, etc.)
- General health
- Systemic enquiry (for general medical screening)
- Past medical history, including previous investigations and treatments
- Past and present drug history
- Family history
- Social history

examination and is an integral part of the case history analysis.

This fourth dimension is critically important to the osteopathic model, as it brings together many fundamental principles, and puts them to practical use.

The fourth dimension
Analysis of this chronological component is done in order to better appreciate the loading of

dysfunction, stress, strain and illness within that person. The osteopath is trying to appreciate the number of possible inter-relations between the 'diverse' disease or pathological categories identified, and to develop and rationalize some idea of progressive relationships (over time) between dysfunction in one area and subsequent dysfunction in another. (Don't forget that 'pathological' here also relates to such things as injury to muscles, and fatigue syndromes and early degenerative conditions of the connective tissues.)

This concept of inter-relatedness has been introduced as one of the fundamental components of osteopathic principles.

It is at this point that all the preceding chapters of the book come together. Here we integrate all the discussions as to the nature of health and disease, and the development of dysfunction within the body. Here we can utilize the concepts of communication between body parts, the hypothesis of disease and dysfunction as a breakdown in communication. Here we can analyse the existence of the various tissue changes, injuries, emotional states and pathological processes within the body and discuss how they could have been (or still are) barriers to communication. We recall that these barriers could be neural, mechanical and fluidic, and we realize that their presence means that dysfunction in one part can be dispersed both to local and distant structures.

These tissue barriers form part of the aetiological analysis of the patient's presenting problems and allow us to reflect upon the chain of events that may have led to presentation.

Using this type of reflection within the case history enables the osteopath to develop a working hypothesis that might explain or shed light on why that person is suffering from that particular problem at that particular time. It is necessary to identify such things, as one of the aims of osteopathic practice is to help the person move into a state where they are less likely to continue to progress through the same cycle of cause and effect and so continuously end up functioning at a less than optimal level. It enables the osteopath to identify things (tissue barriers) that may have **predisposed** to that situation, or

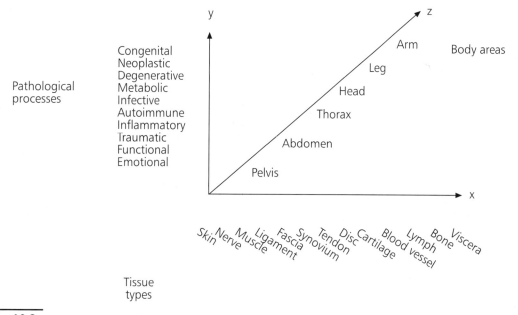

Figure 10.3

The osteopathic sieve in three dimensions. Pathological processes are listed on the vertical (y) axis, tissue types on one horizontal (x) axis and body areas on the other horizontal (z) axis. The body areas referred to here are much more 'broad' than those used in practice. For example, one body area could be the cervico-occipital junction, another could be the right mid-foot, and even smaller anatomical 'groupings' can be used if necessary. Now, one can plot a patient's problems on each of these three axes to give a highly individualized picture of the various states of various tissues within various areas of the body. These 'points' become the basis for developing 'working hypotheses' about the overall nature of the patient's problems.

may be **maintaining** it, so preventing the person from effectively engaging their own self-healing and self-regulating mechanisms.

One should always remember that the practitioner never 'heals the patient'. The practitioner simply attempts to remove as many barriers to effective and efficient function within the tissues of the patient as s/he can identify, so allowing the person to use their own self-healing and self-regulating mechanisms more readily, thus allowing the patient to move themselves towards health.

Additionally, the type of reflection and analysis discussed within this section allows a development of the osteopathic model, which can then be explored during the examination and subsequent management of the patient.

To illustrate some of the ideas reviewed so far, a simple case is given, which covers the case history stage, the formulation of working hypotheses and the examination plan.

Case

A 60-year-old married housewife presents to the clinic (in spring) with generalized lumbar spine aching, mostly across the low lumbar area, radiating into the left sacroiliac and posterior buttock region. She has noticed the symptom for the past 6 months, but a little more so in the last 4 weeks.

The symptom is intermittent, and there are no reported sensory or motor phenomena. She is a little stiff first thing in the morning, which eases after a hot bath, and then throughout the day the symptom can come and go in a variable pattern. Sometimes it hurts when she gets up from a chair or when she gardens, but sometimes it is present when sitting or standing doing the washing up, for example.

She gets up twice in the night on average to pass water. She is usually constipated, certainly over the last 10 years. On occasions she reports melaena, but this is infrequent. She is not sure if it is more prevalent over the last 4–6 months.

She has two healthy grown-up children (with an uncomplicated obstetric history), and three grandchildren, aged 4, 7 and 8. She is apparently healthy, happy and has no financial or marital troubles.

Her past medical history reveals an appendectomy at 20 years of age and a total hysterectomy at 45 years of age for menorrhagia related to fibroids. She takes no medication and does not consult her doctor very often at all. She has always gardened, and has therefore had an intermittent history of low back pain over the years, and is active in the Church in her spare time.

Other questioning reveals that she once broke her left arm (when she was about 30 years old); this took a long time to heal and she was left with an adhesive capsulitis in the left shoulder. She has an ongoing problem with sinusitis and frontal headaches, which have both been going on for many years.

Possible differential considerations
One needs to consider the nature of her presenting symptoms, and some possibilities are listed below.

- Degenerative lumbar spine – osteoarthritic changes;
- Osteoporosis – bone pain and possible pathological fracture;
- Referred from the viscera – possibly the lower bowel.

Justifications
There are several pointers that could lead to these ideas, and examples are given below.

Degenerative lumbar spine is indicated because of the site of the pain, because it is occasionally triggered by movement and because in this case it is more unilateral than bilateral. She gardens a lot, and so might have suffered several microtraumas over the years, leading to increased susceptibility to degenerative change. The fact that it is recently aggravated may be related to the start of the gardening season (she presents in spring). Her lifestyle may be a predisposing factor to her presentation.

Osteoporosis is indicated because of the past history of total hysterectomy. The loss of the ovaries may have led to osteoporosis and,

because there is no reported hormone replacement therapy, this may be important, if not for her current symptoms then for her risk of future pathological fracture and the underlying state of her bones when we come to consider technique. This could be educational both for her and for the osteopath in determining any overall management plan/strategy of care.

Visceral referral is indicated because, despite her long history of bowel symptoms (constipation), there may be a gradual change in this chronic condition from a benign situation to a malignant one. The history of melaena may be relevant, as may the suggestion that this is possibly changing in the last 4–6 months. The fact that she suffers no night pain and that her symptoms are not constant may not rule against this idea. Referred visceral pain is usually more constant in its presentation than musculoskeletal pain, which may lead away from this hypothesis.

Potential examinations
To explore these ideas, one needs to develop an examination to confirm or deny them. Some suggestions are listed below.

- Degenerative lumbar spine: active and passive movements of the lumbar spine; compression may be helpful, but the quality of feel from the soft tissues would be more so;
- Osteoporosis: percussion of the bony aspects around the site of pain, and compression tests of the spine would be useful;
- Visceral referral/pathology: palpation of the abdomen, to look for irregularities and lumps, for example.

Medical tests
There may be aspects of examination and exploration that the osteopath cannot conduct him/herself, but which are considered useful in coming to a more accurate opinion of the problem. Again, a few possibilities are suggested below.

- X-ray for degenerative lumbar spine, to look for loss of disc space and potential neural encroachment;

- Bone scan (and possibly X-ray), the first to assess bone density, the second to investigate pathological fracture;
- Barium enema (with X-ray) to look at bowel outline; possibly, blood tests to assess anaemia with respect to the melaena.

Other factors to beware of

As a primary healthcare practitioner, the osteopath is concerned with any factors within the patient's history that might indicate problems in need of attention, which the patient may not have appreciated. Despite the fact that the patient has not presented complaining of her bladder symptoms, these do not appear to have been investigated so far. They could relate to a medical condition and require treatment, or they could relate to other factors, requiring different intervention strategies.

So, are these as a result of her gynaecological and obstetrical history – i.e. some sort of irritable bladder or prolapse? Are they possibly related to poor pelvic floor tone, with respect to her obstetric history and possible altered pelvic and low back mechanics? Or, are they an indication of a cauda equina syndrome? Is it possibly polyuria and late-onset diabetes? These factors should be borne in mind through any ongoing reflection of this case.

This is not where the osteopathic analysis ends though.

There are many other important and interesting aspects to this lady's case that need to be identified, so that a better perspective of all her symptoms and dysfunctions can be developed.

1 Some of the 'tissue legacies' (**barriers**) from factors in the patient's history may relate to the development and progression of her presenting symptoms.
  a Her obstetric history may have left her with restriction and tension within the pelvic floor muscles and pelvic joints, which over the years have led to an adapted pattern of motion within her low back, which could now be placing mechanical strain at this level and adding to any symptomatology. There-fore, the pelvic tissues may need treating in order to prevent the low back dysfunction from recurring so readily when the patient resumes her normal routines and lifestyle.
  b Her gynaecological history (menorrhagia and fibroids) may have led to a viscerosomatic irritation within the upper lumbar spinal cord, leading to a restriction in the somatic structures receiving efferent supply from this segment, i.e. the upper lumbar paravertebrals and soft tissues. Over time, this reflex may have led to long-term contracture and restriction in the upper lumbar spine, so altering its biomechanics and function. This could be quite relevant for her low back pain if the low lumbars have had to 'move more' over the years because the upper lumbars have 'moved less' (been chronically and reflexly restricted). In this scenario the low lumbars are likely to have developed strain over the years, leading to her current symptoms. Also, in order to allow the low lumbar spine to recover, it would be useful if the upper lumbar spine began to move more efficiently and so reduce load on the low lumbars. The upper lumbars therefore need assessment to evaluate this hypothesis and to determine how much treatment they might need to release.
  c Other mechanical factors may have contributed to the development of poor adapted movement of the spinal column and therefore added to the strain development at the low lumbar spine. There are at least three possibilities here:
    i The shoulder/arm problem. This may have compromised spinal mechanics, particularly in the upper thoracic and cervical areas. We have seen before that affecting movement in one part of the spine will cause change in other areas, and it may be

that the long-standing restriction in the upper spine has compromised low lumbar function. Additionally, if we want to ensure that the likelihood of her symptom pattern redeveloping is reduced, then we should consider treating any restrictions found in the arm, shoulder girdle and upper back, to improve overall spinal mechanics.

ii The chronic constipation and possible pelvic organ prolapse. This is interesting because it may indicate that the dynamics of the abdomino-pelvic cavity are quite adapted. For example, there could be long-term pressure on the abdominal walls and pelvic floor because of the constipation and the straining she performs to help her evacuate the bowel. Altering the function and tension of the abdominal walls will affect the way that these structures engage the thoracolumbar fascia, which is supposed to support the erector spinae muscles and reduce strain at the lumbar spine. She may thus have a chronically undersupported lumbar column, leading to relative instability and subsequent strain. In this situation, any treatment to the lumbar spine is likely to have short-term effects if the abdominal cavity mechanics are not somehow improved.

iii The sinusitis may have complicated the biomechanics of the cranium and cervical areas, leading to dural tension patterns (reciprocal tension) and general spinal curve adaptation, which may have accumulated at the pelvic area and compromised lumbar spine function. Again, to help improve lumbar function these distant areas (the head and neck) may need to be treated to bring long-term resolution.

There are still more possibilities:

2 Her shoulder problems may have led to/be related to her sinusitis problem and headaches. The arm fracture and subsequent adhesive capsulitis may have altered the mechanics of the thoracic inlet area, causing problems with tissue drainage from the head/neck to the thoracic inlet. The tissue tensions may have affected the soft tissues of the anterior throat and jaw, as well as the posterior muscles such as trapezius and levator scapulae. These may have led to mechanical tension developing within the facial bones of the skull and the cranial base, which could be complicating sinus function. Additionally, movement problems in the cervicothoracic, cervical and cranial regions may have affected, through somaticovisceral reflexes, the effective function of the cervical sympathetic ganglia, so further compromising the mucous membrane function and immunity within the sinuses. All of these movement problems could cause muscular tension to develop in the head, or might irritate the nerve supply to the dura, causing the headaches that way, for example.

3 Her low back and pelvic problems may relate to her sinusitis. Mechanical restriction in the pelvis and low back (from the gynaecological and obstetric history and her long history of low lumbar pain) may have adapted spinal mechanics from the bottom to the top, thus giving upper cervical and cranial restrictions that add to the head/neck dysfunction discussed just above, so complicating the sinus function.

4 Her poor abdominal cavity mechanics (affecting bowel support and transit) and related constipation may have led to a chronic nutritional and 'toxicity' problem that may be complicating her sinusitis and headaches. The poor cavity mechanics may also be affecting diaphragm function, which in itself may adversely affect thoracic cage mechanics and so function at

the thoracic inlet, thoracic ducts and tentorium cerebelli, for example, all of which may relate to her sinus and headache pattern.

5 Her various possible spinal restrictions may be compromising the function of the autonomic nervous system and so be related to poor neural control of gut function (and so to her constipation problem). Upper cervical and cranial restriction may affect the parasympathetic supply (vagus); thoracolumbar and upper lumbar spinal restrictions may affect the sympathetic supply to the large bowel; and any pelvic restrictions may affect the pelvic para-sympathetics to the large bowel.

This list of considerations is by no means complete, but one can now see that there are at least a number of possible inter-relations, which we need to explore and which (if identified) we might need to work on in order to resolve the lumbar spine mechanical problem. But we could also consider that, in so doing, we might be able to help some of her other problems if she wanted us to.

This type of list recognizes tissue barriers (neural, mechanical and fluidic) and identifies them as the predisposing and maintaining factors for her presenting state (and whatever myriad symptomatology that involves). Identifying predisposing and maintaining factors gives the patient insight into her problems and suggests reasons for her complaints. They also give insight to the practitioner concerning the number and site of areas that will need exploring in the examination and may subsequently need treatment during management. Hence, these factors have an educational role for both the patient and the practitioner.

This type of compilation of inter-relations is an also an expression of A. T. Still's plea for us to **find it and fix it**: if you don't look, you can't find, and therefore you can't fix!

So, in the case just given, our possible examinations now involve the whole spine, the cranium, the abdominopelvic cavities, the diaphragm and thoracic inlet, the shoulder and arm, as well as all the other things we listed before, to help us appreciate the extent of the local tissue change at the lumbar region and confirm or deny the hypotheses relating to the nature of her presenting symptoms.

Examination strategies

This may seem a lot to do – and it is, which is why examinations have to be prioritized, and why one might in fact explore the many and varied inter-relations within the patient's history and biomechanics over several consultations before gaining the more complete picture. Any prioritization must ensure that, at the very least, an examination is performed to identify the nature of the person's symptoms with respect to tissue damage or disease process, so that in-appropriate care is not given (or appropriate treatment withheld).

Also, if you don't have a global view of inter-relations, you might not think to explore all the above considerations (as you would not have identified them in the first place). Therefore one would be left with management confined just to more local factors, which may or may not be enough to resolve the symptom presentation of the patient.

If treatment does not achieve the desired outcomes, the patient is upset, the practitioner is upset and both may not know why treatment has failed. This can have many negative outcomes such as: the practitioner may blame it on him/herself (poor technique for example); s/he may blame it in the patient, for not stopping gardening, or for being 'difficult to treat', or something else; rather than realizing that it is simply a question of having treated the wrong bits and/or not treating extensively enough.

It does not need much time in practice to realize that treatment of local areas only resolves a small proportion of presenting problems. This is the conundrum of all practitioners.

Having a global view should lead to better treatment outcomes and greater satisfaction and education all around! This is the osteopathic advantage.

The next stage, then, is the examination.

The examination

As implied, this is one of the most important parts of the case analysis. It serves to confirm or deny the hypotheses indicated by the case history and it also allows for a general exploration of the person and their tissues, so that a broad and holistic view of the person's problem (as represented through their physical body) can be determined. The exploration of the state of the tissues is the fifth dimension of the osteopathic sieve discussed above, which we will review in detail later.

As the discussion of the case above should have shown, osteopathic examination follows principles that are different from those followed by other manual therapeutic practitioners. This is not to say that there is not much common ground; there is, but osteopathy does not just reflect upon the extent of the local injury or pathological condition. These things must be considered only as part of the whole person's biomechanical state and therefore functional state, as without this global view we cannot appreciate how to best help our patients.

All of these things therefore relate to an appreciation not only of the number of factors that may have summated to lead to the presenting situation but also of what might be limiting that person's own recovery and what might help recovery and healing if treated/'removed'/'minimized'.

It is still necessary to be able to identify the actual problem, though: to identify the tissues causing the symptoms and to gauge the extent of any damage, pathology and injury. Without this type of consideration, one cannot be said to have made a diagnosis. This ensures that osteopaths are clinically safe and able to talk to external practitioners in terms they will understand. It is also important for the patient to have their symptoms recognized and 'categorized'. This helps them to understand the subsequent management plan that is given, and can lead to better cooperation between patient and practitioner.

Note: It is important to remember that, even if the osteopath finds a number of inter-relations and wants to treat them, the patient has the choice not to have a general treatment and in such cases the osteopath must either accept the patient's view and treat the most immediately relevant factors or, if s/he doesn't want to treat in such a way, refer them to someone who will.

Recognizing the state and extent of any change, adaptation or damage, not only within the local tissues (giving the presenting symptoms) but also within the tissues throughout the body, also gives an appreciation of prognosis. This then helps to determine what might be necessary to 'reverse' that change, in terms of treatment style, or to more effectively accommodate those changes if reversal is not possible. We will return to this point when we discuss the fifth dimension.

To appreciate these points in more detail, examination considerations are reviewed in more detail.

Remember that one aim of the examination is to confirm or deny various hypotheses from the case history. One must therefore know how to evaluate each of the different possible scenarios and how to attempt to reproduce the symptoms depending upon the potential hypothesis being tested.

Site

One of the ways of doing this is to consider the site of the tissues that may be giving the symptoms. It is important to note whether the tissues causing the symptoms are **local** to the site reported, or are **referred**. A careful local analysis of the tissues should indicate this.

Example

Someone with pain in the knee might (after due consideration of case history details as well as examination findings) be diagnosed as having an overstrain of the medial collateral ligament, with respect to the following, for example:

Tenderness over the site of the ligament and some swelling within the tissues. Pain on medially gapping the articulation. Slight (or marked – depending on the amount of damage) protective spasm in the quadriceps muscles, for example, on general mobility testing of the knee. Stability within the end of range findings for the remainder of the knee movements.

This will be quite different from someone who has pain on the medial aspect of the knee, walks with a limp and has associated pain in the low back. They might have no findings local to the knee but movement testing of the low back might provoke the symptoms, indicating some type of irritation of the obturator nerve (a branch of the lumbar plexus), which serves the medial aspect of the knee. In this case there might well be a variety of findings in the lumbar spine, such as:

Reduction of movement in the apophyseal joints of the mid-lumbar spine. Tenderness and reactive muscle spasm of the para-vertebral muscles local to the affected area.

One needs to know, then, how to provocatively test for medial collateral ligament strain, and for referred pain to the knee due to obturator neuritis from a low back injury (in the above examples). A cautionary note is timely here: in very many clinical situations, the onset and aetiology of pains and symptoms is not clear. There may have been no obvious active injury to the knee to focus the mind on a local cause, and any back pain present may well have preceded the knee symptoms by some time and therefore not be associated with the knee pain by the patient. It is always the practitioner's job to explore all likely and relevant avenues.

Thus one aims to locate the problem, and quantify it to a degree, and therefore establish a prognosis for healing. Depending on the state of the tissues it may be possible to say that the joint should recover its normal anatomical and physiological integrity and thus pose no long-term problem for the patient, or there may be some long-term instability and perhaps predisposition to early degenerative change, due to the ligaments having been damaged beyond their normal elastic limit, meaning that the joint is therefore unable to recover its previous strength and integrity.

Inter-relatedness of parts

One might say that this sounds like standard orthopaedic practice, and how is it thus special to osteopathy? Well, apart from the finesse with which an osteopath can perform this type of analysis (which should not be underestimated), the job of evaluating the patient has only just begun, as the injured area must be placed 'in context' before a more complete and thus more accurate prognosis can be made. This is the other main aim of the examination.

This point has been made above, but reinforcing it is useful. Considering the whole – the fact that a body is not just a collection of bits strung together but works as a very finely tuned and coordinated structure – is something that is very basic to osteopathy. The nature and extent of the injury is one thing to consider but **one must also judge what might hinder the area from healing in the most efficient and complete manner.** This is a most important point. This means the practitioner must have some sort of concept of inter-relatedness between parts, to prompt him/her to explore the body more fully in order to better appreciate the context of the presenting condition.

The preceding chapters discussing the inter-relations between parts of the body (the spine, the limbs, the head and neck, the body cavities and so on) should have given the reader some idea of the extent of the osteopathic perception on the inter-relatedness of parts and should have set the stage for a very global view of assessment to be incorporated within effective osteopathic practice.

Different models of osteopathic thought may lead to different emphases as to which areas the osteopath thinks are inter-related, but all osteopaths think (or should think!) globally. One benefit of this is that treatment will be individually tailored to the individual patient: people who present with the same injury will not receive the same treatment.

To illustrate this we can consider two people, both with medial collateral ligament strains from injury sustained playing football.

One has a mildly arthritic hip, and so has a slightly altered orientation of the femur, thus giving a slightly different tracking of the femoral condyles in relation to the tibial plateau. One has a slightly lax ankle into inversion, due to a previous injury at this site, meaning that when running and twisting the stability of the lower leg is less than ideal. One was only playing football with the children from next door as a one off, and can afford not to play again for several weeks if required. One has an important series of five-a-side games to play within the next few weeks and absolutely will not countenance not playing. One is a plumber, who crouches all day and every day in all sorts of odd positions. One is an office worker, who does not have to move farther than the printer for the computer and back again. One is 50 years old, the other 25.

Each of the two above patients will have a different set of 'findings' in their structure (the other joints and soft tissues of their lower limbs, pelvis and rest of body) as well as lifestyle and age constraints. They could clearly react quite differently to their 'injuries' even if the actual strain local to the knee is identical. The job of the osteopath is to identify which combination of factors relates to which patient, as the specific combination will then influence recovery and the prognosis for their complaint.

Also, the osteopath must assess the underlying state of the local tissues and not just remark upon the injury recently sustained. Thus, in addition to all the above type of variations, someone whose knee is arthritic, for example, will heal much more slowly and less efficiently than someone whose knee was normal, intact and healthy prior to the injury.

Further considerations could also be required in this analysis. What happens if one has an appendix scar affecting the tension and contractability of the psoas muscle influencing hip mobility? What happens if one is suffering from the flu, or has a stiff shoulder on one side (affecting overall gait patterns)? What happens if they happen to suffer from osteoporosis or have peripheral vascular disease (e.g. atherosclerosis)? What influence do all of these types of factor

have on the progression of their problem and on the style of treatment programme suggested?

Thus the examination considers many aspects and is necessarily broad, both with respect to the mechanical efficiency of the whole body and also to the substance and lifestyle of the person (patient) themselves.

Part of the working hypothesis about these two medial collateral ligament strain cases depends on identifying the number of anatomical sites of dysfunction that are combining to affect the knee mechanics, and the nature of the tissue state in these areas (including the knee), which determines how reversible these factors are and what style of treatment could be applied to them to induce change.

With all of this relevant information gleaned from all stages of the case analysis so far (case history and examination), the osteopath is then in a position to consider a management plan, which is based upon all the above and on their concepts of treatment and their skill repertoire.

Another benefit from a global view is that one can help break into the cycle of many 'chronic' conditions and repetitive episodes of dysfunction that can affect and compromise a person for many years, giving them a long-term poor quality of life and a reduced potential for expressing themselves to their full potential and living their lives as they would wish. There are many possible cause-and-effect cycles that the osteopath needs to explore to appreciate how to move the patient on towards better overall, and better long-term, function.

Cause-and-effect cycles

Very many patients present with no immediately obvious cause for their symptoms. These patients say such things as 'well it came on gradually', or 'each time it comes on I don't know what triggers it, and this makes me very frustrated as I don't know what to do to avoid it returning'.

We have discussed many aspects of communication and inter-relatedness within the human form and one of the aims was to get readers to appreciate that, as cause and effect are not usually linear, the combination of compromising factors (barriers to good function) will summate and lead to a network of fluid dynamic distortion, a network of neural 'discoordination' and a network of stiff, tense, poorly elastic and compliant tissues that will compound further communication through neural and fluidic channels.

The concepts of tensegrity, synergy, movement inter-relation and communication networks that we have discussed give a picture of an individual summation of cause and effect within one person that depends upon their individual history and will lead to individual outcomes of function (and dysfunction) within their systems. Universal strategies of care will not work in these situations, as only removing what is a barrier to function within the individual will lead to a resolution of the networked cause-and-effect cycles that have given them their poor function.

The various injuries and disease that they have suffered from will take their toll, and certainly one can predict where in the body one might find some of these restrictions (effects/legacies). However, once an area is compromised, this will set off a chain of reactions that pervade the body on a level that the patient is not aware of. Adaptation can begin 'silently' and spread throughout the body, and often the person only becomes aware of these things when they have summated in whatever area of the body, leading to symptoms of soft tissue distress, circulatory or neural irritation, poor tissue health and possible disease. One cannot therefore only consider the 'obvious' areas of restriction, such as the reported sites of trauma and disease arising from the case history questioning. One needs to explore the whole body, looking for the hidden reactions and adaptations that have developed from the insults, stresses and strains the person has endured, so that one can appreciate how the body is now globally compromised and so how the person may have developed their subsequent problems.

Finding all of these 'hidden' factors gives the individual assessment and management plan that is relevant for that person.

This is what osteopathic examination is all about.

It is the osteopath's job to explore, appreciate and release whatever barrier to function is within that person. These terms form a useful acronym, **EAR**, which is very appropriate, as osteopaths 'listen with their hands' in order to do this!

A quote from *Visceral Manipulation* by Jean-Pierre Barral and Pierre Mercier is very illustrative of an osteopath's palpatory skills:

> *The osteopath is a mechanic in the noblest sense of the word – really a micro-mechanic. We all have two hands but who among us really knows how to use them? No one argues with the wine taster who, by using his palate, can tell us the characteristics of a wine – its region, its vineyard or even its vintage. The education of touch can go at least as far.*
>
> Barral and Mercier, 1988

In order to complete our understanding of osteopathic examination, one must have still more detail as to the analyses used during soft tissue palpation and joint mobility evaluation; if one is to appreciate the osteopathic model, one must have an appreciation of the fifth dimension within osteopathic analysis.

As indicated before, it is also the state of the tissues that helps to develop treatment strategies within management plans, and so we cannot discuss these things without knowing what is meant by 'tissue state'.

The fifth dimension

Different tissues each have a different quality when they are palpated.

In a previous chapter we suggested that the osteopathic tenet 'structure governs function' would be better written as 'motion relates to physiology'. We also suggested that appreciating the dynamic anatomy of a tissue will help appreciate how microstructure relates to homeostasis and how changes in soft tissue biomechanics can relate to pathophysiology within the tissues. The fifth dimension – palpation – allows us to interpret tissue function.

Dynamic anatomy

Different histological make-up brings differing amounts of inherent pliability and elasticity; because of this a muscle feels completely different from a ligament, a bone or an organ, for example. Thus there is a 'normal' feel to healthy tissues that is different for each tissue. This has to be learned through repeated exploration of 'normal' and the practitioner builds up his/her own vocabulary of what 'normal' is.

Once someone is trained to use palpation efficiently, then finer and finer differences between tissues can be felt. This is vital, as one must be able to differentiate when something has changed from being 'normal' to being 'not normal'. There are lots of things that could be considered 'not normal', as we shall see.

Changes in anatomy

'Not normal' can include various 'pathological states' within those tissues. In this context, inflammation is a pathological state; as is 'laxity' (for example, in a damaged ligament, or a muscle affected by a peripheral neuropathy leading to lack of tone); as is increased collagen content, 'fibrosity', which can come with chronic shortening due to lack of activity, with ageing or in association with inflammation. 'Not normal' can also include emotional tension within a tissue and degrees of irritability within the tissues, because of various aspects of excessive neural activity, for example.

An arthritic knee will thus feel quite different from a healthy one that has sustained a medial collateral ligament overstrain. This will feel different again from one in which there is a bursitis or an infection. Also, one can feel if the inflammation is mild or severe; if the arthritis is simply minor degenerative change or a massive disruption of the articular surfaces with gross bony adaptation from altered load-bearing forces. Such refinement of touch certainly takes practice and it can be very helpful to make use of whatever X-rays or scans a patient has to hone one's skills against actual recordings. However, once the skill is acquired, then it can be used to further the assessment of the patient in a material

way. Palpatory skills are part of an osteopath's diagnostic repertoire, in much the same way as blood tests and ultrasound scans are part of a medical practitioner's repertoire.

Palpation then enables one to assess whether there is in fact some sort of pathological change in the tissues or not, which is a part of the confirmation and denial of hypotheses that is an integral part of case analysis. Palpation also gives a view of the extent of the pathological/traumatic/functional change (when coupled with the information gained during the case history analysis) and helps appreciate the potential for change (thus leading to ideas on prognosis) and also to the type of treatment style that might be most usefully applied to bring that tissue state back towards the normal.

Different practitioners will have a different repertoire of technical approaches, which are designed to induce change within the tissues and will therefore suggest slightly different management plans based on this skill base. However, they will all be using the same appreciation of tissue change, pathophysiological involvement and understanding of tissue remodelling/adaptation, as these are all based on a common understanding of tissue histology, tissue function and pathological change.

Osteopathic physical evaluation incorporates testing all tissues of the body, not just those relating to the articulations (joints) within the musculoskeletal system. Muscles and joints, when they are tested/evaluated, are assessed by using both active and passive movement. Other body tissues, such as connective tissues through the body and the organ systems of the body, are not under 'voluntary' control and are therefore evaluated not by getting the person to perform active movements but using 'passive' strategies. Passive testing means that the patient does not perform the action, the practitioner does.

Active testing, where appropriate, can reveal interesting factors but it is often the passive testing that can be the most interesting and revealing. Indeed, most of the above palpatory analysis within the fifth dimension of the osteopathic sieve can only be achieved through passive testing, as it is only when doing so that tissue state and reaction to movement can be fully evaluated.

Link to previous information

Before going any further, there are important links to previous information given about osteopathic models and practice, which need pointing out.

In Chapter 6, there was a lot of discussion concerning 'reductionist' and 'revised' models of spinal motion testing. These centred on evaluating joint mobility by referring to tissue reaction within that motion testing, rather than relying on a simple analysis of relative joint position.

In that chapter, the important gains made within the profession by changing to a model of using tissue responses within motion testing were discussed, but there was no comment made on what the tissue responses were, nor of their clinical relevance. It was stated that all this would be discussed in detail later, which is in fact what this next section is all about.

Evaluating tissue responses, and what this means for technical intervention during treatment, is a complex subject and the profession must pay tribute to Professor Laurie Hartman for his work in the field of articular evaluation and diagnosis.

To guide the reader through this analysis of the fifth dimension, it may be useful to start by revising what may ordinarily be felt with a normal healthy joint.

Movement and tissue responses in motion testing

We will be discussing many aspects of subjective analysis of tissue feel during movement testing and palpation. By its very nature, this type of comment is initially open to much dissatisfaction, as one cannot be specific about what is clearly a subjective 'science', with interuser reliance open to question. However, regardless of the descriptors individuals choose to adopt, they all build up their own library of sensations that they have correlated from exploring the tissues of many people within their professional training and subsequently throughout their practice lives (as

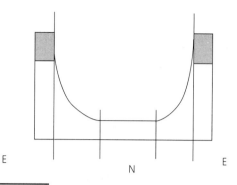

Figure 10.4

The normal range of a joint from, for example, full extension to full flexion. The range of motion is shown on the horizontal axis. The curve represents the resistance in the tissues and articular structures, which increases towards the end of each range of movement. Tissue resistance is shown on the vertical axis. E = end; N = neutral.

mentioned earlier). Thus the ways to recognize the difference and meanings of one tissue state within an articulation/structure from another are carefully passed by qualified practitioners to a student within the undergraduate teaching clinics so that experience is passed to those learning the skills for the first time.

It is important to stress that one cannot simply read such a list of palpatory findings and expect to diagnose from them with no supervision. It is not possible to learn such a skill properly without full training, in both theoretical and practical aspects.

Motion testing: the normal joint

In Figure 10.4 a normal joint is represented. From E to E (end to end) represents the normal amplitude (in whatever direction, say from full flexion through to full extension). N is the midrange, and can be thought of as when the joint is in a neutral position.

From a neutral position the joint can be moved in one direction or another (for example, the left or the right in the diagram) and, as the joint approaches its end of range, the resistance in the soft tissues increases until the articulation is brought to a natural halt. At this point, if the joint is pushed gently a little more against this 'stop' then a little extra 'give' is normally still perceived. This extra give is represented by the shaded boxes in the picture. The increasing resistance as the joint moves towards end of range is referred to a joint 'bind' and the resistance when the joint comes to a natural halt is called the 'tissue barrier' (in other words the barrier to further movement). The perceived extra give is called the 'end feel'. In mid range, the articular surfaces normally come in close contact and, if these cartilaginous structures are healthy, they will glide over each other in a relatively slippery and friction-free manner. Thus there are several 'natural' palpatory possibilities, depending on what part of the joint's amplitude of movement is being assessed, which are part of the feel of a 'normal' joint. These palpatory findings (end feel, bind, tissue barrier and so on) are illustrated in Figure 10.5.

A normal joint will not be red, hot or cold, or swollen, nor will there be any protective muscle spasm associated with its movements (active or passive). When the joint is moved towards end of range the tissue barrier (resistance) will come on slowly and progressively and the end feel will not be reactive – there will be no 'kick back' in the muscles when the joint is passively pushed a little further into the tissue barrier (unless this is done too violently or to too excessive a degree!). If all of the normal amplitudes of movement are tested, there will be a uniform feeling to the tissue barrier found with each range, and the mid-range (neutral) will be smooth and supple. There will be also be a certain feeling of vitality of the tissues within a healthy joint.

Note: Vitality is a difficult concept to describe with words but if one imagines feeling a young child's skin, and pictures this with one's 'minds fingers', so to speak, then the skin will feel soft yet strong, warm and springy, fit and healthy. Now if one imagines feeling an old person's skin, the texture will be quite different. The skin will be sagging and loose over the underlying muscle and there will be much less inherent elasticity. There will be less spring and, although the skin may be as warm as before, it will not feel so fit. Another analogy, but one that not all readers may have felt, is the sensation in the tissues of a quite

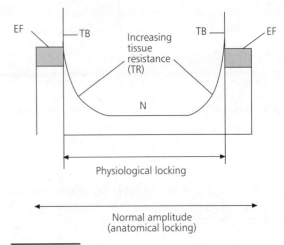

Figure 10.5

A normal joint, with characteristic changes in tissue resistance at different points within the joint range and at the end of the joint range. Joint range is show on the horizontal axis and tissue resistance is shown on the vertical axis. EF = end feel (should be elastic); TB = tissue barrier; N = neutral (should be gliding and smooth); TR = tissue resistance (should be non-reactive and evenly progressive).

sick person. Here there will be less spring, the temperature may be different and there may be excessive dryness or 'clamminess' (sweating). There may be a little swelling in the tissues, such that they are slightly 'puffy' (oedematous): the tissues may feel 'boggy'. The tissues will feel much more inert and unresponsive to pressure and stroking. They will literally feel less healthy. These can all be expressions of vitality, or lack of it, and constitute a subjective analysis of health within the tissues.

In the normal joint, although there may be naturally more amplitude (amount of movement) in one range (direction) than another, due to differing anatomical considerations in and around the joint, one 'range' should not be more 'lax' or 'limited' than another and should not have a different end feel, unless the anatomy dictates this (for example, in the elbow, flexion is limited principally by the bulk of the flexors getting in the way of the approximation of the humerus and the forearm, whereas extension is limited by bony contact between the olecranon fossa and the ulna). Any accessory movements

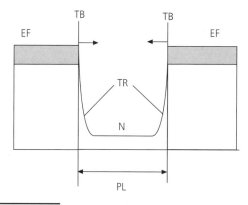

Figure 10.6

The changes in palpatory findings when muscle reaction is more active than normal. TB = the tissue barrier now occurs earlier in the joint range; TR = tissue resistance builds up much more sharply and quickly; EF = the end feel is now more 'aggressive' and the muscle 'kicks back' as it is tested; N = neutral (mid-range) is still smooth; PL – the overall joint range is reduced and physiological locking comes earlier than before.

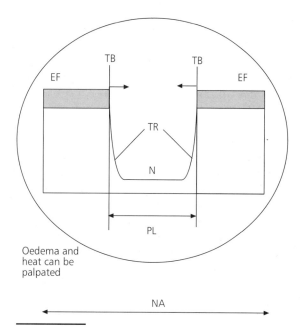

Oedema and heat can be palpated

Figure 10.7

The palpatory changes in a joint with a degree of soft tissue trauma. TB = the tissue barrier now occurs earlier in the joint range; TR = tissue resistance builds up much more sharply and quickly; EF = the end feel is now more 'irritable' and the muscle 'kicks back' in a protective manner as it is tested – muscle spasm can be palpated; N = neutral (mid-range) is still smooth; PL – the overall joint range is reduced and physiological locking comes earlier than before; NA = normal amplitude has not been affected but cannot be effectively assessed because of the muscle spasm.

should not feel unstable. Throughout all of the induced movements there should be no pain nor any unpleasant or uncomfortable feelings reported by the patient (or owner of the joints!).

Motion testing: the 'not-normal' joint

There are many aspects of joint motion and feel that change when the joint is 'not normal' in some way, and for some reason. We will start by discussing 'basic' changes. These changes are illustrated in Figures 10.6–10.10 and can be compared against Figure 10.5. The reader should carefully compare such things as the size of the neutral range, the angle at which tissue resistance builds up, the point within the range at which tissue resistance creates a barrier and the size and quality of the tissue end feel. These points are all discussed within the text and captions of the figures listed.

More active muscle reaction

The first change is when muscle reaction is more active. This is shown in Figure 10.6.

Such things as minor muscle injury; an adapted 'holding' and tension of the joint and soft tissues, such as might be found if posture or bio-

mechanical action is slightly adapted; or if the person is 'nervous' or 'bracing' their muscles through subconscious emotional association; could account for such a finding. Such findings might be expressed through isolated ranges of motion, with the remainder of the joint performing 'normally' or the restriction may be universal throughout the joint.

More severe soft tissue injury (through trauma, for example)

The findings shown in Figure 10.6 are now added to by the presence of oedema and heat, as signs of active inflammation. The extent of the swelling, muscle spasm and irritability of the tissues is a guide to the severity of tissue damage but, if the injury has not caused instability (i.e. significant disruption of the capsuloligamentous

Figure 10.8

The palpatory changes in a joint that has become unstable through injury. The vertical dotted line indicates where the normal tissue barrier would have been found and the horizontal dotted line indicates that the normal joint amplitude has been increased in one or more ranges. The tissue barrier within the range that has become extended has quite different characteristics. If there is not too much muscle activity 'guarding' the lax range then the tissue barrier will not be progressive, but feel as though it comes to an abrupt halt, unless the ligaments are ruptured, when the end feel will be missing. If there is a degree of muscle guarding the tissue barrier might be more aggressive, initially limiting the range, bringing physiological locking much earlier. NA = the overall anatomical range (normal amplitude) of the joint has been extended, usually in one direction, implicating one ligament, but may be through several ranges – instability may therefore be in one or more directions; TR = the tissue resistance may build up quite differently in different directions/ranges tested. In the direction of ligamentous damage, there may be very little resistance, and consequently the TB (tissue barrier) and EF (end feel) may be limited and not strong. In other directions the TR and TB may be as for the mildly injured joint in Figure 10.7 – i.e. bringing PL (physiological locking) nearer neutral range in those directions. TR and TB may feel relatively more resistant than in the injured range. N = neutral (mid-range) feel should still be normal.

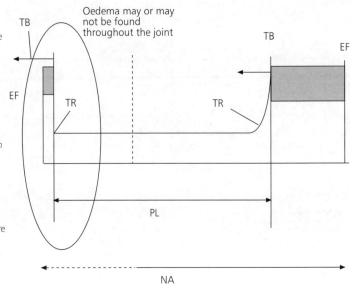

arrangement), the joint will probably feel as described below. These new palpatory findings are illustrated in Figure 10.7.

Important note: These types of finding may be present in a joint that has not been injured, but is expressing the consequences of 'acute' spinal cord 'facilitation', as was discussed in Chapter 4.

One of the ways of determining whether the joint in question is adapted as a result of injury or as part of a neural reflex response is (1) to discover if there has been a trauma that might account for the condition, or (2) to see if there is any visceral dysfunction that might be triggering this reflex response. One needs to know which organ is segmentally related to the joint in question and then one can evaluate that organ. This is done through the history – where organ disease might be identified. But the viscera may not be presenting symptoms in its own right (perhaps if it is an early presentation of disease, or the dysfunction is relatively mild and therefore 'subclinical'), in which situation the case history questioning might not reveal its presence. One

needs therefore to 'double-check' by palpating the organ in question, to evaluate whether it is dysfunctional at some level and thus still capable of reflexly disturbing the spinal articulation that was originally being explored.

Returning to our analysis of injury to joints: if there is instability, then the joint will feel different again. This is shown in Figure 10.8.

This type of joint disruption is interesting, as the individual characteristics will change depending on the extent of the injury.

Degenerative joint disease

In degenerative joint disease, there are other changes. These are shown in Figure 10.9. In late degenerative change, some of the findings reverse. These are shown in Figure 10.10.

There will be a whole variety of subtleties based upon these types of image, depending on the extent, and on the combination of injuries and changes. Readers should not forget that often many states are superimposed as dysfunction and injury accrue chronologically.

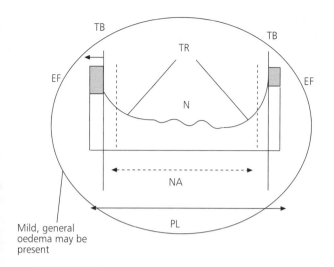

Mild, general oedema may be present

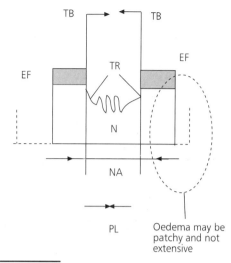

Oedema may be patchy and not extensive

Figure 10.9

Palpatory changes in a joint with early degenerative change. The joint can feel as though it is slightly unstable in all ranges. PL = here, due to disruption of tissues, there may be a slight overall increase in range above neutral – denoting a slight general instability of the joint (physiological locking extends beyond the normal amplitude of the joint); TB = the tissue barrier will have moved 'outwards' and the end feel may be slightly reactive and aggressive in this situation, but not too much, as the ligamentous disruption is not as severe as in Figure 10.8; N = the mid-range/neutral feel may be slightly adapted and may denote changes in intra-articular fluid levels, early cartilage change or early damage to intervertebral disc tissue, for example.

Figure 10.10

Palpatory changes in late degenerative joint disease. NA = the normal amplitude may be quite limited but this may not be expressed uniformly through all ranges; PL = the physiological locking and TB (tissue barriers) will have moved towards mid-range; EF = the end feel is likely to be less reactive than in all other examples and to be less elastic, and more 'fibrotic' and 'bony', than in normal joints; TR = tissue resistance may not build quickly and end feel could be arrived at quite 'abruptly'; N = the mid-range (neutral) feel will be quite different and will depend on the extent of change in the articular surfaces, menisci, discs and so on.

This type of motion analysis then gives a window into the state/degree of damage and compromise within a joint and its surrounding tissues. It is therefore part of diagnosis. Then, depending on the state of the tissues, a variety of treatments/techniques can be applied, to restore more normal motion and tissue responses to the joint complex. Thus, this type of motion testing can help determine treatment choice.

We will be returning to these analogies a little later to discuss treatment choices, but first we need to look at motion testing in other tissues.

Motion testing is more than evaluating joints

Other aspects of tissue state, which are applicable to all tissues, not only joints and their immediate structures, need to be evaluated and can be discussed using these types of image.

Tissues can be thought of as springs, oriented around an embryological fulcrum giving the tissue an inherent natural orientation, with a rhythmicity (from neural activity/involuntary motion/whatever cause) and will have several palpatory features. Figure 10.11 aims to show a palpatory analogy similar to that used for joint testing, as above.

When joints are tested, soft tissue evaluation comes into play – and creates the tissue barriers, tissue resistance and end feel characteristics that we have been discussing. However, it is worthwhile discussing soft tissue evaluation in its own right, as there are many areas of the body where soft tissues are not intimately involved in joint mechanics and need to be assessed individually.

Springs

Each individual structure can act a little like a spring, which can be stretched and compressed, with each direction of movement having a different palpatory 'conversation' with the person

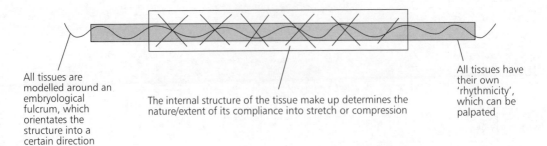

All tissues are modelled around an embryological fulcrum, which orientates the structure into a certain direction

The internal structure of the tissue make up determines the nature/extent of its compliance into stretch or compression

All tissues have their own 'rhythmicity', which can be palpated

Figure 10.11

The broader rectangle represents the structure of the tissue being tested. The cross-hatching denotes the internal architecture of the tissue (for example, collagen fibres in connective tissue, trabeculae in bone, contractile fibres within muscle and so on). The wider, shaded box indicates that, because of natural physiological activity within the tissues, there will be a basic rhythmicity that can be palpated. The wavy line indicates that all tissues in the body are basically oriented around an embryological fulcrum – and any tissue damage will be repaired in such a way that the tissues are remodelled around this original fulcrum.

monitoring/'listening to' the tissue responses. One can 'pull' on a tissue, take up any 'slack' within it and see how compliant the whole structure is and what quality of resistance it offers during stretch, as you take up the slack and also as you test out the limits of its stretch and compliance. One can also 'push' on the structure, thus 'closing down the coils' of the spring, and follow the tissue sensations as it 'concertinas' into a compressed state. All of these types of 'push and pull' actions can be structured into particular evaluation techniques. These evaluation techniques can also be used in a therapeutic context, and become treatment modes and styles.

Motion testing by 'pulling'

Motion testing within one muscle, or one ligament, or one organ, or one bone, for example, cannot be done in isolation. As you pull on one structure, motion will be passed to other tissues that are attached to it. The motion characteristics of whatever structure is being tested will be reflected on to chains of muscles, interconnections of tendons and ligaments, general fascial planes and so on, throughout the body. The motion characteristics of distant parts can also feed back and influence the more local structures as well. There is always a reciprocal influence between tissue types and their relative mobilities.

This leads to a three-dimensional vision of motion testing. One takes up the 'slack' in one

component first, thereby evaluating it, and then one continues to pull, thus engaging the next component. This next component is evaluated 'through' the first one and then, once that slack has been taken up, one continues to pull again, taking up the slack in yet more distant components. In this way, you can test multiple components from the comfort of your armchair, so to speak: in other words, from one point of contact. This makes global testing more efficient and enables many things to be evaluated in a short space of time. Time can often be a premium within evaluation and it is useful to be able to get a general overview of what is going on within the body: global screening tests such as this can be handy – they quickly direct the practitioner to areas of the body that need more detailed examination/exploration.

As all tissues within the body are networked together in a three-dimensional way, the 'chains of tension' and the 'pulls' you create will be in several directions at once. It is difficult to move one part without moving anything else simultaneously. This is the principle of tensegrity that we discussed before. This means that you need a sharp mind and a good knowledge of anatomy to follow all the tensions and see if they are as elastic as you expect and if they are occurring in a normal pattern/direction. Figure 10.12 shows what happens as you evaluate tissue tensions by 'pulling'.

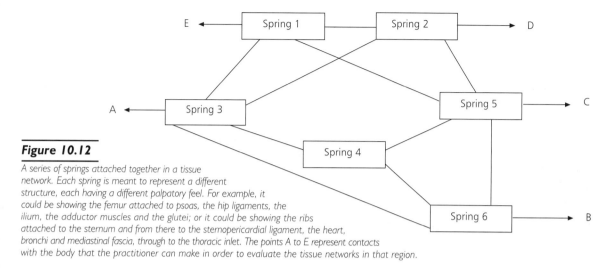

Figure 10.12

A series of springs attached together in a tissue network. Each spring is meant to represent a different structure, each having a different palpatory feel. For example, it could be showing the femur attached to psoas, the hip ligaments, the ilium, the adductor muscles and the glutei; or it could be showing the ribs attached to the sternum and from there to the sternopericardial ligament, the heart, bronchi and mediastinal fascia, through to the thoracic inlet. The points A to E represent contacts with the body that the practitioner can make in order to evaluate the tissue networks in that region.

You are assessing the compliance and elasticity within the soft tissues, and you are looking for differences in resistance to movement that might be adapting the normal biomechanical activity in that part of the body. The tissue at fault will be the one that is offering a resistance that is different from normal.

Looking at Figure 10.12, it can be seen that you can test the whole web from any of the points, e.g. A – E. The person testing should know what the whole structure should feel like if you pulled on A as opposed to B, for example, and you should be able to tell if the response from spring 2, as you pull on point B, via springs 6, 4, 3 and 5, is as it should be. Each of the springs could be a ligament, or a bone, or an organ, or a fascial sheath, and will each have its own 'feel'. So, as you take up the slack in each, you will have to continuously retune your palpatory awareness to pick up what is happening in each spring as you engage it through the one before, and avoid getting lost in the noise, so to speak. Also, it is easy to pull too much at once and so take up all slack in the whole web, and therefore not be able to tell which spring was the component that expressed adapted movement as it was engaged!

This gives global testing from a single contact.

Motion testing by 'pulling' is what osteopaths are doing within joint testing, for example, and if you move one joint and evaluate the tissue responses as you test that joint, you can follow the pulls that are created to sites distant from the joint, so that you can perform a global test within your normal joint testing, if you wish.

For example, if you extend the knee, then eventually the hamstrings should tighten and limit joint range. You may feel that the hamstrings are tight, because the extension is limited compared to what you would expect normally. However, if you now carry on testing the knee by moving the hip into flexion, then through the hamstring pulls, the pelvic structures will be engaged and the ilium will begin to rotate backwards. This is shown in Figure 10.13.

Now, as the ilium rotates backwards, you can immediately tell if there is the normal amount of movement coming from that area – by the response you get through the whole leg. If the ilial articulations and structures are normal and not compromised, then, once you have created enough motion at the knee to extend the whole movement behind the hamstrings, you are simply testing the ilium as though you were holding it directly.

If the ilium is restricted, you will pick this up just as well as if you were holding it directly. And so, in this case, you know just from your knee extension test that there is also something wrong with the hip/ilium, for example, which might

307

Figure 10.13

The leg being tested. Initially, the patient lies on their back with the hip and knee slightly flexed. The practitioner first extends the knee and then, keeping the knee extended, raises the whole leg further upwards (flexing the whole leg at the level of the hip). In this way, several structures from the knee ligaments and hamstrings to the iliolumbar ligaments, sacroiliac ligaments and low lumbar spine can be screened 'collectively'.

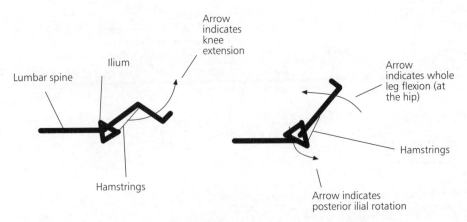

need to be treated in order to resolve the hamstring tensions so that the knee can recover. The chicken and egg question of which came first (and therefore where to direct treatment), the ilium problem, the knee problem, or indeed the hamstring problem, will be returned to later.

This is a simple example, and most motion tests within the body are in reality much more complex than this: biomechanical appreciation means having a good understanding of how structures are linked together and how they move three-dimensionally in an integrated manner. There can be many very subtle and very complex changes to overall movement patterns when one or more parts of the whole are moving in an adapted manner.

As stated, this type of testing is not just for joints: if you are looking at bones, or large muscular structures that have many fascial attachments to them (such as the diaphragm, with its many pleural, peritoneal and visceral relations/ attachments) or at organs, then the tensegrity web analogy above comes into its own and, again, allows you to evaluate complex three-dimensional movement conundrums from relatively few movements and contacts.

Motion testing 'into compression'
In order for the body to move as a springy, integrated whole, for every oscillation of movement that stretches out a tissue there is a following one that compresses it. For example, there is the load-

ing and springing of the arches of the foot during walking; or the contrary rotations of the shoulder girdle and pelvis during motion (torsioning/compressing the thoracolumbar region); or the longitudinal lengthening and shortening of the spinal curves (opening and closing of the vertebral articulations); and so on.

This compliance into compression, whether it is within a disc, a bone, a blood vessel, an organ or whatever, is a necessary component of the whole biomechanical and physiological function of that part/tissue.

As you put movement through one part, this begins to create a compression, a wave of pressure, a concertina effect, through the adjacent tissues. If you push just a little bit, the compression wave only passes through a few tissues before its effect is dissipated and becomes difficult to feel. If you push a little more, then you will be able to follow/observe the wave permeating through tissues further afield. As you push, you are monitoring the resistance to compression within those tissues and comparing it to what you consider is normal.

For example, if you push/compress the leg longitudinally through the foot, you should feel the leg gradually concertina and the motion pass through the ankle, knee, hip and into the lumbar region. Normally you would expect this to happen evenly, and for the forces created to cause a slight shift in the pelvic articulations and tissues and end up causing a sidebending/rotation in the lumbar spine, which pivots at a certain point. However, if there is a restriction somewhere, a part of this chain of tissues that will not compress as it should, then the motion passes unevenly through the limb, which has to buckle to accommodate these changes, and so the movement in the lumbar spine (for example) ends up pivoting around a different point. Now you know that something is wrong and you can explore more specifically to find out at which level it is to be found.

Please note: one should not develop the impression that osteopaths go around pushing harder and harder on various bits of their patients' bodies to see what happens at the other end. This is not the case. In the same way that you can 'overpull' during tensional testing, so too can too much compression be inadvisable. Apart from causing the patient pain, it will not allow the practitioner to observe the gradual accumulation of compression through the component parts, to discern which individual component was at fault. To overcome this, rhythmic oscillatory movements are put through the tissues, which allows the waves of compression to be more accurately resolved without placing too much force on any one particular part. This style of motion testing is very like 'manual ultrasound scanning' – putting a wave of motion through will cause ripples of force, which will be reflected back to the practitioner's hands, where they can be interpreted and analysed.

This is one aspect of what occurs within the general osteopathic treatment (GOT) routine that was first introduced in a previous chapter. It requires skill and a lot of practice to create effective motion testing using this concept. However, once learned, it gives a very useful and interesting analysis of body motion.

Why look three dimensionally?

This point has been raised many times, but here is another analysis, based on the above motion principles, to give further insight.

Multiple areas of dysfunction will recreate a network of tissue tension acting upon and through any particular component of the chain, which will not act uniformly through the whole structure as it is supposed to do (tension and compression forces are not balanced: some components will be overstretched and some will be overcompressed). This then places strain on component parts. If one component, one spring – one muscle, for example – begins to become fatigued or strained as a result, then one can massage it locally, for example, but the shifting web of tensions will re-establish that tendency to strain and compromise as soon as the practitioner's hands are removed from the patient. That is, it will unless several factors are worked on so that, when the practitioner lets go, the same network of tensions is not recreated – and so the previously compromised component now 'sits' in a better environment and the adverse tension/compression is either diminished or shifted somewhere else!

While we are discussing these things, do not forget all the discussions on fibroblasts, and how they react to tensional forces; and also, do not forget the neural control of balance and co-ordination, which relies on feedback from myriad proprioceptors throughout all the tissues of the body. Movement changes create barriers to communication and function.

If tension/compression builds in one part, the nervous system detects this and then directs one of its contractile components (a muscle/a group of muscles) to alter the tension in the whole structure by contracting, with the aim of reducing the adverse forces in the original area. After a while, the nervous system will 'let go' of this adaptation; hopefully the failing component will have healed, so the tensional web should revert to normal balance and integration, and all information streaming in from the proprioceptors will have returned to normal. (Apologies for the rather 'loose' discussion, but at least this way the overall ideas should come through, without getting lost in detail.)

However, if the component has not healed, then the nervous system will be aware of this and will have no choice but to continue to keep certain muscle(s) contracting to keep the forces away from the compromised part. Unfortunately, this often leads to a chronically shifted dynamic within the web, with all the other neural reflexes adapting and all the fibroblasts remodelling the internal fascial/tissue frameworks (ECM and cytoskeleton), to fit with this 'new' distortion of the web. Thus tension accumulates at another point, another component fails, the web shifts again, and adaptation is endless, with the web getting more and more inefficient every day.

Now all the neural reflexes are so confused they don't know how to move anything properly any more and, if they do, all they get is a harsh resistance from lots of remodelled tissues that won't allow compliance and movement any more; all the fluid dynamics will be compromised, the neural confusion will spill over into the autonomic nervous system and the neuro-endocrine immune system, and the whole body will grind to a halt, and declare itself diseased. This is where the body also screams 'get me to my osteopath quick!'

Before discussing how to treat this poor body, let us continue with our discussion of motion testing within tissues.

Tissue changes and their palpatory effects

In the same way that we analysed joint motion testing, we can illustrate how adapted/altered tissue may feel on testing. Remember that we are talking about 'passive' testing (i.e. the practitioner does the movement, and not the patient). Osteopaths can evaluate a whole variety of tissues in this way, including hollow organs (smooth muscle tubes), solid organs (with an internal connective tissue framework), fascial sheaths and mesenteries, dural and membranous structures, bones, ligaments, tendons and, of course, skeletal muscles.

As stated before, each tissue will have a different feeling/elasticity and compliance because of its natural histological make-up. Each tissue will have a different normal compliance from its neighbours. Each tissue will operate around a different embryological fulcrum, and each will have its own expression of rhythmicity. This is illustrated in Figure 10.14. Note: The size of the boxes and the curve patterns are not meant to

reflect accurately real-life differences, but may give some hint of normal variation between tissues.

When evaluating rhythmicity and orientation around the embryological core/fulcrum, then the osteopath becomes passive as well and 'listens' without inducing movement in the tissues. Readers should note this difference between passive testing and listening skills.

Each different tissue type has a different structural and histological make-up. This is indicated by the different fillings in the broader rectangular shapes. Each structural type allows a degree of internal movement within the tissue, and each one will act as a type of 'spring', as introduced earlier. As each of these pictograms is looked at, you can imagine the various 'sliding elements' or 'couplings' or 'elastic components' within each of the tissues. These are depicted by the straight, wavy or dotted lines. (The 'sine waves' indicate the embryological fulcrum and the shaded boxes the rhythmicity.)

These elastic couplings/sliding elements are formed by such things as the actin and myosin components of muscle; or the trabeculae in bone; or the proteoglycans, collagen molecules and fibronectins in fascia; and so on.

Because of these differences, the amount of:

- internal stretchiness;
- tissue resistance towards the end of stretch, and end feel;
- compressive resistance;
- torsional resistance;

will be individual to each tissue, and must be learned by the osteopath. They will each have a different palpatory quality.

Amplitude, end feel, tissue resistance

As one can compress or stretch a tissue in three dimensions, it will therefore have a three-dimensional vector quality for each of these types of feel. The way all the components slide over each other, or resist movement and stretch, is determined by their make up – and so the internal mobility or **tissue resistance** of the structure can be assessed.

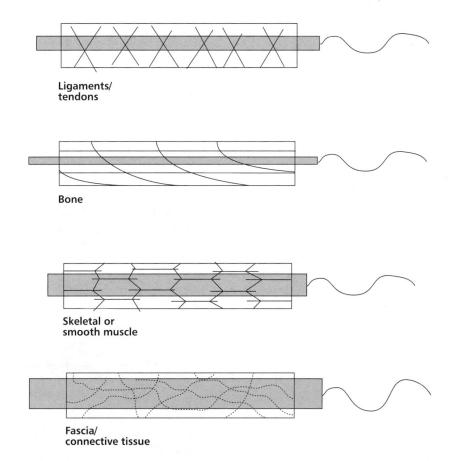

Figure 10.14

Four different tissues. The different fillings within the broad rectangles aim to show the individual histological make-up of each tissue. An attempt has been made to make these rectangles reflect the palpatory differences between the tissue types. The wider, shaded rectangles represent the rhythmicity of each tissue. The relative size of these rectangles aims to show the differences in the quality of these natural rhythms (thinner rectangles showing less 'active' rhythms than thicker rectangles, for example). The wave-like or sine waves indicate that each tissue is oriented around an individual embryological fulcrum.

Ligaments/tendons

Bone

Skeletal or smooth muscle

Fascia/connective tissue

As one moves the tissues into either stretch or compression, they will each have a different amount of movement available, therefore determining the natural **amplitude** of either stretch or compression.

As one reaches the end of available movement, the tissues will express bind/resistance, giving an idea of **end feel**.

Changes
Now, if the tissue is injured, becomes oedematous or scarred, or has adhesions and increased connections between its sliding elements or connective tissue components, or has its motile elements directed to contract, or receives no nerve impulses and so becomes atonic, and so on, each of these scenarios will leave a different palpatory legacy.

Now, when the torsional, tensional, and compressive vectors, core fulcrum and rhythmicity are palpated, then all the palpatory responses will be different. Examples of the above tissue changes are illustrated in Figure 10.15, and one should reflect on the possibilities for movement within these adapted tissues that these lead to.

The shaded rectangles depicting the core fulcrums are shown as discontinuous, which indicates that all of these changes may lead to the tissue being 'torsioned' around its natural fulcrum and so less able to express normal function as a result. Rhythmicity within the tissues will also adapt and its rate, amplitude and quality can all change, leading to a fast, irritated and 'tight' rhythm, a slow, ponderous and pendular rhythm, or no rhythm at all, for example. There are many possibilities.

The osteopath now puts all these things together.

Figure 10.15

The four tissues as before, after they have suffered some type of trauma or undergone some sort of structural change. The changes in the palpatory quality of each of the tissues will vary according to the type of adaptation present, and this has been indicated by altering the fillings within the broad rectangles (compared to Figure 10.14). Each tissue type is shown adapted in two different ways, so that a number of examples of palpatory responses to motion testing can be shown. These are shown on either side of the vertical line running through all the tissue types. With the structure of the tissues having been changed by oedema, increased bone deposition, contraction, fibrotic changes, scarring and so on, each time the histological change can give recognizable changes to palpation and so one can begin to categorize tissue changes as they occur. This can form a type of tissue diagnosis.

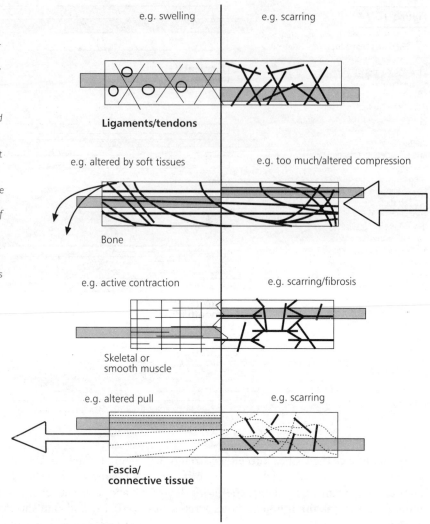

e.g. swelling   e.g. scarring

Ligaments/tendons

e.g. altered by soft tissues   e.g. too much/altered compression

Bone

e.g. active contraction   e.g. scarring/fibrosis

Skeletal or smooth muscle

e.g. altered pull   e.g. scarring

Fascia/ connective tissue

Completing the examination and compiling examination findings

So far, then, during the examination, we have looked at:

- global tension and compression testing, to pick out block areas of dysfunction within the whole body – motion testing within the 'whole web';
- specific joint testing, with an eye on local tissue responses;
- local testing of soft tissues/other structures (bones and organs), considering them as

springs and as structures oriented around a fulcrum, expressing rhythmicity;

(the last two representing local testing of component parts of the web).

Global testing

Global testing is a key starting point as one simply cannot examine everything minutely in one consultation after having taken a case history and before giving the patient (hopefully) some treatment, all within the space of 30–45 minutes, including booking them in for a next appointment and writing up their notes. It is too much all in one go, and so the examination is refined by having a general evaluation that picks out the main areas of interest for further/more detailed analysis. The other factors can be explored in later sessions.

From the case history the osteopath has part of the examination already mapped out – by the need to confirm or deny hypotheses, for example. Various sites may also be implicated by a history of trauma or disease, which need to be followed up. However, the rest of the examination needs to take into account all those 'hidden' factors that are so important to gaining a biomechanical and physiological impression of inter-relatedness between dysfunctional and symptomatic areas.

The osteopath must always allow him/herself to find what is evident in the patient and not what s/he expects to see or hopes to find.

This is where global screening comes in.

Global screening includes:

- observation;
- standing movement tests and other active tests;
- global motion tests (tensional and compressional);
- global 'listening' tests (webs and general fulcrums, and general rhythmicity).

Observation is just that: the osteopath observes the patient standing and looks for asymmetry in their form. S/he looks for differences in head tilt, spinal curves, thoracic shape, upper and lower limb torsion and so on. S/he looks to see if the person is standing evenly with respect to their centre of gravity: are they shifted slightly forwards, backwards or slightly to one side? These and many other observations point to areas of the body that are holding tension and may not move appropriately.

Next come the active tests. This is where the osteopath asks the patient to bend in various directions and watches what happens to the spine and other body areas – for example, are the movements uniform or adapted, are they evidently in pain, are the movements stable or

unstable? These active tests are always performed with respect to patient comfort. Any symptoms (pain, neural radiation and so on) that are provoked by these movements are important indicators for whatever working hypotheses the osteopath is exploring and can contribute to the eventual diagnosis. Active tests also include resisted muscle tests (such as are also used within orthopaedic evaluation), which can help determine tissue dysfunction.

Next come various special tests, such as blood pressure, compression tests, neurological examination and ophthalmology, that might be necessary to explore the working hypotheses. Then come all the various motion tests, both global and local.

The main approaches to global motion testing have been described, but two – global 'listening' and general fulcrum evaluation – have not. The basis of these tests is quite simple, but their efficient interpretation requires advanced palpatory awareness.

Global listening

To understand this test, we return once more to our idea of the body as a tensegrity web. Imagine the body as a series of contractile and elastic elements, rather like a spider's web. Imagine how, if one part of the web is dysfunctional, this will create a focus of tension, which will 'pull' on all the various strands of the web (body tissues) and, if you place a hand on any part of the web, you should feel the tension acting in a direction that is towards the site of dysfunction. This is how the spider 'knows' where its prey has landed as it is caught in the web. All roads lead to Rome, so they say, and if you place your hand at different points around the web (body) the direction of pull will always be towards the same spot. Thus you will be 'attracted' to the main area of dysfunction in the body by 'listening' for these 'attractive pulls'. If there are a few areas of dysfunction, the direction of the pulls and where they are leading to may become a little confusing, and so the osteopath 'listens' at various points and gradually 'hones' down on the position of the various sites of tension. This can be a very quick and effective way of identifying areas for further exploration.

Global fulcrum testing

This is a test that relates to the rhythmicity and general orientation of body structures around their embryological and tissue tensegrity fulcrums.

Now the osteopath moves on to local testing of the areas identified by all the tests so far (reflecting on their relationship to the working hypotheses and case history details as s/he goes).

The concept is that there is a continuous shifting of movement throughout the body, which can be called involuntary motion or a general shifting of tension throughout the tensegrity tissues of the body (the dural membranes, the fascial planes and connective tissue structures). This 'inherent motion', which continues whether the patient is moving or not, occurs in a cyclical and rhythmic way, and should follow an established pattern and oscillate around various fulcrum points. The movement is expressed throughout the body and the osteopath can 'listen' and evaluate if this motion is being properly and effectively expressed. If it is not, the fulcrums around which it is oscillating will have shifted, and the movement becomes oriented around sites of dysfunction or will have shifted in such a way that the osteopath can determine the origin of that shift – i.e. the site of dysfunction. This again gives the osteopath a broad overview of the main sites of dysfunction within the body.

Local screening

This includes:

- local testing of joints and all other tissues/structures (tensional, compressional);
- local 'listening' tests (web 'areas', local fulcrums and rhythms).

Local testing is of the joints and the other tissues of the body as already described, and all the time the osteopath is looking to explore the sites of dysfunction already identified, to appreciate the actual extent of these changes, which

then allows him/her to understand the immediate cause of the symptoms. It also allows him/her to appreciate the way all the factors have summated and are forming barriers to the body's own self-healing and self-regulating mechanisms.

Where, why, what?

At the end of all this, the osteopath should have identified a number of dysfunctional areas. S/he should have noted the quality and extent of soft tissue change, and should be able to state what level of injury or dysfunction those tissues are expressing. S/he should be able to discuss the various cause-and-effect relationships that these restrictions have, both within themselves and the relevance they have for body physiology and self-healing. The osteopath should therefore know at this stage if s/he can help the patient in some way or not.

So, the osteopath knows **where** the problems area and **why** they are contributing to the patient's problems, and s/he finally has to decide **what** to do with them all.

Such a simple little thing!!

'What' is determined by:

- the state of the tissues (which has already been assessed);
- the models of practice that the osteopath adheres to;
- the individual skill repertoire for various technical approaches that each practitioner has.

The 'what' choices that the practitioner has to make are 'What style of treatment should be applied?' and 'What order should the various factors be approached in?'

Technical approach will be discussed in a moment, and this leaves a discussion on the prioritization of examination findings.

Prioritization

Many of the spinal models discussed before have their own ways of prioritizing where to start/direct treatment. Readers should revisit those for a reminder. Most of these, though, centre on the idea of determining 'chronicity' within the restrictions and deciding which ones came first and which ones are 'secondary' (adaptations) to those 'primary' factors.

There will of course be a chronological pattern of primary and secondary findings but some early problems may not have left as important a legacy as some later problems and therefore 'time chronicity' is not the most important thing. It is the 'tissue chronicity' that is the most revealing.

Tissue chronicity

All the palpatory changes that we have discussed so far, whether they are in joints and their surrounding tissues or in any other structure (organ, fascia, ligament, bone and so on), will give the osteopath an idea of the reversibility of the tissue change that is currently being expressed. Areas that are important primary areas to the dysfunction are often the ones that are the most 'fibrotic', the most 'scarred', the most profoundly immobile, and those with the least rhythmicity and most out of alignment with their fulcrum.

It may seem strange to say this, as surely the most damaged or inflamed or recently injured part should be labelled as the primary area for concern? Well, yes and no. Yes, in the sense that this had to be evaluated so the patient can appreciate the nature of their condition and the osteopath can know what s/he may or may not be able to do to that tissue directly. No, however, in the sense that the reason for the presence of the symptomatic site of dysfunction/development of the injury is because it adapted to the pre-existing changes in the body, and therefore these pre-existing changes are the primary ones. These pre-existing (predisposing and maintaining) factors are the most important to change if the person is going to leave the consultation room less likely to suffer a recurrence of their problem.

However, having decided which are the primary areas and which are the secondary areas still does not give an iron-clad choice for treatment. The tissue changes in the primary areas may be so extensive that reversibility is questionable or negligible (and so may take months or even years of treatment), or they may be impossible/inadvisable to change at all. This may mean that some things should be left 'in situ', with the osteopath left pondering how to make the rest of the body function more effectively around them. This means the less primary areas, and the secondary and symptomatic areas, are treated. Note: It is usual that some form of treatment is always given to the symptomatic area, although if the injury or change in the presenting area is not too great, then it can be released by working solely on the other areas of restriction within the body.

This is perhaps where followers of the Littlejohn model and its variations, and those who look to three-dimensional mechanics, fascial models and the involuntary mechanism have the advantage, as these models inherently guide the osteopath to a wider appreciation of cause and effect.

Another choice is necessary though, one which, like all treatment choices, involves the patient. Patient expectations are often very particular things and it is the osteopath's job to discern what it is the patient is aiming for from their visit to the osteopath. If it is a 'quick fix', then they will not be happy with a management plan that requires extensive treatment, when local treatment to the secondary/presenting area will reduce their symptoms and 'get them going again' until the next time. 'Tomorrow is another day' is a very common philosophy in patients, and needs to be respected.

Indeed, this may not always be seen as a negative option, as there can be very good reasons why short-term treatment is best – because of work, home, sporting or other pressures, for example. The patient can always return for more extensive treatment once the 'crisis' has passed. Thus, short-term treatment can be very valuable.

However, many patients, once they have had all the factors explained to them, are often very happy to have a more extensive course of treatment, to address the underlying causes of their problems, as they would like to return to long-term good health and function if at all possible.

Thus prioritization depends on the contract of care that the patient is happy with, which is developed from the individual osteopath's models and approaches to management.

Management: technical approaches

There are many things involved in managing a case, and treatment to the tissues is just one (albeit an important one!). Advice to the patient, exercises, strapping of unstable joints, referral to another healthcare professional are all others, as is the decision not to treat. These things are universal in many professions and so we will devote the following discussion to exploring the particular contribution that is osteopathic: the various technical approaches that we have.

As was stated at the beginning of the book, many manipulative professions use similar techniques (identical in some cases) but the point to appreciate is that techniques are never applied arbitrarily. They are always applied in accordance with principles.

In deciding which technical approach to use, several things are important.

- **What is the state of the tissue** (e.g. fibrotic, oedematous, inflamed, fractured, infected, malignant, fragile, in spasm, torn, degenerative, etc.)? What is the best way to treat tissue in this state? Is stretch the best, is inhibition, is muscle energy, is functional?

- If a certain technique is chosen, **is there any general contraindication (relative or absolute) to it?** For example, if the cervical spine has a joint with muscle spasm around it, high-velocity thrust techniques may be very effective but they would be inadvisable if the person happened to be suffering from vessel disease, e.g. vertebral artery atherosclerosis. Such things as gentle stretch and functional techniques would be more advisable. There are a whole variety of 'risk–benefit' equations that must be considered when deciding on treatment style, and only sound and broad training will ensure this.

- **Will the technique be acceptable to the patient?** They may not like thrust techniques, or they may not think they have had a treatment if these are not used. Some people will prefer techniques that are less invasive or intrusive, and others are happy to receive whatever the osteopath suggests. One never knows until one asks, and informed patient consent to each and every procedure is vital.

That said, the biggest determinant of treatment choice is tissue state.

Direct and indirect techniques

Many treatments are categorized under the heading of direct or indirect techniques. These terms need clarification.

In the preceding section we spent a long time discussing the exploration of tissue tensions and the types of response and palpatory feeling within tissues that are possible. That discussion is clearly only the tip of an enormous iceberg, but should give us some of what we now need.

These terms are all about how one engages the tissue tension that one has identified, regardless of where in the body it is and which actual tissue type is being treated.

The tissue analogies explored all give an indication of how to test for such things as tissue resistance, decreases in elasticity and reduction of range, end feel and so on. One of the key elements within evaluation is to find a sense of limitation within normal tissue or joint mobility. When a tissue is dysfunctional there is always some sort of barrier to movement, whether this comes at the beginning, middle or end of the range of movement or in stretch/compression testing.

Finding the tissue barrier is the first step to deciding technique. The quality of that tissue barrier is the next.

Direct techniques are those that will engage the tissue barrier – push against it in some way to make the tissue/joint release. Indirect techniques are those that move away from the tissue barrier – into a direction where the tissue/joint does not express tension.

Important points:

- One can have a direct contact on to the tissue, yet still use an indirect technique.
- One can use an indirect contact, i.e. distant to the tissue in question, and still use a direct technique within that tissue. One example of this is long-level high-velocity thrust techniques applied to the spine. Here, the forces applied to the spine are first directed at points somewhat distal to the affected articulation. The motion passes through the spine and eventually directly engages the tissue barrier within the joint, so achieving a direct technique to the tissue tension, but from an indirect contact.

Direct techniques include:

- high-velocity thrusts;
- articulation of joints;
- soft tissue techniques such as stretching and massaging of tissues;
- inhibition of muscles;
- muscle energy techniques;
- fluid drive techniques.

Within these techniques the quality/nature of the reaction in the tissue barrier as you engage it determines the exact delivery of the technique.

Some examples:

- If a muscle is in spasm, then harshly engaging the barrier will only irritate it more and cause greater pain and further reflex contraction. This makes the joint/muscle more tight, not less tight. So, one works in the available mid range and performs the stretch at the beginning of the tissue barrier, just as the tension begins to mount. Now, one can either gently nudge against the barrier or one can hold the barrier steady, and both scenarios should lead to a gradual relaxation of the muscle, allowing the barrier to diminish and amplitude of movement to improve.

- If the tissue is fibrotic or scarred and the end feel is less reactive and more 'hard', then gentle nudging at the beginning of the barrier may be insufficient. Here, the technique should be applied later in the amplitude of available motion – further along the curve of mounting tissue resistance. The barrier can be engaged a little more firmly and, if the barrier is very stiff, sustained firm pressure can be used at the end of available movement – right up against the barrier.
- If a tissue is oedematous, but its structure underneath is 'normal' and elastic, then gentle rhythmic mobilization can be given that engages the beginning of the barrier, to help promote fluid flow. If the underlying tissue is more contracted or fibrotic, then slightly firmer techniques may be necessary to mobilize/open and close the internal fascial components of the tissue to enable the fluid to disperse.

Indirect techniques include:

- functional techniques;
- various involuntary motion techniques such as induction;
- balanced ligamentous tension techniques.

There is not space to discuss all of these direct and indirect techniques, but two are important and widely used, and will therefore be discussed. These are high-velocity thrust techniques and the functional technique. They are not being discussed because they are in any way more important than the others, as this would be profoundly untrue. In fact, articulation and soft tissue techniques are sadly underused, and many practitioners perhaps use thrust techniques too readily and forget the powerful effects properly directed articulation, for example, can give. Also, the other indirect techniques are not less effective than the direct ones, and in some cases are infinitely more effective than thrust techniques.

To illustrate this point, consider that the spine is oriented in position and movement by the soft tissues that act upon it. This includes all the tissues that act on/influence the spine (and all the balanced shifting of tensions within these structures, and the mechanics of the cavities and other body structures). Thus the locally acting paravertebral muscles are just one component in the forces that influence spinal motion patterns. Now, if a spinal joint becomes dysfunctional, thrusting it will do nothing to affect the other tensions that usually have accumulated and led to the spinal dysfunction developing in the first place. Therefore the thrust technique could be considered a poor choice of treatment if one is looking at global patterns and inter-relations. Many of the indirect techniques are much better placed to address these wider issues and so release the spine more effectively than a thrust.

That said, thrust techniques are very useful, and to appreciate their subtleties (for subtle techniques they should be) a few points are discussed below.

Techniques are very precious things to osteopaths and there are probably as many versions of the various techniques as there are stars in the sky! To be serious, though, each technique is an adaptation of the tissue state found within the patient and therefore they **should** be unique to that situation and that person. This does lead to many ways of doing things, though, and one should not be prescriptive but realize that technique is, at its best, a fluid event that is never the same twice.

High-velocity thrust techniques

High-velocity thrust techniques use highly controlled fast movements to engage the barrier and cause a reflex relaxation of the muscles that are limiting the motion within that joint. They are not techniques that push through the barrier arbitrarily, and they are not about 'putting the bone back in'.

A joint that is dysfunctional will have tissues within it that are stressed and damaged, and are therefore often weaker and more fragile than normal. Even a chronically restricted joint that is as stiff as they come is not strong. The tissue changes may be binding the joint very effectively,

but they are changes that mean the normal integrity of the tissue is compromised. In this case, the tissues are no longer strong and should still be respected as much as where the joint is sprained/the tissues are torn or overstretched.

The method that will be described relates to the revised model of spinal mechanics and is not the Fryette model. The Fryette model dictates that the positional relations of the vertebra are assessed and one decides what combination of sidebending, flexion/extension or rotation the two adjacent vertebra are held in. The thrust is then made in a direction that will reverse these components. The revised model does not follow this method and here the direction of thrust is determined by tissue feel and not position relation. (However, it must be stated that those that use the Fryette model are not 'unsafe' or 'less effective' compared to those using the revised model.)

In the revised model, one takes the joint in question and starts motion testing in three dimensions to get an overall picture of where the tissue barriers are and when in the ranges of movement they come on. The idea is not to find the biggest barrier and thrust through it.

Warning: this is not a technique class. The information given is not sufficient to enable readers to use these skills from scratch. One can never learn technique from a page. Proper, supervised teaching is essential.

The purpose of describing the technique only is to demonstrate some of the palpatory comparisons and analyses osteopaths use within these procedures.

Motion barriers

The barriers to motion will have left the joint with a diminished and slightly adapted mid-range of motion in which there is usually a little 'play' left in the joint. This is shown in Figure 10.16.

In the compromised joint, if the practitioner now uses just one direction of movement to create bind, s/he might need to take the joint towards the end of its normal range before engaging the tissue barrier enough so that there is sufficient bind in the joint to make the thrust

Figure 10.16

Motion barriers within a joint. Refer to the text for a full explanation.

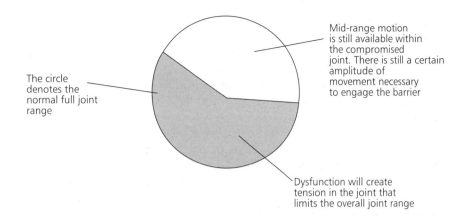

The circle denotes the normal full joint range

Mid-range motion is still available within the compromised joint. There is still a certain amplitude of movement necessary to engage the barrier

Dysfunction will create tension in the joint that limits the overall joint range

effective. (One needs to create bind in a joint to effect a thrust.) However, this might mean that, when the thrust is performed, the joint is taken beyond its normal range of motion, which could damage the joint.

To avoid this, the practitioner starts by finding this remaining mid-range, which usually means moving the joint in a direction away from the barrier to find the more neutral position. The joint is also usually more comfortable in this position, which is better for the patient and easier for the practitioner, as the tissue responses are not so 'aggressive' in this position. With the joint in this position s/he has a little more freedom of movement available in which to perform the technique.

Now, the practitioner moves the joint minimally in one direction to start to engage a little tissue resistance. This creates a little 'bind' in the joint but does not engage the original barrier full on. It does not necessarily matter which direction this movement is in, but it must be in one that creates a little 'bind' – not much, just a bit.

The practitioner now introduces another component of movement within that joint, which increases the tissue resistance and bind but still does not fully engage the original barrier. Now, the joint is held in a degree of tension but the movement introduced means that the dysfunctional joint has still not been taken beyond the mid-range of its compromised state.

The idea is to move the joint in such a way that 'bind' is created in the joint, but within the mid-range of movement created by the original barrier combination. One can see from Figure 10.17 that, by adding small components of movement, the bind in the joint will increase/accumulate and now the joint needs to be moved much less in order to create enough tension for the thrust. This means the thrust can be performed in mid-range, and not towards end of range, which is safer, and more comfortable.

When the thrust is now performed, the amplitude can be minimal but the speed must be quick enough and the movement of the thrust must be halted before normal joint range is reached. To stop a thrust is as important as to start one.

As indicated above, this is not a full description of thrust techniques and apologies go the practitioners who follow other models, for not discussing their methods.

Functional technique

This is an indirect technique, and one that moves the tissues away from the tissue barrier, away from accumulating bind and towards ease. It still works on the integral proprioceptive reflexes within and around the joint, but uses different methods to achieve a release.

In functional technique, it is still useful to palpate the nature and extent of the tissue barrier so that you know what you are attempting to release. This way, once the procedure is completed, the original barrier can be retested to evaluate the success of the technique. This is in fact true of all techniques, but sometimes, when using indirect

Figure 10.17

Adapting motion barriers within a joint to aid treatment efficacy. Refer to the text for a full explanation.

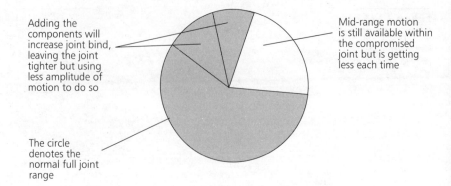

Adding the components will increase joint bind, leaving the joint tighter but using less amplitude of motion to do so

Mid-range motion is still available within the compromised joint but is getting less each time

The circle denotes the normal full joint range

techniques, one may be tempted to just 'get on and release the tensions' without fully analysing them in advance. This leads to poorly directed technique and it is poor practice not to make a proper tissue diagnosis before treating.

In the tissue being treated (whether this is a joint, an organ, a fascial structure, a bone, or a muscle for example) the tissue is oriented in such a direction that one moves away from the tension in the tissue and towards a direction of ease. One can start the procedure by gently testing the tissue in three dimensions, to find the direction that is 'easiest'/offers the least resistance. If one simply moved the tissue into that direction and kept going, then, of course, some other tissue tension would be found – probably the normal end range of that joint. This is not the aim of the technique.

When the tissue is dysfunctional there will be a variety of torsions passing through and within that tissue, so that it is expressing a three-dimensional tension pattern. Somehow, if the tissue is oriented correctly, then those tensions can be 'unwound', and the tissue will be able to rest 'unhindered' by those conflicting forces. So, there is a pattern of motion that will wind up the tissue more and make it more tense, and a pattern of motion that will unwind the tensions and make it relax. The aim of the functional technique is to find this direction(s)/orientation, and so lead to a release of the problem. There should be a pathway of ease that one can follow within the tissue that should release it.

So, when one has found one direction of ease, the tissue is only moved into that direction a little before the next part of the pathway of ease is

tested for, found and followed. It sounds simple, but this is motion evaluation in many directions at once – one must be able to follow all the shifting patterns of tension at once so that the best pathway of ease is identified. Once the pathway has been followed, one should arrive at an orientation of the tissue where all the diverse tensions have been balanced out, and the tissue rests in an easy state. At this point, the tissues may release immediately, 'wriggle' out from under the practitioner's contact and re-establish their normal orientation, free from tension. The practitioner may need to hold the orientation for some moments, though, before this occurs, and the sense of tissue release may be quite subtle and easy to miss.

When the functional technique was originally described, people were directed not to repeat any one component/direction of movement in their search for the pathway of ease. However, as time has gone by, others have felt that to follow whatever seems to present itself is equally effective, even if this does mean repeating movement directions in the overall re-alignment/orientation of the tissue.

Summary

It is hoped that this chapter will have given some insight into the thought processes and evaluatory procedures that osteopaths use in their management of cases. It could never describe everything, but hopefully some of the concepts used have been illustrated, to give a window into the art of osteopathy.

The last chapter reviews a number of cases, which it is hoped the reader will find of interest.

REFERENCES

Barnett, R. (1997) *Higher Education: A Critical Business*, Society for Research into Higher Education/Open University Press, Buckingham.

Barral, J.-P. and Mercier, P. (1988) *Visceral Manipulation*, Eastland Press, Seattle, WA.

Education Department (1993) *Competences Required for Osteopathic Practice (C.R.O.P.)*, General Council and Register of Osteopaths, Reading, Berks.

Fish, D. and Twinn, S. (1997) *Quality Clinical Supervision in Health Care Professions*, Butterworth Heinemann, Oxford.

Osterman, K. F. and Kottkamp, R. B. (1993) *Reflective Practice for Educators. Improving Schooling Through Professional Development*, Corwin Press, Newbury Park, CA.

Reason, P. (ed.) (1994) *Participation in Human Inquiry*, Sage Publications, London.

FURTHER READING

American Osteopathic Association (1997) *Foundations for Osteopathic Medicine*, Baltimore: Williams and Wilkins.

Beal, M. C. (ed.) (1989) *The Principles of Palpatory Diagnosis and Manipulative Technique*, American Academy of Osteopathy, Newark, NJ.

Beauchamp, T. L. and Childress, J. F. (1994) *Principles of Biomedical Ethics*, Oxford University Press, New York.

Brookfield, S. D. (1987) *Developing Critical Thinkers*, Open University Press, Milton Keynes, Bucks.

Chaitow, L. (1987) *Soft Tissue Manipulations*, Thorsons, London.

Chaitow, L. (1991) *Palpatory Literacy*, Thorsons, London.

Hartman, L. (1997) *Handbook of Osteopathic Technique*, Chapman & Hall, London.

Heron, J. (1996) *Co-operative Enquiry. Research into the Human Condition*, Sage Publications, London.

Stoddard, A. (1983) *Manual of Osteopathic Practice*, Hutchinson, London.

11 FULL CASE STUDIES

In this chapter 20 cases will be reviewed, some in more detail than others. They aim to show the wide range of patients who present for treatment and to give an indication of the treatments that were applied to achieve symptom resolution. Such a list of patients cannot be indicative of all work done by osteopaths and, for example, the treatment of children and sports injuries is underexplored here. However, these cases may give some indication of the application of the osteopathic approach and it is hoped that they will illustrate a number of the points raised during the book. I hope that they are of interest and, like all practitioners, I would like to thank all my patients, and the students to whom I have tried to help explain the osteopathic approach, as it is they who have taught me most of what I know.

The following cases are illustrated:

- 53-year-old woman with low back and left sacroiliac pain
- 42-year-old man with prostatodynia
- 36-year-old woman with bladder and urethral dysfunction and chronic pelvic pain
- 38-year-old woman with pelvic organ prolapse and a uterine fibroid
- 31-year-old woman with left sacroiliac pain and ovarian cysts
- 54-year-old woman with pain in the abdomen and difficulty eating
- 72-year-old woman with stress incontinence of urine
- 47-year-old woman with brachial neuritis and back pain
- 36-year-old woman with peptic ulcer
- 52-year-old man with right flank pain and low back pain
- 65-year-old man with femoral nerve compression
- 66-year-old man with brachial neuritis
- 53-year-old man, on renal dialysis, with right shoulder and cervicothoracic pain
- 60-year-old woman, treated postoperatively for poor drainage following breast lumpectomy
- 49-year-old man with headaches and left low back pain
- 34-year-old woman with coccydynia
- 50-year-old man with left elbow pain and 'generally achy arms'
- 40-year-old man with recurrent ear and eye infections and headaches
- 31-year-old woman with abdominal and pelvic pain, treated before and during pregnancy
- 12-year-old boy with knee pain and poor coordination

CASE 1   53-year-old woman with low back and left sacroiliac pain

This case should illustrate the relationship between the compartments of the erector spinae/multifidus muscles and the stability and function of the lumbar spine and pelvis.

Patient
53-year-old female beautician.

Presenting symptoms
General low back discomfort, and left sacroiliac pain, intermittently. Also, bilateral knee problems (retropatellar aching, with some crepitus). The pattern was intermittent over the years and was often aggravated by her sitting activities at work, or if she went on long walks (she had several very large dogs, which need a lot of exercise). Over the preceding few months the symptoms had also started to bother her at night in that she found it uncomfortable to get to sleep – her back felt quite 'restless'.

Onset
This occurred 30 years ago, following her two pregnancies. In the first pregnancy there was no discomfort until the delivery, where the birth was normal although she had an episiotomy. The problem arose when she was left for a very long time with her legs up in stirrups, waiting to be stitched up. Consequently, her legs were abducted, flexed and externally rotated for some time, placing quite a strain on the posterior ligamentous apparatus of the sacroiliacs and lumbar spine. In her second pregnancy 1.5 years later, she had quite a degree of low back pain and a very lordotic posture. The birth process was less complicated, though. Subsequently she was left with a very weak back for a number of years and never felt that she could walk very evenly afterwards, because of having to 'guard' her low back.

Over the years, her back was intermittently uncomfortable and she gradually began to suffer knee pain, as she was walking quite awkwardly because of her back. She had tried various manipulative practitioners before over the years and had always gained short-term relief. She had had one recent upset, which had caused quite an acute reaction in her low back – she had been hitching a trailer to her car when she tripped, caught her non-weight-bearing leg on the towbar and twisted around the other, weight-bearing one. Since then she had had quite constant aching in her back, which worsened whenever she tried to do anything.

On examination
The patient had quite a flat spine overall, but especially in the lumbar region. She had limited flexion in the lumbar spine and the lumbar region tended to move as a block rather than in any sort of graduated way. There was a strong pelvic torsion, where the whole pelvis seemed posteriorly rotated, but the right sacroiliac was acutely held in posterior rotation. All the pelvic joints were very limited in movement, and the soft tissues from the buttocks up to the thoracolumbar region were very 'fibrotic' and tight. There was very little elasticity of the thoracolumbar fascia and very little elasticity in the bulk of the erector spinae muscles on palpation. Both knees appeared slightly degenerative and the whole spine was somewhat chronically restricted.

On closer examination, the patient appeared still to be 'stuck' in the original stirrup position and there was quite a degree of strain within the sacrum and stiffness in the sacroiliac ligaments. The sacrum was very compressed and the level of strain had passed internally, such that there was an intraosseous strain to the sacrum. There was no normal 'floating' of the sacrum between the ilia and the whole pelvis was quite 'frozen'. Consequently, the knee articulations had had to adapt quite a bit, and a lot of the thigh musculature had tensed into a strain pattern, thus causing the patellar movement to be limited on both sides. On the whole the left sacroiliac was more chronically restricted than the right, although the right side, as stated, showed signs of a recent acute stress, and was posteriorly rotated.

Opinion

Considering the very tense and chronically restricted nature of this lady's back, it seemed that the whole bulk of the erector spinae, and the ligamentous arrangement of the pelvis that these merged with, were not functioning well. It seemed that the original strain caused during the pregnancies and deliveries, especially the first, caused a general disorientation of the deep fascia of the posterior pelvis, from which she was not able to fully recover. Her pattern of pain with activity, when the muscles would normally bulk up, is not inconsistent with a type of compartment syndrome, and also the fact that she was increasingly finding it uncomfortable to settle at night suggested that the circulation within these tissues was not as efficient as it might be. The altered shape and tension of the erector spinae fascia would have caused a limitation upon the normal function of the muscles within it. The recent torsion pattern induced by tripping over the towbar had caused a general shift in the orientation of the insertions of the deep fascia of the lumbar spine and posterior pelvis, and had consequently distorted the fascial support of the lumbar soft tissues and ligamentous arrangement of the low back, causing further distress to the erector spinae muscles. Over a protracted period of time, as she did not have freedom of movement in the posterior pelvis, her gait would have accommodated, leading to the knee problems that were latterly manifesting themselves.

Treatment

This consisted of two main approaches: (1) deep soft tissue massage and neuromuscular techniques to the posterior soft tissues of the lumbar spine and pelvis; and (2) functional release of the intraosseous strain of the sacrum, to allow it to float a little more between the ilia and also to be a little more malleable, allowing greater adaptability over the face of the sacral articulations with the ilia. She responded well after six or seven treatments, and then proceeded to gain further relief with intermittent treatment and a programme of yoga exercises to try to stretch out the fascial structures of the posterior pelvis. Gradually, her knee symptoms also subsided, although no direct work was done on them.

CASE 2   42-year-old man with prostatodynia

This case should illustrate the usefulness of osteopathic manipulation in this type of case, which so often proves unmanageable for the orthodox medical profession.

Patient
42-year-old, fit and healthy actor and writer.

Presenting symptoms
Heat, pressure and aching in the perineal area between the anus and the penis; occasional urinary frequency and slower flow of urination; pain in the penis with the sexual act at climax and sensitivity in the epididymis, with bilateral tenderness, right worse than left.

Associated symptoms
Debilitating tiredness, especially in the mornings; and a general feeling of nausea on some occasions, with very occasional disturbed bowel habit.

Onset
The first episode was 10 years prior to presentation. It started just with pain in the right testicle. Urological examination revealed nothing, and the symptoms gradually faded, leaving the patient with an occasional ache in the testicle. The second episode started 3 years prior to presentation. The symptoms were then as listed above. The symptom pattern was variable and intermittent for 6 months and thereafter was more or less constant, especially when under stress. Further urological screening revealed a possible chlamydial infection (although all subsequent cultures have proved negative) and a congested prostate – detected by transrectal ultrasound.

Urological diagnosis and treatment
Congested prostate and prostatodynia. Treatment was by repeat-prescription antibiotics. The patient has gained very little relief from this medication over the last 3 years prior to presentation.

Other history
Low back pain since the age of 14 years. Used to play a lot of rugby, where he suffered several compressive injuries to the lumbar spine. Symptoms are much less frequent than in his 20s. X-rays have previously revealed a narrowed disc space between the L4 and L5 vertebrae. There are no classic sciatic or femoral neurological signs with this lumbar condition. Some 11 years prior to presentation the patient suffered a ruptured right Achilles tendon, which was stitched, and recovered well. Paradoxically, this seems to have led to a compensated gait (giving disturbed motion through the left leg) and he now gets discomfort in both his knees, the left more than the right. The discomfort is at the superior tibiofibular articulations. This discomfort has been prevalent over the 2 years preceding presentation.

No other medical history was revealed.

On examination
Overall posture was of a flattened spine, roughly symmetrical, apart from a mild torsion at the level of the thoracic inlet, and a strong torsion of the pelvis, accompanying a flexed left knee stance.

There were restrictions throughout the right thoracic inlet and the cervicothoracic regions. The T4 area, lower thoracic spine and T/L areas were also restricted chronically. The sternum was also quite tense and immobile over the anterior chest, and the patient additionally reported a feeling of pressure here when his prostatic and other symptoms were prominent. The low lumbar spine was generally restricted, as one might expect from the X-ray findings. The pelvis was twisted and not moving freely, with the left ilium being forwards, and the left sacroiliac joint being very limited in movement. The sacrum was very compacted, with a right-sided sacrococcygeal restriction. Poor motion was noted through the sacrum and cranial base. The right inguinal region and spermatic cord were tense and tender, as was the perineal region, and the prostate was less mobile and more tender than usual (on external evaluation). Oedema through the perineal region could be palpated. Note: This patient had discovered during previous rectal examinations that his anus was a little tight and irritated (not uncommon with male lower urinary tract problems) so was not keen on repeated rectal examinations. There was some limitation in movement at the symphysis pubis, and some tightness in the caecal area of the colon.

Evaluation

This patient had a stiff pelvis, with limited excursion through the perineum and limited mobility of the prostate. The congestion that had been noted on ultrasound could be discerned from the oedema, the increased stiffness of the gland itself and the tenderness of the area. The left sacroiliac restriction seemed maintained by the degenerative state of the lumbar spine and the altered gait following the right Achilles injury. The right inguinal tension and the symphysis pubis lesion were related to the mechanics of the rest of the pelvis and were contributing to tension in the prostate and also the right testicle. The patient seemed to be exhibiting a general autonomic disturbance, in that he was routinely tired and had gastrointestinal symptoms and disturbed urinary and sexual function (which could also be partly explained by the mechanical restrictions in the pelvis). It is interesting to note that the lower thoracic and T/L area restrictions may have related to the autonomic imbalance.

Treatment

This was a varied approach that incorporated management of all of the above areas. Soft tissue techniques, articulation and mobilization of the joints of the spine and pelvis were undertaken every so many sessions. Vibratory techniques and deep soft tissue/neuromuscular techniques were applied to the lower thoracic region of the spine. Functional techniques applied to the sacrum and low lumbar spine were used to decompress the area, as were sacral toggle techniques and muscle energy techniques. Some gentle mobilizing techniques were applied to the abdominal viscera. The most routinely used approach was to articulate and mobilize the perineal area, and to give external massage to the prostate, via the inferior perineal route. External work to the sacrococcygeal joint was also given. Some standard articulatory and soft tissue work was carried out throughout both lower limbs and some functional work was applied to the cranium.

Progress

This patient was seen weekly for about 6 months and thereafter every few weeks and gradually his symptoms became less intense, less frequent and less wide-ranging. After a year of treatment, he became virtually symptom-free and now has intermittent maintenance treatment. The length of time might seem excessive, but one needs to bear in mind the degenerative state of the lumbar spine, the chronicity of the soft tissues and the amount of congestion within the prostate, which had to gradually be reversed and then maintained by the body's own mechanisms. This was borne out by the fact that the patient subsequently still suffered bouts of prostatodynia, especially following infections elsewhere in the body (e.g. a chest infection) or when sitting for prolonged periods (over several weeks).

CASE 3   36-year-old woman with bladder and urethral dysfunction and chronic pelvic pain

This case should illustrate the need for constant ongoing evaluation when managing a complex case with multiple maintaining factors. Management needs to be adapted to the changing focus of tensions that emerge as treatment continues, before the whole pattern can be redressed and the original symptoms addressed. This case can illustrate the complex inter-relations of the internal pelvic soft tissues.

Patient
36-year-old female mortgage manager. Reasonably fit and healthy, apart from her lower urinary tract problem.

Presenting symptoms
Spasms in the urethra; fluttering contractions of the bladder; chronic suprapubic pain and pulling; urinary frequency and urgency. These symptoms were very debilitating: often simply bending over would provoke the spasms of the urethra and her life was dominated by the constant need to be close to a lavatory. General activities, walking, travelling by car and bus were all problematic. Over the past few years these symptoms had also been cyclically related to her menstrual pattern.

Onset
Following a particularly bad infection of the bladder 10 years prior to presentation, the patient started to have quite consistent urgency and frequency; this was relieved while she was on antibiotics, but when she stopped, the symptoms returned. She had had a long history of intermittent bladder infections but they usually stayed resolved for long periods of time until the one 10 years ago, which never really settled. Just after this, she had appendicitis, and had an appendectomy and a partial right ovary removal (history of cysts, for which she had previously had two unsuccessful laparotomies). Following this there was increased difficulty in emptying the bladder. Symptoms carried on intermittently until 6 years prior to presentation, when they became more consistent. Cystoscopy and urodynamic studies 4/5 years prior to presentation had revealed various findings, but the procedure – which included a bladder stretch – induced the urethral spasms.

Urological diagnosis and treatment
Outflow obstruction to the bladder, decreased compliance of the bladder, reflex dyssynergia between the bladder and the urethra, slight irregular elevation of the bladder neck and incomplete bladder emptying were diagnosed. Treatment was repeat antibiotics and medication designed to influence the action of the autonomic nerves to the lower urinary tract.

Other history
The patient had been involved in two road traffic accidents resulting in minor whiplash and intermittent cervical/mid-thoracic aching. Postviral syndrome at 19 years of age. Ongoing dental work, involving treatment for abscesses and a number of extractions.

Evaluation
These symptoms were consequent to a history of lower abdominal surgery and pelvic infection. These factors had left quite a degree of scarring and chronic inflammation in and around the tissues of the lower urinary tract and are contributing to a continued distortion of the tissues and a reduction in their relative

mobility. This was having the effect of disturbing the reflexes governing continence and micturition and also leading to poor local fluid dynamics and circulation, compounding the chronic inflammatory state. There were a number of general mechanical findings within the patient's pelvis, low back and hip articulations/regions that were also adding to the torsion and tension (and hence poor function) of the intrapelvic tissues and organs.

Management and treatment

One of the original over-riding factors was the scarring in the right iliac region following a complicated appendectomy. This was leading to a strong pull of the pelvic peritoneum and a distortion of the bladder and lower urethra to the right side of the pelvis. Whatever other restrictions there were present, they were not as marked (chronic, resistant and 'fixed'), at the outset, as this area. Several sessions of treatment were directed at releasing the structures of the lower abdomen such as the ascending colon, the root of the mesentery for the small intestine and the psoas muscles. Alongside this a degree of work to the low back and pelvis was necessary (general articulation and mobilization) to help the general mechanics of the area.

As the right side started to change, it was possible to begin to explore the more deep aspects of the pelvis, which had been a little too inaccessible and reactive up till then. Some internal work was done to try to access the internal pelvic structures, notably the pelvic fascia and the uterus, which was placing quite a degree of strain on the bladder. The bladder was initially too reactive for local work to be tolerated. To accompany the changes induced by working from the coccyx and the deeper aspects of the pelvis, it was necessary to look at the thoracic spine and the cranial base. The thoracic spine was (and still is to a degree) very restricted, and the paravertebral muscles were very fibrotic all along the thoracic area. The whole thoracic spine was in an extended pattern, which would not help the pelvis and low back to adjust very easily to the local treatment. The cranial base had quite a complicated pattern in its own right, consequent to the dental work. The patient currently had an incomplete bite pattern and was at this stage awaiting dentures to correct this.

Also, as the right side of the pelvis was easing out, an underlying (and previously masked) tension of the uterus to the left was becoming apparent. Also, the left side of the bladder was quite bound down and the urethra was not very elastic (and the urachus was quite immobile). The sigmoid was also quite tense, which was adding to this left-sided pattern (as stated before, this was pre-existing, but masked by the scarring from the appendectomy). Gradually, the pelvis started to respond, and this caused some reaction in the lumbosacral articulation, which needed to adjust to the changing sacral orientation. The sacrum was gradually changing in relation to the uterus being differently mobile, and as these tissues responded it was finally possible to assess the local distortion of the urethra in relation to the symphysis pubis. This again had been present all along but was too strongly influenced by the other tensions to be able to be resolved in the short term. Locally, the urethra had been quite scarred and was kinked along its length. I am sure that this will be contributing to the poor flow and spasms within the urethra itself. Having released off the uterus, the adnexae and (subsequently) along the vagina, it was easier to stretch out the urethra itself. Throughout all this time it was necessary to continue to work at various points along the spine and to do quite a bit of general release through the pelvis, to help it accommodate the more local changes.

Progress

Overall, we are now at a stage where a lot of the external influences on the bladder are reduced, and the bladder itself is gradually re-learning a pattern of micturition. This lady has much reduced pain, better bladder function, fewer urethral spasms and a much better lifestyle, including an increased tolerance to being in the car/travelling. This amount of progress has taken 2 years to achieve, not least because of the scarring, weakness in the chronically inflamed tissues and the patient's fear of having too much treatment in case there was a short-term aggravation of symptoms, which she would not emotionally have been able to contemplate.

38-year-old woman with pelvic organ prolapse and a uterine fibroid

This case should demonstrate the inter-relatedness of the biomechanics of the various pelvic organs and tissues.

Patient

A 38-year-old female opera singer, who tours around the UK and Europe for various engagements.

Presenting symptoms

Stress incontinence and generalized pelvic discomfort. This was relatively mild, and the wet episodes associated with the bladder problem occurred perhaps once or twice per week, but she was constantly aware of the fact that her pelvic organs felt heavy, and this irritated her in a number of ways. In particular, it was beginning to interfere with her normal breathing sensations – being a classically trained singer she was used to breathing down into the abdomen and pelvis. She was also engaged, and found sexual activity a little uncomfortable. When she presented, her honeymoon was 5 weeks away and she was anxious for some relief of her condition prior to this.

Onset

The fibroids had been gradually becoming more prominent over the past 2 years, but were not growing at a very fast rate and she had been advised that she should have a hysterectomy as the quickest way to gain relief. The patient was worried about this operation because of the possible effect on her singing and also on her relation with her fiancé.

Diagnosis

Her stress incontinence was associated with uterine fibroids, which were pressing on the bladder. There was also a mild uterine prolapse, with some probable associated pelvic connective tissue weakness.

On examination

Externally there was a general pelvic torsion, although there was no major restriction in the sacroiliacs or the symphysis pubis. There was a slight unevenness in the perineum and the levator ani muscles and there was a torsion of the sacrococcygeal articulation. The lower abdomen was a little tight and tender in the midline, and there was some tension in the small intestine area. On internal examination, a slight weakness (lack of tone) could be felt in the anterior vaginal wall, and the trigone of the bladder was not as elastic as would normally be expected. The uterus was enlarged and generally oedematous. Its normal mobility was reduced, not only because of the fibroid but also because of the unevenness in the pelvic connective tissue around it. Where it was immobile, it was causing tenseness in the anterior vagina, which was helping to distort the trigone and bladder neck, and the pressure from above downwards was also producing pressure on the bladder.

Treatment

This consisted of general articulatory work to the lumbar spine and pelvis and some mobilization of the sacroiliacs. Some general preparatory work was done on the abdominal viscera – some articulation and functional work. Internally, *per vaginam*, some functional work was applied to the uterus directly and some gentle mobilization of the uterus with reference to the surrounding soft tissue tensions (gentle stretching and balancing). Working on the uterus directly was very satisfactory, as I could feel the size of the uterus gradually diminish and its quality soften (from being quite tense and hard). The oedema was reducing and because of this the effect of having a large, immobile, slightly prolapsed uterus was reducing also. As the pelvis was worked on, the tone in the pelvic connective tissue improved and the uterus was held in a slightly better orientation.

Progress
This patient had four treatments, by which time she was quite a bit better. Subsequently, she had a treatment every now and again to help maintain things.

CASE 5 31-year-old woman with left sacroiliac pain and ovarian cysts

This case demonstrates the potential links between the different urogenital organs and how restrictions throughout the body may affect each other mechanically and physiologically.

Patient
A 31-year-old housewife.

Presenting symptoms
Pain in the left iliac fossa region, with a general aching around this region. There was a sharper pain into the left groin. She always had some symptoms, although the majority of the symptoms came in waves. There were occasional similar symptoms on the right side. There was also some general left sacroiliac joint discomfort.

Onset
The onset had been a few weeks previously and had started with just left-sided symptoms. The patient contacted her doctor, who arranged a pelvic ultrasound scan. This revealed cysts in both ovaries. Some 3 months before the onset the patient had suffered a miscarriage, but her cycle had settled down well again, until just recently when there had been some pain associated with her cycle.

During this recent pregnancy there was also a pelvic scan, but this had showed no abnormalities. The most recent scan, as stated above, showed cysts on both ovaries but the one in the left ovary seemed to be on a stalk, and it was felt that this might be twisting and giving her present iliac fossa symptoms.

As the cysts had arrived so quickly, there was concern that they might rupture and there was talk of removing them surgically. However, the patient was not very happy at this prospect as she would still like to have another child.

Her previous obstetric history revealed a pattern of repeated miscarriages, which were thought to be due to a menstrual cycle imbalance that persisted too much through the pregnancies. The patient's cycle was normally regular, though. She had had one successful pregnancy 4 years earlier.

She had had some osteopathic treatment before, but for minor aches associated with a viral arthritis. She considered herself free of this problem now. There was no history of any mechanical trauma having been sustained. Her one pregnancy was delivered by emergency caesarean section following attempted delivery of a posterior presentation baby. The recovery was apparently good.

Her past medical history revealed a few minor operations on the left knee – where she intermittently had a problem with expanding capillaries. These are easily removed, but can recur. Her general health was fine, and she took a limited amount of ibuprofen to cope with her present symptoms. Her family history showed that her mother had cystic ovaries, and also cancer of the uterine cervix when in her 50s. (The patient had regular smears, which had revealed no abnormality.)

On examination
There was decreased range and amplitude of movement in the sphenobasilar junction and the left temporal. These were quite fixed in themselves, although some of the tension in the cranial base seemed to be coming from the T10 area.

There were chronic upper cervical restrictions on the right and the lower cervicals and cervicothoracic junction bilaterally. There was also a very chronic/fibrotic restriction in T8–10, with lesser restrictions at L1/2 left, L3/4/5 right, the left sacroiliac and the left L5/S1. The left sacroiliac was tender and the soft tissues were not fibrotic but reactive, and in a semiacute state. The symphysis pubis was very tender and in a degree of torsion. There were general restrictions throughout the left leg, particularly the left knee.

Viscerally, the uterus was not too bad, but the left fallopian tube and ovary were very tight and oedematous, much more so than the right. This internal tension seemed to be spreading to the left ilium. The pubis restriction seemed related to the sacral torsion associated with the L5/S1 restriction. When examining the abdomen it became apparent that there was a problem with the left kidney, which seemed chronically tight and restricted. On explaining this to the patient, she revealed that in fact she had a long history of gravel being produced in the left kidney. This history was almost certainly associated with the lower thoracic restrictions.

Treatments
The first treatment consisted of functional work to the left ovary and sacroiliac combined. There was an attempted mobilization of the upper lumbar spine on the left, and inhibition of the paraspinal muscles at that level. There was also functional work to the pubis and sacrum. There was a little less tenderness in the left ovary at the end of the treatment.

The second treatment was 2 weeks later. The patient had been a little more comfortable and an appointment with a specialist gynaecologist had produced the opinion that no radical treatment was needed at this stage and that hormone treatment would be tried, to commence in 1 month's time after the patient's cycle had been monitored.

On examination there was less tension between the left iliac fossa and the sacroiliac joint. The treatment consisted of functional work to the pelvis in general and some to the cranial base. The next appointment was 2 weeks later.

At the third treatment the patient reported that she was symptom free – she had started to really improve from the day after the last treatment. She had gradually become aware of having no symptoms. On examination, there was still tension in the left tibia, which was affecting the pelvis. The pubis was a little tight and there was still some sphenobasilar restriction. The treatment was a functional approach to those structures. The patient cancelled the next appointment, which was to be in 2 weeks time, as she had become pregnant and was going away on holiday!

Discussion
This case was interesting for several reasons. Firstly, it showed the management of symptoms associated with a pathological condition of the ovaries. Next it showed that treatment around the time of conception of a child is not necessarily a hindrance to the process. Next, if one is not in the habit of examining broadly, the restriction in the left kidney might have been missed, especially as the patient did not volunteer the fact of the kidney dysfunction. This kidney restriction will later be seen to be quite relevant in the aetiology of her present symptoms. Also, it demonstrates well the link between structural problems and physiology.

The problem causing the sacroiliac restriction was tension in the pelvic connective tissue and some of the pelvic organs. This was able to be deduced from palpation of the joint, because, although there was a mobility restriction, its quality was not that of being locked or fixed but was still slightly elastic. The soft tissues were reactive to induced movement but not severely so. Also, in globally mobility testing the pelvis, it was apparent that the restriction that was more significant, three-dimensionally, came from within the pelvis.

There was a more chronic soft tissue restriction in the piriformis and sacrum, with a sacral torsion. This may well have come from the left leg biomechanics being altered from the minor operations. The pelvic connective tissue restrictions will also have contributed to the sacral torsion as these tissues connect to the sacrum. The tension in the left kidney (and the left psoas, underlying this) related to the sacroiliac joint dysfunction by restricting movements of the upper thoracic spine by mechanical links and also the lower thoracic spine via viscerosomatic reflexes. The left kidney restrictions may well have led to some ovarian congestion over time, as the left ovarian vein goes to the left renal vein and not the inferior vena cava, as on the right. Thus its route is more vertical and long. The sacrum and diaphragmatic (upper lumbar) restrictions will have contributed to the problems in the involuntary mechanism and the restriction at the sphenobasilar junction. This is turn may affect the sella turcica and hence the hypothalamus–pituitary axis, and contribute to the hormonal problems that the patient was experiencing. Finally, her recent pregnancy, miscarriage and associated stress might well have been the precipitating factor for her presenting symptoms.

The patient responded well to treatment, and symptoms disappeared before any drug therapy was initiated. The fact that she became pregnant was particularly pleasing both to her and to myself.

CASE 6   54-year-old woman with pain in the abdomen and difficulty eating

This case should illustrate the mechanics of the abdominal cavity and how restriction in the subdiaphragmatic viscera can influence lower rib cage biomechanics.

Patient
A 54-year-old housewife.

Presenting symptoms
The patient was suffering from a variety of gastrointestinal symptoms. She had difficulty in eating, there was poor appetite, and a decreased functional volume of the stomach. She often felt sick after having eaten and regularly suffered from constipation or diarrhoea. There was some associated right flank pain. This was not similar to the occasional episodes of 'mechanical' back pain that she had had in the past, which was related to childbearing and to a childhood accident where she fell on her back doing acrobatics.

Onset
These symptoms started some 2.5 years ago, following a cholecystectomy. There were no complications of the operation itself. There were slight symptoms of discomfort after a few days. When the patient consulted her doctor, she was advised to restart the low fat diet that she had been on for her gallbladder dysfunction. She eventually had a barium enema, endoscopy and sigmoidoscopy, as her symptoms had progressed. There was a diagnosis of inflamed intestines and no treatment was suggested.

Her symptoms had reached such a level that they were really interfering with her lifestyle. Her mobility was quite restricted by the pain and she had had to give up dancing, which she and her husband had been doing for years. Her vitality was also decreased and she did not have the quality of life that she had before the operation.

She suffers from osteoarthritis in the cervical spine, which gives some radiations into the arms. She receives no treatment for this.

Her previous medical history revealed polycystic ovaries, which had been removed some 25 years ago. She has also had bilateral carpal tunnel operations. Her general health was all right at the time of presentation, but she did have some increased discomfort associated with her menstruation since the operation. She had been taking hormone replacement therapy for the previous 4 years. Also associated with the pain, when it was bad, was some increased frequency of urination.

On examination
There was a lot of tension around the liver and associated ribs, and throughout the thoracic spine, especially the mid to lower parts. It was initially very difficult to assess the mobility of the viscera because of extreme tenderness. The mobility of all organs in the upper right quadrant of the abdomen was decreased, especially around the liver and the duodenum. It was not possible to assess whether the right kidney was at fault in its own right or just as a consequence of the duodenal tension. (The patient complained of increased frequency of urination whenever the pain was particularly bad.)

It was apparent that there was some degree of adhesion around the cholecystectomy site, which had resulted in some chronic inflammation in the surrounding tissues including the stomach, liver, duodenum and kidney. Due to the fascial pulls created within the peritoneum around these organs associated with the adhesions and inflammation, the mechanically connected areas of the musculoskeletal system had also become restricted. Immobility was also due to an emotional protecting of the painful area.

Treatment

The first treatment consisted of soft tissue work to the right thoracic paravertebral muscles and an attempted mobilization of the T9 area. The motility of the liver was worked upon.

At the second treatment, the patient reported feeling slightly less sick and more inclined to be more active. She still had a lot of aches through the right side. On examination the area was slightly less tender. The patient was also less wary, although she still guarded the area considerably. On palpation the area felt very slightly less inert.

(I associate a feeling of inertness in the tissues with parts of the body that have been proprioceptively quiet for a long period of time. In effect these parts have stopped sending information to the central nervous system and, as a result, the CNS is not controlling body movement in such a way that mobility passes through these inert areas, thus compounding the problem. When you put your hands on such an area and attempt to move it, you do not get a sense of reaction in the surrounding tissues. It does not seem to be connected to/conversing with the rest of the body.)

The treatment consisted of more soft tissue work – functional work to the duodenum, liver and right kidney and ascending colon area. The tissues responded slightly more than before.

At the third treatment the patient reported that, after some initial aggravation, she had had some relief, which was now wearing off. Overall, though, she was not as bad as originally. She was still not eating very well but was 'less afraid' of her 'stomach'. On examination the area was definitely less tender – and it was possible to palpate the organs much more directly. The mid to lower thoracic spine was still congested and very restricted.

The duodenum was still very tense, and although the liver and stomach area was still tense, it was more 'active'. At this treatment the patient also complained of some cervical pain with radiations down the right arm, and a little low back discomfort. These had both, apparently, been mild intermittent ongoing problems that she had not reported in the initial case history. Further examination revealed a thoracic inlet problem and some low lumbar spine restrictions.

Treatment consisted of soft tissue work, mobilization of the right lower lumbar spine and the mid thoracic spine, functional work to the thoracic inlet and work on the motility of the stomach liver and duodenum.

The fourth treatment was 2 weeks after the third, and the patient reported that the first week and a half had been good, although the appetite had still not recovered. The arm was a little better, but the low back was still niggling with sitting. The treatment consisted of a general articulatory approach.

At the fifth treatment she was quite a bit better. She had definitely been able to be more mobile and was even going to try dancing again (something she thought that she had had to stop for ever).

On examination it was definitely easier to get nearer to the liver, although the epigastric area was still a little tight.

Treatment consisted of soft tissue work to the abdomen and functional to the organs. A liver pump technique was used, and work on the motility of the liver was done. There was a general soft tissue and articulatory approach to the thoracic inlet area.

At the sixth treatment, the patient was feeling very good. Treatment followed the general plan and consisted of a functional release of the abdomen and thoracic spine. The patient was then going to leave treatment for a while, to see how her symptoms stabilized.

Progress

Some 6 months later her husband (also a patient) reported that she was still feeling very much improved overall on her presenting state and was so much more outgoing and positive than she had become because of her chronic symptoms.

Discussion

This case is interesting osteopathically, as it shows to a degree the need for working in stages. It was not until later treatments that direct articulation of the liver was possible. Also, with visceral work, it is sometimes necessary to wait, to gain the 'trust' of the patient, when working in this emotionally sensitive area. Also, this patient was helped with some fairly simple work on the viscera and surrounding musculoskeletal system – and it made a huge difference to her lifestyle. Treatment along these lines is something that most osteopaths would quickly become adept at and it is perhaps less difficult to expand your scope of practice into these areas than you might think.

CASE 7	72-year-old woman with stress incontinence of urine

This case should illustrate that, even when tissue adaptation has been present for a long period of time, change is still possible.

Patient
A 72-year-old lady who tried to remain as active as possible.

Presenting symptoms
The patient suffered incontinence of the urinary bladder when it was full. She noticed the problem most first thing in the morning and towards the end of the day. She was sometimes woken at night with the desire to urinate. She also had some urgency but restricted her fluid intake to cope with this.

Onset
The problems started some 40 years earlier with the birth of her second child. She has had pelvic torsion ever since, and has received intermittent osteopathic care over the years to cope with associated spinal and pelvic symptoms.

Her symptoms gradually accumulated over the years and 13 years ago she had had to have a genital prolapse repair. Although there was some relief, the operation was not as successful as it might have been, and her symptoms gradually returned.

She also got occasional bladder infections, for which she had a cream to apply locally.

Her general health is good, although she had recently had a year-long spell of haemorrhoids, which now seemed fine. She did yoga exercises and swam regularly, and she felt that these activities had helped the haemorrhoids. She got some paraesthesia in the right arm, mostly in bed. These symptoms were associated with using a computer (she did some writing) and had persisted for about a year.

Her previous history revealed several bad falls on the coccyx, one of which gave her an out-of-body experience. She had an appendectomy at 8 years of age, hallux-straightening operations bilaterally and a left carpal tunnel operation (not very efficient nor 'tidy').

Her obstetric history was four successful pregnancies and one miscarriage. In the first, the third stage of delivery was difficult and she had to have a general anaesthetic to deliver the placenta. The patient had whooping cough during her second pregnancy and also coughed a lot during the labour. The labour was very long, as she was very tired. Although she had difficulties, she didn't have any stitches. The third and fourth pregnancies were normal.

On examination
Externally, the pelvic floor palpated very lax and there was a very bad coccyx/sacrum/L5 lesion. There also seemed to be a significant left ilium lesion. This whole bony complex was very compressed indeed, and I felt that I didn't have to look much further for the root of her problems. There were undoubtedly other restrictions within the pelvis and body, but they were nowhere near as marked as those in the sacral area, and it would be fruitless to treat these other areas without getting some release in the sacral area.

Treatment
Treatment consisted of external articulation of the coccyx and an attempted sacral toggle.

The second treatment was I week later. At this stage there was no improvement (but this was not surprising in view of the chronicity of the tissue tensions).

We started by considering the right arm symptoms, which seemed to be due to a mild nerve root irritation of the right C7 nerve. This was not severe, as neurological reflex testing revealed nothing significant. There was a chronic restriction throughout the right side of the cervical spine and the upper thoracic spine. There was a marked T6/7 restriction, which seemed to be interfering with the upper spinal mechanics quite strongly. None of these problems were helped by the patient's working position in front of her computer.

Treatment consisted of soft tissue and articulation through the above areas and advice on working posture. An internal adjustment was made to her coccyx, *per vaginam*, followed by some work to the pelvic floor muscles (the left being a little tighter) and some examination of the bladder area. The urethra was found to be a little bound down and this was gently stretched.

The third treatment was 2 weeks later, and the patient felt a definite improvement: she couldn't stop the flow yet, but was definitely getting more awareness of any 'warning' signals that she needed to urinate. She could also do her pelvic floor muscles a little more successfully (which she was in the habit of doing when she remembered).

The treatment was to the left obturator foramen (to affect the pelvic floor) and a lot of articulation to the left hip, with an attempted mobilization of the joint. The pubis was mobilized and there was a general functional release of the supra-pubic area and stretch to the left medial umbilical ligament. There was some general work to both feet.

The fourth treatment was 2 weeks later, and the patient reported that she was definitely improving. She still had occasional wet episodes first thing in the morning, however. The treatment was to the left obturator membrane again, and the pubovesical ligaments. There was some functional work to the sacrum and coccyx.

The fifth treatment was again 2 weeks later. She was continuing to stay improved, although this time, the relative improvement was not so marked. Treatment was to the left leg in general, to help the left hip and pelvic floor. We decided to leave treatment for 2 months to see if the improvement was maintained or not, before deciding on further action.

Discussion
This case demonstrated the effects that mechanical restrictions can have on visceral function. Through working primarily on the musculoskeletal structures, the bladder function was improved. Also, even after a 40-year history, it is still possible to affect change to some degree (and in this case, quite a lot of change).

Whenever there has been a restriction for a long period of time, the proprioceptive signals in and around the soft tissues and articular structures of that area become reduced. As a result it seems that the spinal cord and the cortex are not stimulated as much and as a consequence seem to 'forget' that that area is there. In other words, decreased movement leads to decreased cortical awareness through reduced proprioceptive input. The effect of this is that general and local biomechanics are now altered and movement is not directed through these immobile areas in the same way as before. This compounds the restriction and the body gets into the habit of not using certain areas. Consequently, doing exercises such as those for the pelvic floor may have little effect, as you need good cortical awareness to initiate movement.

With this patient once some movement was restored, this increased the cortical awareness and the patient reported being 'more aware of sensation in the bladder and an increased ability to perform her usual activities'. I feel this demonstrates the importance of articulation and increasing range of movement even in very stiff areas. Also, despite the fact that she had had quite a bit of osteopathic treatment to her pelvis over the years, she had not previously had any relief of the urinary symptoms.

The previous treatments did not deal directly with the coccyx and pelvic floor restrictions and this case serves to show that examination must include all structures and not those that are simply the most easily accessible.

CASE 8   47-year-old woman with brachial neuritis and back pain

This case should illustrate the way that a variety of problems can summate to compound a case of repetitive strain within the cervicothoracic region. It also highlights how a variety of tissue tensions can affect neural compression syndromes.

Patient
A 47-year-old right-handed female hairdresser (of average height and build).

Presenting symptoms
- Occasional aches in the cervical spine, due to her working posture (osteopathic treatment had helped her in the past);
- Sinusitis, which is easier if the cervical symptoms are easier;
- Intermittent lower brachial neuritis, which is predominantly right-sided but can occur on the left. This is complicated by the presence of bilateral cervical ribs. These episodes have previously been related to her workload, and have been relieved by rest and osteopathic treatment. She presented primarily with a recurrence of the right-sided lower brachial neuritis. This had not settled as previously. She had a heavy aching in the posteromedial aspect of the right arm, with subjective numbness in the C8 distribution. She had a slight motor loss within her hand – her grip was occasionally weak.
- Residual lower thoracic spine aches, due to viral pneumonia 18 months prior to this current presentation.

Onset
Her hairdressing has not always caused her cervicobrachial problems. In fact, it was only after a period of heavy lifting at home around 3 years before this current presentation that the problem emerged. She was sent for X-rays by her general practitioner, which discovered the cervical ribs. Subsequent to this the episodes were around every 4–5 months and would resolve after 2–3 weeks of rest and general osteopathic treatment.

However, following a bout of viral pneumonia 18 months before the current presentation, the cervico-brachial symptoms returned and were ongoing. The pneumonia had also left her with a lower thoracic ache (bilateral around the T10/11 area), which was mostly apparent on deep inspiration, and a sensation that 'the whole chest feels tight' – especially the anterior (retrosternal) area; she complained of being unable to take a full breath in as a consequence. She was now often a little breathless. She had a chest X-ray 10 months after the pneumonia but nothing abnormal was revealed. Note: She had an enlarged heart at the time of the pneumonia.

Associated symptoms
She had been aware of a little indigestion subsequent to the pneumonia and a 'decreased stomach capacity'.

There were no other relevant facts in her history.

On examination
General: She had a slightly kypholordotic posture, although the mid-thoracic spine was locally extended. The second ribs were both quite prominent.

Active mobility testing provoked no major symptoms and did not reproduce the brachial neuritis. However, bilateral rotation was reduced and uncomfortable in the lower cervical area. Sidebending was limited bilaterally throughout the thoracic area. The cervical spine was more restricted and uncomfortable locally, on the left more than to the right.

Compression of the cervical spine did not aggravate any symptoms and Adson's test was positive on the right.

Neurological screening revealed a C8/T1 segmental level paresis with slight motor weakness in the right hand.

Passive mobility testing: The sternum was generally restricted and many of the ribs were in a degree of tension and expressed uneven movement. The 12th and second ribs bilaterally were particularly tight. The thoracic inlet area on the right was generally more immobile than the left. There was chronic contracture through most of the cervicothoracic paravertebral musculature. The cervical spine expressed uneven movement, the C0/C1 articulation was markedly restricted and the atlas seemed slightly subluxed (in a functional not pathological sense) to the left, which may have been associated with the patient's work posture.

With 'listening' (feeling for any tension in the deeper tissues of the body): the area around the pericardium and central tendon of the diaphragm seemed very tight. The right hilum of the lung region seemed more restricted than the left during respiration, and general listening of the lower mediastinal area was exaggerated (with inspiration).

Treatment
The patient received several treatments centred on soft tissue work to the thoracic spine; functional release of the sternum, diaphragm and central tendon, and recoil techniques to the sternum; functional release around the pericardium and mediastinal structures.

She also received some soft tissue work, articulation and functional release of the cervical spine, with a high-velocity thrust to the C0/C1 articulation, towards the end of her treatments. Her brachial neuritis and her breathing problems both cleared within six treatments.

36-year-old woman with peptic ulcer

This case demonstrates how it is possible to work with a patient who has a medical condition, and that this is not necessarily contraindicated.

Patient
A 36-year-old female management consultant (who was treated before the importance of bacterial infection in many gastric ulcers was established).

Onset
The ulcer had been diagnosed 2 years previously by endoscopy, following a couple of months of epigastric pain and discomfort. She has had periodic flare-ups of her symptoms and she might have melaena when her problem was acute. Treatment had been cimetidine, relaxation and trying to eat properly.

General information
The patient had always been a somewhat tense and nervous person, and any emotional tension that she had expressed itself 'in her stomach' (even before the ulcer was diagnosed). Her episodes of more acute pain were often set off by emotional upsets. She had been to her general practitioner several times following the initial diagnosis, but the management is the same and, apart from the medication, she just had to 'wait it out' while her symptoms gradually improved. A friend of hers studied osteopathy but, although she had had manipulation before for cervical pain 'of a muscular origin', she had not mentioned her ulcer problem to the practitioner: she wondered if she could now be helped in some way.

Other relevant history
The patient had had tropical hepatitis 9 years before the current presentation. She had had to stay off alcohol for 1 year, but could now tolerate it fairly well, although not during a flare-up of her ulcer. She had had two minor operations for anal abscesses during the last 6 years.

There was also a fall onto the right shoulder that just preceded the onset of the ulcer, which also coincided with a split up with her then boyfriend. This fall precipitated the cervical symptoms for which she had previously had osteopathic treatment. Since the fall, she has had intermittent aches in the cervi-cothoracic region (perhaps every 6 months, with no particular triggers). These usually pass within a few days, without treatment. However, if she swims she can precipitate some aching into the right anterior deltoid.

On examination
General: A thin lady with a compressed-looking anterior rib cage, rounded shoulders, slightly kypholordotic cervicothoracic area and a narrow waist with a small lower abdominal ptosis.

Active mobility testing: No spinal symptoms were triggered. All the junctional areas of the spine were restricted bilaterally (O/A, C/T, T/L, L/S). There was a visibly facilitated T7/8 area in the spine (being quite red, oedematous, sweaty and tender to the touch).

Passive mobility testing: There was restriction throughout the thoracic spine, which was generally fibrotic but exhibiting a classic facilitated segment at the T7/8 area (as above). The rib cage as a whole was also restricted, right more than left, and the diaphragm was tight. The thoracolumbar region was a little torsioned, which seemed to be related to the pelvis and the liver/diaphragm/visceral pattern (see below). There was a sacral torsion and the right sacroiliac joint was restricted (chronically). There was a general poor vitality within the involuntary mechanism but no over-riding cranial lesion pattern. There was a very chronic restriction in the left C2/3 articulation.

Visceral findings: The liver was generally immobile and a little tender to palpation. The capsule seemed a little tight (the liver felt 'stiff'). There was irritation and restriction within the pylorus and the first part of the duodenum. The lesser omentum was tense, increasing the tension on the lesser curvature of the stomach. The tension in the duodenum seemed to be related to the upper lumbar spine torsion.

Treatment

This was carried out in 'stages' – to accommodate the irritation and tissue weakness within the stomach as a result of the ulcer. Functional work to the stomach and duodenum eased some of the initial tenderness. When this had reduced, it allowed a little deeper contact, so more direct work on the liver and duodenum could be carried out. Stretch to the diaphragm and the lesser omentum was also carried out to try to ease out the drainage of the stomach and the cisterna chyli. The torsion in the lumbar spine was addressed with articulation and high-velocity thrust work, after general preparation. This allowed a more pliable spine, such that movement here could now pass towards the area of the coeliac plexus. As the area began to relax and become less irritable to the touch, the facilitation within the spine also reduced but not completely; thus it was necessary to apply a local thrust to free this articulation more completely.

As the patient was generally tight, quite a bit of general mobilizing and articulating was done in a rhythmic manner to try to get her to relax more generally. To help this process some work was done within the involuntary mechanism.

She ended up feeling that she was much more in control of the whole situation, and this as much as anything led to a pattern of decreasing frequency of episodes over the following 6–8 months, and now she presents without having such manifest symptoms.

CASE 10 52-year-old man with right flank pain and low back pain

This case illustrates the way that visceral problems may mimic a musculoskeletal presentation.

Patient
A 52-year-old office worker who used to be quite fit but has been much less so over the last few years. He was generally healthy and did not suffer from undue stress at work or home. His past medical history revealed nothing of interest.

Onset
One week before presentation, his 20-year-old daughter came to stay and they went out riding together. This is something that they had done before, but not for a few years.

The patient was anxious to 'keep up with' his daughter and they had a reasonably hard 2-hour ride. He felt no problems anywhere at the time (apart from an increasingly 'bruised' bottom!). Within a few hours of finishing the ride he became aware of a stiff aching in his left side, which overnight became quite uncomfortable. He would get occasional spasms in the upper lumbar (right lateral area) with movement or the odd deep breath. There were no neurological or urological symptoms.

On examination
General: The only thing of note was a scoliosis in the thoracolumbar area, which had a 'protective' appearance.

Active testing: Most movements induced a degree of tightening in the area, but sidebending both right and left were the worst, reproducing the pain.

Passive testing: There was a degree of puffiness in the tissues in the right flank, but nothing very substantial. The right 12th rib was sensitive to movement and there was a spasm in the quadratus lumborum, with apophyseal restriction at the thoracolumbar junction. However, although this articulation was tender and surrounded by irritated paravertebral muscles, it was not completely locked and if I moved it minimally it did not really react as would be expected if the problem were local to that joint.

Visceral palpation: Following on from the above, if the lumbar spine and 12th rib were carefully moved, then a sensation of heaviness on the anterior aspect of these parts could be discerned. On palpation of the abdomen, a tender and slightly inflamed right kidney could be felt, and if it was gently pressed, it reproduced the symptoms. So, despite there being no urinary symptoms, because of the palpatory findings of flank heaviness, and a tender kidney, a diagnosis of referred pain could be made. The kidney had been irritated by the jolting movements of the riding and become somewhat 'bruised' and inflamed.

Treatment
Some local functional work was done, to try to accommodate the kidney a bit better and help drainage through the area. A very gentle articulation was done through the area and, at the end of the treatment, the 12th rib spasm and painful movements were reduced by about 50%. The patient was advised to go to his general practitioner for urine screening, as this was not available on site. A week later he was much better.

CASE 11 65-year-old man with femoral nerve compression

This case demonstrates that a number of 'minor' aetiological factors can summate, leading to neural compression without obvious traumatic onset. It also illustrates that neural compression can occur at a number of sites along the nerve pathway – in this case foraminal encroachment and compartment compression within the lower limb.

Patient
A 65-year-old retired man whose hobby was gardening (he had 2 acres of plot to care for).

Presenting symptoms
Anterior right thigh pain that spread around the patella and radiated down the anterior shin. There was occasional numbness in the anterior shin (the previous numbness in the right hallux had now gone). There was no pain as such in the low back, but the patient was aware of some sort of discomfort sensation in this area.

Onset
Approximately 2 months prior to presentation, after going to bed with a slightly stiff low back, the patient woke the next day with severe pain in the leg. There was no remembered aetiology – the patient was not aware of having 'done' anything, although he had been doing a reasonable amount of gardening recently and had not long come back from visiting relatives in Australia.

Progression
The leg pain eased over the first 3 weeks after onset, then became bad again for no particular reason and for 4 out of the last 6 weeks prior to presentation, the symptoms had been very bad – with the pain progressing to numbness in the anterior shin and hallux. Walking was very difficult and most movements were compromised because of the pain. He visited his GP, who referred him for investigations at his local hospital. X-rays and an MRI scan revealed degenerative changes in the mid-lumbar spine, which were consistent with his age and history of activities. There was no indication of central canal stenosis due to degenerative change and no other findings were noted. A diminished L3/4 reflex was noted on neurological screening. On the way back from hospital, lying on the back seat of the car, the patient reported that 'something had shifted', and he began to feel a little better. This was 2 weeks prior to presentation, during which time the symptoms, although not as bad as before, had not improved further. Walking remained very uncomfortable, as was going upstairs. The right ankle swelled slightly on walking. There was no reported change in bladder or bowel activity.

Previous history
The patient reported that he had suffered from low back pain before but not for the last 15 years. He had never suffered any leg pain previous to this current episode. He had suffered no major trauma, had never been ill and his general medical history was insignificant apart from a left-sided inguinal hernia, for which he had been successfully operated on 7 years ago.

On examination
Neurological testing revealed a diminished L3/4 reflex on the right, a positive femoral nerve stretch test and some aggravation of his symptoms during a sciatic nerve stretch test on the affected side. The foot everter muscles and the knee extensor muscles were weaker on the right.

There were very restricted movements throughout the lumbar spine articulations – particularly the mid-lumbar region. Both sacroiliac joints were very tight, as one would expect in a gentleman of 65 years. The soft tissues of the anterior abdominal wall were slightly tethered because of the scar in the left groin, following the hernia repair. There was also a marked restriction of the symphysis pubis associated with this. This restriction seemed more marked than one might expect from age-related changes.

The right hip was slightly restricted into extension and the right psoas muscle was tight and quite fibrotic. The right foot was generally restricted, the medial arch was dropped and the muscles of the leg and the intraosseous membrane were tight. There was some slight non-pitting oedema around the malleoli. There was perhaps a very slight delay in pulse testing between the femoral and popliteal arteries in the right leg. Blood pressure was within normal ranges. It appeared that the fascial compartments within the lower limb were very tight, and that this could be inducing a degree of pressure on the nerve during walking. This compression might also be affecting fluid movement within the lower limb, contributing to the ankle swelling (although cardiovascular system changes could also account for this).

Discussion
The fact that there was no traumatic aetiology in this case is not unusual. Many patients end up with symptoms after a combination of factors that summate to give problems some time later. It is likely for this patient that the recent trip to Australia, coupled with 'catching up' with the gardening jobs that had consequently been put off, are both implicated in the onset of his problem. The problem in this case is one of peripheral neuropathy, which could be related to compression within the spinal canal, in the intervertebral foramen or along the course of the nerve, although two sites of compression were particularly involved.

The restrictions noted in the examination in the hip and lumbar spine were both consistent with degenerative change. As a result of this, the biomechanics of the lower limb and pelvis had become adapted and the right psoas muscle was chronically contracted as a result. This patient was always very active, doing lots of gardening all the time, and this level of exercise would be effective in keeping a reasonable level of relative suppleness in the low back and pelvic region, which helped to offset the effects of the degenerative changes present. Thus his condition had been stable for some time (and he had not suffered back pain for some considerable time).

However, during the trip to Australia, not only would he have sat for long periods during the flights but his general activity while abroad was less than he was used to. This meant that he was not stretching out the degenerative joints and contracted muscles, especially psoas, with the effect that the lumbar spine became more biomechanically inefficient as a result. This was enough to 'tip the balance' and, with little room for manoeuvre in the already constricted intervertebral foramina, the nerve roots would have become quickly irritated from the increased pressure. The tension in the psoas muscle may also be relevant in the sense that this may also be affecting the normal mobility of the femoral nerve as it courses along the posterior abdominal wall. The psoas fascia and deep soft tissues of the abdominal cavity around the nerve, being tight as a result of the psoas muscular contracture, could well affect the mechanics of the femoral nerve, adding to its irritation.

Additionally it seemed that all the changes induced by the extra stiffness also affected the leg, which could not adapt to the slightly changed mechanics in the hip and pelvic girdle. Hence the compartments of the lower leg became more tense than before, leading to local soft tissue distress and slightly poor fluid drainage.

Treatment
Treatment consisted of a series of articulations, soft tissue stretches and general mobilizations to the hip, pelvis and lumbar spine. The foot and intraosseous membrane were mobilized and the thoracic spine was given some articulation to enable change to pass throughout the spine. Direct soft tissue massage was given to the right psoas and the mid-lumbar spine was manipulated. These treatments were carried out over a period of seven treatments. At the end of this time, the reflexes were almost normal, he had no swelling in the foot, there was no leg pain and only very slight numbness. He was 80% improved and was discharged with some exercises to rehabilitate his spine before getting going with the gardening again.

66-year-old man with brachial neuritis

Patient
A 66-year-old retired doctor who keeps very active, particularly with 'DIY' work.

Presenting symptoms
Right cervical spine pain and bilateral arm symptoms. In the right arm he had pain in the deltoid region, with weakness on elevating the arm and elbow flexion. In the left arm he had paraesthesia in the C3/4 distribution.

Onset
These problems had been present for a few years and had been investigated. The symptoms could vary over time, depending on the patient's level of activity, and could be aggravated by his penchant for DIY. He often wakes with cervical pain at night, and one or both arms could be generally numb on waking or when holding his arms above shoulder height.

The diagnosis from X-ray and MRI scan was that there was severe degenerative change. Decreased disk height was noted at C2/3 and C5/6, marked anterior osteophytes at C7, posterior osteophytes at C5/6 and facet degeneration in most levels. The scan did show the presence of cerebrospinal fluid all around the cord, despite some central 'crowding' of the cord within the spinal canal.

There was no other significant medical history.

On examination
The brachial neuritis was confirmed by neurological screening and the cervical spine was examined. It was very quickly evident that the level of tissue change within the cervical region was very extensive. Movements were very limited and there was very little elasticity left within the soft tissues around the joints.

With the amount of tissue change present, it was decided to focus treatment just at the level of the cervical spine. So, despite the fact that many other restrictions were obvious from observation (such as the thoracic spine and rib cage) and there were undoubtedly many interlinked mechanical factors throughout his spine, the cervical spine was too stiff to be able to respond to work done elsewhere. It seemed that the only way to achieve sufficient release of the neural compression was to release the nerve roots from the tension in the deep cervical fascia and the muscular entrapment within the scalene muscles, increase foraminal mobility and reduce constriction at these points. General mechanical assessment was therefore put to one side, to see how the patient would respond to local treatment.

Treatment
Soft tissue stretch and gentle functional treatment to the cervical spine was given, as well as controlled traction and gentle articulation. Although there was some aching initially after treatment, the neural compression quickly eased and within two treatments the patient was definitely improved. He responded well despite the level of degenerative change present and was still improved over a year later (although he could still suffer short-term aggravation when he overdid the DIY).

Comment

This case is interesting as despite all the discussion of the need to look throughout the body before commencing treatment, sometimes local work only can be of benefit. However, not all cases respond as well as this and it is when change does not follow on from local work that some practitioners become 'unstuck' through lack of observation of other factors within the patient.

CASE 13 — 53-year-old man, on renal dialysis, with right shoulder and cervicothoracic pain

Patient

A 53-year-old man, who had been on renal dialysis for 3 years at the time of presentation. Consequently, he was not working.

Onset

For 2 years prior to presentation the patient had been increasingly aware of right shoulder aches, which had progressed, giving him pain underneath the medial scapula, radiating to the tip of the right shoulder and down the lateral aspect of the right upper arm. He also suffered from right cervicothoracic pain. He had not been aware of any particular aetiology. The progression had been gradual but was now quite often very acute. He had fairly constant symptoms most of the time when he presented, which had become manifest around 4–5 months before presentation.

Renal history

This patient was born with polycystic kidneys, although this had not been diagnosed until 12 years ago. Around 3–4 years before the kidneys were undergoing end-stage failure, and he started dialysing three times a week 3 years ago. He was suffering from hypertension and anaemia consequent to the kidney disease. He had diseased arteries in the legs (atherosclerosis and calcification), which was partly smoking-related. Arteriovenous grafts in the legs had aggravated this problem and complicated the resultant intermittent claudication. His bone density seemed well maintained and he was not aware of problems related to this.

Because of the vascular problems in the legs a subclavian graft had been prepared for the dialysis. However, this had become unusable following a complication of left jugular venous thrombosis. Consequent to this, he had had a right subclavian graft prepared around 8 months prior to presentation. He noted that this procedure had aggravated some of his right shoulder symptoms.

Other history

Asthmatic for the last 20 years.

Two minor operations for cancerous growths above the right eye within the last 5 years.

Medication

Co-proxamol and warfarin.

On examination

This patient clearly had a number of factors within his history that might complicate a manual approach. His symptoms could be related to metabolic factors such as calcium deposits in the soft tissues, neural and muscular irritation due to the renal failure and nerve compression due to degenerative change. His vascular history meant that manipulative procedures to the spinal column might be relatively contraindicated and his history of carcinoma might give cause for concern with respect to metastases. However, he could also have various biomechanical restrictions that could account for his presentation.

Exploration of these revealed that he had a complex pattern of restrictions in the right thoracic inlet and lower cervical spine. These included a clavicular torsion following the graft insertion, pectoralis minor tension, restriction in the upper ribs on the right, a restricted glenohumoral joint and tension in most of the shoulder girdle and cervical muscles. His spinal mechanics were affected generally but the lower thoracic/thoracolumbar area was affected mechanically by tension in the psoas and diaphragm from the kidney problem and also neurologically via the renal sympathetics. This lower spinal tension was complicating the mechanics of the upper thoracic area and shoulder girdle. The rib cage and the lungs were also generally compromised because of the history of asthma.

There was a concern that he might react to treatment if too much was done, so a minimal approach was taken, which would also mean that only gentle techniques were used (respecting the relative contraindications). Over 3–4 sessions of treatment, gentle soft tissue techniques and a functional approach to the area were used. This resulted in very minimal relief of his symptoms. The tissue tension would not release given this non-invasive approach and the patient was getting quite distressed because the pain was still severe and he seemed to be gaining no benefit. At this point, there was quite a discussion with the patient about the merits of and concerns about a more direct approach but in the end it was decided to perform a stronger treatment.

Soft tissue massage and articulation was given to the thoracic spine and shoulder girdle and a manipulation to the upper thoracic spine and upper rib on the right, and this finally resulted in a reduction of symptoms. However, this approach was only taken after considering the relative state of the tissues consequent to the renal disease and how treatment styles might affect this.

CASE 14   60-year-old woman, treated postoperatively for poor drainage following breast lumpectomy

Patient
A 60-year-old housewife who was undergoing treatment for carcinoma of the right breast.

Presenting symptoms
Swelling postoperatively, which was not draining despite the chest drain *in situ*. The patient was seen 2 days postoperatively.

Operative history
The patient had undergone a right-sided lumpectomy on the breast, accompanied by a latissimus dorsi transplantation (creating a flap joined into the pectoral tissue) to replace lost breast volume and give a good cosmetic outcome. The incision was from the right axilla and around the inferior margin of the breast. Various lymph nodes had also been removed from the right axilla for investigation.

On examination
The right shoulder girdle was generally tight and there was a degree of guarding in the tissues, as would be expected. The tissues were generally oedematous, but particularly so along the inferolateral aspect of the breast, around the axilla and along the lateral chest wall. It quickly became evident that there was marked tension in the latissimus dorsi and that this might be adding to the chronic soft tissue tension around the chest wall, which was not helping the drainage of the postoperative oedema.

On further examination, other relevant points in the history came to light. She had a chronic low back problem and a restriction of the right hip. She had a slightly adapted gait and her right leg was generally less mobile than the left. She had had gall bladder surgery and exploratory surgery to the lower abdomen 20–25 years previously. She had also had an operation for bowel carcinoma 2 years previously, which had gone well. The present cancer was not thought to be related. She suffered from a degree of asthma, and indigestion due to a hiatus hernia (present since having children).

The upper abdominal and chest restrictions would have made the breast tissue and pectoral tissues less easily drained but, when the latissimus dorsi was transplanted, it did not have sufficient elasticity to accommodate its new position easily. The latissimus was chronically in tension from the right hip and low back problems the patient had suffered for a number of years. (The internal components of the chest would also have been restricted because of the history of asthma and hernia.) It was felt that the adverse tension in the anterolateral chest wall that all these factors had created, coupled with the torsions from the surgery and the incision healing, was complicating soft tissue drainage in the area.

Gentle functional treatment was given to the right hip, low back and latissimus, and to the right chest in general. Gentle soft tissue treatment was given to the right posterior shoulder and cervical region. Within an hour, the chest drain had become operative and the patient was losing the oedematous fluid much more effectively. Indeed, when it started, it was reported to more or less 'rush out' for about half an hour, as opposed to gently flowing out, which it subsequently did.

Discussion

This case is interesting, as it is only very occasionally that one can see a patient so soon after an operation. The gentle techniques should not have been contraindicated and it was not due to the removal of the axillary lymph nodes that the tissues were not draining. This patient subsequently had no problems with lymphoedema. The surgical team could not comment either way as to whether they felt the treatment had been related to the drainage improvement, but the patient was certainly relieved.

49-year-old man with headaches and left low back pain

Patient
A 49-year-old building contractor.

Presenting symptoms
Headaches, which were like a ring/tight band all around the head, with some aches into the left cervical area, radiating occasionally into the right shoulder, and some general aches into the left shoulder.

Lower back pain. This was predominantly on the left but could present on either side, or centrally. The pattern of the back pain was variable over the years and the patient did suffer from generalized muscular pains at various times.

Onset
Most of the symptoms seem to have arisen about 6–7 years prior to presentation. The patient was not clear exactly – because of his job in the building trade, he had had various twinges over the years but, on the whole, the head and low back symptoms had definitely been more prevalent over the previous 6–7 years. There was no specific aetiology. The symptoms had grumbled along for a few years and got particularly bad about 3–4 years before. At this time he had tried various complementary therapies, which did not seem to help much. He had tests for rheumatoid factor but these were negative. Over the preceding 2 years things had calmed down but were now brewing up again, which had prompted him to come for treatment.

Previous history
Appendectomy 7–8 years ago.

Bilateral hallux metatarsophalangeal joint removal and replacement 2 years ago. This was done for arthritis within the joints. This took about a year to settle properly and he now had no symptoms in the feet.

He had had various fractures and minor traumas to the legs and ribs, and various compressive strains to the back, all mostly due to his rugby-playing past.

On examination
This gentleman had a variety of restrictions, which were due to his various traumas and to a postural accommodation to the foot operations.

He had a marked spasm of the left quadratus lumborum, associated with a pelvic torsion and a very restricted thoracolumbar region. This was compromised by a restriction of the left 12th rib and arcuate ligaments and was also related to previous fracture to the lower left ribs. The upper lumbar spine was also quite tight. The thoracic spine was generally immobile and slightly scoliotic, with particularly chronic restrictions in the T9 area and the T4/5 area. The mid cervical spine was restricted on the left, and the O/A joints were bilaterally restricted, the right more than the left.

The pelvic torsion had left him with a left sacroiliac restriction and both legs had an adaptive pattern of tension within them. The right mid-foot and right superior tibiofibular joint were markedly restricted and the tibia on the right had a degree of intraosseous strain.

The cervical region seemed compressed into the upper thoracic area and the right thoracic inlet was tight. The involuntary mechanism was unbalanced and there was tension through the tentorium, thoracic diaphragm and sacrum.

Comment

The restrictions noted all seemed fairly well established. It seemed advisable to look briefly at several factors rather than concentrating on one particular area. As we shall see, during treatment, the restriction pattern was further complicated by a road traffic accident, requiring a slight change in emphasis during treatment.

Treatment

Treatment started with a soft tissue approach to the thoracolumbar region and a fascial unwinding of the tissue strains in this area (which was initially too tight to adjust 'cleanly'). This was followed by functional work to the lower left ribs and left sacroiliac joint and some soft tissue work and articulation to the cervical spine. Symptoms began to improve but then returned. This is not unusual in long-standing cases – tissues that are recovering will still be prone to fatigue and may need further treatment to help them 'settle into' a new pattern of movement. Treatment continued with manipulation to the mid thoracic spine, recoil work to the left 12th rib and involuntary mechanisms release around the 12th rib and arcuate ligaments.

At this point the low back and headaches were both improving and treatment continued with manipulation of the left sacroiliac joint and functional unwinding of the cervical spine into the upper thoracic compression pattern. Work continued with manipulation of the upper lumbar spine, release of the sacrum and articulation of the right foot and superior tibiofibular joint. The patient was given exercises to help maintain the mobility of the foot and lower leg. At this point many of his symptoms were very much better.

However, he then had a road traffic accident, a head-on collision. He did not go to casualty and there were no symptoms for a week. He gradually developed a left cervical spine pain, affecting the left shoulder more than previously. There were no neurological signs and testing did not reveal any neurological damage. He had oedematous tissues around the left cervicothoracic region and strain to the C6 area. There was also tension in the right C2/3 articulation. The compression within the upper thoracic spine had become noticeable again and was compromised by tension within the sternum and diaphragm. These had probably been induced by the seat belt pressure during the accident. The thoracolumbar and pelvic torsion patterns had also been reinstated to a degree.

Following this episode, treatment was directed to the cervical spine, with manipulation, soft tissue work and cervical traction. Release of the involuntary work via the cranial base eased a lot of the cervical tension and recoil and functional work to the sternum and anterior chest released the thoracic inlet and thoracolumbar regions. Manipulation was given to the right upper cervical spine and to the lower thoracic spine. Finally, as the low back pain was responding less well than the cervical spine at this stage, a functional release of the sacrum was done, coupled with deep soft tissue massage to the lumbar erector spinae and manipulation of the thoracolumbar spine. Following these last couple of treatments the patient was significantly better, and he maintained a much better level of comfort and mobility than he had done for some years.

Patient
A 34-year-old office worker, who sits a lot. She also plays a lot of badminton and tries to keep generally active to offset the 'inactivity' of her work.

Presenting symptoms
Bilateral coccygeal pain, which was worse on the right. It was aggravated by sitting and was particularly worse when trying to rise from a sitting position. It was generally worse towards the end of the day.

Onset
She had had two falls on to her lower back and bottom and felt that the symptoms stemmed from the second fall. The first was 7 years before, when she had slipped while ice-skating. There were no real symptoms following this episode. The second fall was 4–5 years before, when she had slipped down a ramp on to her bottom. Gradually she had become aware of symptoms, which were initially intermittent, but now much more constant.

Progression
For the first year of symptoms, she had put up with things, She eventually went to her doctor, who referred her to a consultant. She had a cortisone injection, which eased things for a few weeks. In the end she had five separate cortisone injections, all of which provided temporary relief but no lasting resolution. She tried some manipulative treatment but again there was no real change. It was at this point that she presented for osteopathy.

There were no other significant factors in her history.

On examination
She had a kypholordotic posture, with an impacted lumbosacral area. There was a marked sphenobasilar symphysis compression and tension throughout the dural membranes to the coccyx. The left C4/5 was restricted, as was the T2 area and the lower thoracic spine. The clavicles were under a degree of torsion and the sternum was tense. The right pelvic floor muscles were tight and the pubis and the right foot were restricted. The coccygeal tension seemed to be maintained much more strongly by the dural and cranial restrictions than by those within the pelvis and pelvic floor.

Treatment
This started with a manipulation to the T2 area, functional work to the cranial base and sacrum. The pubis was mobilized and muscle energy technique was given to the right obturator and pelvic floor muscles. This was followed by release of the clavicles, the diaphragm and upper lumbar spine and work to the diaphragm and left occipitomastoid suture. As the sternal area was being treated she commented that she did get some chest pain. This had been investigated, with no pathology noted, as there was a family history of early myocardial infarction. Treatment continued with functional work to the cranial base and pelvis, recoil work to the sternum and manipulation to the mid and upper thoracic spine. At this point she was maintaining a good degree of symptom relief.

Treatment was spaced out, but she still required some work to the left temporal bone and maxilla and to the soft tissue tensions remaining in the pelvis. The right foot was also treated with articulation and manipulation of the cuneiform joints. Following this she became symptom-free.

Discussion

This case is interesting as it shows that, despite symptoms being in one particular area, treatment can be successful when more generally applied. It shows the relationship between the cervical and thoracic spine and pelvic mobility, and indicates the way that dural tensions can maintain general biomechanical torsion patterns.

CASE 17   50-year-old man with left elbow pain and 'generally achy arms'

Patient
A 50-year-old electrician, who did as much 'DIY' at home as he did at work.

Presenting symptoms
Left arm symptoms, consisting of generalized aches and forearm stiffness and a painful left lateral elbow, with 'cracking and crunching' within the left elbow. The right arm was generally 'achy'. The patient had ulnar distribution paraesthesia in the left hand, and occasionally the left.

Onset
Some 3–4 months before the patient had been lifting a lot of bags of sand and gravel and he felt he had strained his left arm somehow. Since then he had been 'putting up' with the symptoms, which were gradually getting worse. He had not been to see his doctor, and came for treatment as he could not get on with all of his jobs at home as well as at work.

Previous history
A 20-year history of low back pain, for which he had intermittently had osteopathic treatment. This had been related to his work and also to his darts playing – he standing with the right foot forwards. He had also had a fall on to the back, fracturing a few lower ribs on the right, which still 'twinged' on occasions.

On examination
This patient had restriction in the left elbow – at the ulnohumeral joint and also the radiocarpal joint. The intraosseous membrane of the left forearm was tight and radial mechanics in general were affected. This was complicated by a pisiform restriction and tension in the medial carpus. The cervicothoracic region was generally restricted and there was torsion at the C7 and C6 articulations. The thoracic inlet on both sides seemed a little compressed and was probably not helped by his work (involving a lot of arm activity and pressure when screwing and drilling, for example).

There was some general thoracic spine stiffness, but particularly in the T3/4 area and the thoracolumbar junction. The right lower ribs and diaphragm were restricted. His low back and legs were not examined in the first session, apart from observation (which revealed some tension but nothing very dramatic).

Neurological screening was inconclusive and it seemed that the ulnar irritation could be coming from the thoracic inlet and also from the lateral elbow. The compartments of the left forearm were very tight, which would be related to the muscular aches and stiffness in this region.

Treatment
This was directed primarily at the upper thoracic spine and left arm. General soft tissue work was given to the shoulder girdle and a manipulation to the upper thoracic spine and left elbow was performed. Articulation and functional work was given to the lower cervical spine and deep soft tissue work was given to the forearm muscles. This was followed by muscle energy technique to the forearm supinators and pronators and articulation to the shoulder. His symptoms initially took a couple of treatments to relieve but, following a little more treatment, including articulation to the upper thoracic spine, left first rib and carpus, he gradually became much more comfortable. Progress was slowed somewhat by the amount of work he was doing, which was slightly reactivating the tissue irritation between treatments.

However, as the restrictions eased, he became able to carry on as before, but with the warning that he may suffer a repetition of the original strain if he did not adapt his working pattern slightly.

Discussion

This patient did not want his low back examined or treated. So, although the rib restrictions, diaphragm tension and possible lumbopelvic tension present would relate to the thoracic inlet and shoulder girdle/arm torsions, treatment had to be directed to more local factors, to accommodate his wishes.

40-year-old man with recurrent ear and eye infections and headaches

Patient
A 40-year-old sales engineer, who did a lot of driving and computer work.

Presenting symptoms
Bilateral ear and eye infections, and bad headaches. The ear infections could be in either ear or both simultaneously, and mostly affected either the middle ear or external ear (where the skin was affected). He could have inner ear infections, which gave dizziness and nausea, which caused him problems when driving. The eye infections could be on either side also. These were a little like episodes of conjunctivitis, affecting the whole eye and eyelid. The headaches were predominantly occipitofrontal and over the orbit and eye. They could be either side.

Onset
The patient had had a long history of headaches over the years, which were probably originally set off by dispatch riding by motorbike. His subsequent driving and work using a computer did not help. However, it was not until the previous 5 years or so that the headaches had become really bad and it was not until about 18 months before that he had started to have all the ear and eye problems. He had been investigated by his doctor and a consultant, neither of whom could find any particular problem or account for the repetition of the infections.

Previous history
Operation for Meckel's diverticulum about 7 years ago.

Eczema as a child.

Penicillin allergy (he uses some homeopathic remedies at present to try to combat the infections rather than the antibiotics he has been prescribed, as these don't seem to clear the infections very well).

He had a fall through a glass roof as a child, in which he hit his head on the edge of a tank. He brushed this off when asked about it, but he had sustained a 'minor chip' fracture somewhere in the skull and was left with a 10 cm scar over the right parietal region, just off the midline. He subsequently suffered numerous bumps and bangs to his head over the years, none of which he paid much attention to.

On examination
There were a lot of cranial base, vault and facial bone restrictions, which were too complex to fully assess on the first visit. These were coupled with a very chronic restriction to the upper cervical region, a facilitated state in the mid-cervical region and a complex pattern of tensions within the thoracic inlets and shoulder girdle.

The upper thoracic spine was 'quite disjointed' – the vertebrae were all rotated in different directions and there was a marked local kypholordosis at the cervicothoracic junction. The right clavicle was depressed and the right shoulder internally rotated. There was a slight fullness in the left supraclavicular region and he had a positive Adson's test on both sides. The mid to lower thoracic spine was restricted and there was tension over the left lower ribs and spleen. The upper lumbar spine was restricted on the left and the right sacroiliac joint was in torsion. The lower sternum was very bound down and the second ribs were very restricted anteriorly and posteriorly. The tension in the diaphragm was not as bad as might have been expected.

Discussion

The tissues over the face and neck were oedematous in patches, particularly around the eyes, and the general tissue quality was poor. The restrictions noted in the head and neck region were complicating soft tissue drainage of the face and ENT structures, and the tension in the thoracic inlet areas would also compound lymphatic drainage. The original intestinal problem may have irritated the vagus nerve, leading to tension within the upper cervical region, complicating the pattern of mechanical tension in this area. The operation to resolve this had led to tension within the abdominal wall, affecting the lower sternum.

The patient seemed to have an imbalance within the autonomic nervous system and the areas of the spine that were in tension correlated segmentally to the autonomic nervous system components for the ENT structures affected by repeated infection. The thoracic and cervical restrictions related to the sympathetic fibres and the cranial and upper cervical region restrictions related to the parasympathetic fibres. Because of adverse irritation of the nervous system from these restrictions (many of them originally trauma-related), the tissue function in and around the ears and eyes was compromised and general immune system function was probably impaired by the thoracic cage and spleen restrictions. Many of the thoracic spine and anterior rib cage restrictions would be maintained by the abdominal scarring following the intestinal operation.

Treatment

This began with soft tissue work along the spine, manipulation along the thoracic spine, and to the lower cervical spine. This was done with care to avoid provoking episodes of dizziness. Recoil and functional work was applied to the sternum and anterior chest, and articulation to the thoracolumbar region.

As some of the tissue congestion and tension began to be resolved, closer attention was paid to the cranial restrictions. The ethmoid was completely rigid and was affected by restriction throughout the facial bones, maxillae and orbits. The temporal bone movements were asynchronous and the right parietal bone was impacted, affecting the falx, ethmoid and tentorium. Work continued with these restrictions as well as to the areas listed above.

Gradually his symptoms receded, with the headaches becoming much less and the infections less frequent and less severe each time. The restrictions in the cranium were very chronic and took repeated treatment to begin to change. Over several treatments, work was extended throughout the body to integrate the changing tissue tensions that followed release of the cranial structures. (Manipulations were applied to the lower spine and pelvis, and articulation and mobilization were given to the pelvis and lower limbs.) Every now and again, symptoms would return, or move to slightly different areas, as the tissues learned to move in a different pattern. After several months of treatment, he was considerably better and the ENT symptoms were considerably diminished. He continued to have intermittent treatment to maintain the changes, and remained relatively symptom-free.

31-year-old woman with abdominal and pelvic pain, treated before and during pregnancy

Patient
A 31-year-old office worker who does a lot of swimming and riding.

Presenting symptoms
This patient had had period pain for many years, and had a history of right shoulder and low back pain for a number of years (following a fall off a horse). The back pain was also related to a congenital hip problem and bilaterally short Achilles tendons. She began to have treatment for her low back and pelvic symptoms, and to see if any of the soft tissue restrictions within the pelvis could be related to problems she was having conceiving. During the course of treatment she did actually become pregnant and continued to have care for her ongoing symptoms (relating to her previous history, and in association with the pregnancy).

Previous history
She had been diagnosed with endometriosis and had a retroverted uterus, with both fallopian tubes torsioned behind the uterus. She had laparoscopy and laser surgery to remove adhesions, which freed up the right fallopian tube, although the left was still quite constricted. As stated, she had a bilateral congenital hip condition and short Achilles tendons, neither of which had been operated on. She had fractured her right wrist (and had had two corrective operations on this) and had fractured the left tibia, which had healed well.

She had been prone to constipation for many years and had had tests for thyroid function (as she also had dry skin, easily felt the cold and was prone to putting on weight). These were not conclusive. She had also suffered various episodes of head trauma a number of years before.

On examination
Initially, it was noted that she had tension in the left ilium and a sacral torsion. The coccyx was very tight on the left, and the left cardinal and uterosacral ligaments and fallopian tube were very tight and congested. The uterus was very severely retroverted and it was difficult to feel any part of the fundus. The cervix of the uterus was very tense.

She had bilateral psoas tension, associated with the hip condition, and the right 12th rib was very restricted. The ascending colon and small intestine were also quite tight and immobile. There were some restrictions in the upper thoracic spine, right shoulder and cranial base, which were briefly noted.

Treatment
This was first directed at the visceral restrictions within the pelvis and to the ascending colon, bilateral psoas tensions and cranial base. Over several treatments, which concentrated on the release of these tensions, her period pain began to diminish, ovulation pains decreased and she became much less 'wary' of having her abdomen and pelvis examined and treated. In general her gait had also changed a little and she could walk a little more freely than she had done for the last few years. Work was carried out through the lower rib cage and around the liver and intestines to help her digestive tract to function more smoothly.

Work continued on the pelvis and cranium, with some attention to the general restrictions noted above, and 8 months after commencing treatment she found that she was pregnant. When she was about 6 weeks pregnant, she began having lower abdominal pains, which were a bit like period pains, and she was quite concerned about this. The sacrum felt more torsioned than it had and the right psoas was in a degree of spasm. The uterus was rotated and sidebent to the right but was expressing some normal motion and did not feel too 'agitated'. There was also a marked torsion of the right occipitomastoid suture (which had not been apparent before) and which seemed related to the psoas tension. At this stage, minimal functional work was given to the right psoas, small intestine (surrounding the uterus), right occipitomastoid suture and temporal bone. The patient was a little more comfortable at the end of treatment and was seeing her consultant within the next few days.

When she next came for treatment a month later she was still suffering from lower abdominal pain, and some of this felt quite deep – like period pains. Sometimes the pains came in waves, and she noticed some suprapubic 'pulsations' and 'pricking sensations'. She also had a new problem – bilateral facial pain, left more than the right. This had started 10 days before, and had been diagnosed as atypical fasciitis. On examination the uterus was not quite so sidebent (its mechanics will naturally alter as the baby and placenta enlarge) and felt more central. However, the tension in her lower abdomen and liver was quite noticeable, and there was a lot of tension in and around the lumbosacral junction. The tensions in the upper abdomen and the lumbosacral area were treated and some release was directed again to the occipitomastoid suture and cranial base.

Following this she felt much better and the pregnancy progressed well, with scans indicating no problems. Over the next few months, she continued to have some headaches and some episodes of abdominal pain, although this was reduced compared to before. The uterus was expanding more freely, although it still felt tight along its right side, and there was a slightly uneven balance between the left and right uterosacral ligaments, giving a degree of sacral irritation. The right temporal restriction was persistent, as was a chronically restricted T3–4–5 area, which was not allowing the thoracic spine to settle into flexion to accommodate the postural changes of the pregnancy; these areas were addressed on an ongoing basis with soft tissue work and articulation. Treatment was also directed to the rectus muscles (and to the xiphoid and symphysis pubis, to help the abdominal muscles expand evenly).

Through the pregnancy she remained reasonably comfortable, with some abdominal pain on an occasional basis. Towards the end of the pregnancy she also suffered from some pubic pain, which was due to the expanding pregnancy and was complicated by a fall as she was climbing over a stile. This was treated with external soft tissue work to the pelvis and some gentle functional work internally to the cervix of the uterus, vagina and pelvic floor muscles. These were a little tight, as they had previously been adapted to the congenital hip problem, but now needed to accommodate the changing sacral mechanics associated with the pregnancy. Note: Gentle articulation and mobilization had been given to the hips throughout.

She completed her pregnancy without real further complication and gave birth to a healthy baby. (She was not seen for subsequent treatment, due to the practitioner moving house!)

Comment
Treating women during pregnancy is natural to many osteopaths and although there are some ethical and medical considerations to obstetric care, there is also much that can be done to help the person adapt to the changes occurring at this time. (Some discussion of obstetrics was given within the chapter on the pelvis and lower limb.)

CASE 20   12-year-old boy with knee pain and poor coordination

Patient
A 12-year-old boy, who was suffering from knee pain during sports at school and often at other times. He was also generally uncoordinated, with a somewhat ungainly running style, poor hand–eye coordination and slightly below average reading ability. He had two siblings and got on well with his mum and dad. His dad played a lot of sports and was generally very good at them.

Onset
He had been having some pains in both knees for the last couple of years, which came on most during and after sports. His parents had taken him to be examined and the problem had been diagnosed as apophysitis of the tibial tubercle (Osgood–Schlatter's disease). No treatment had been offered, except to reduce his sporting activities and to 'wait for him to grow out of it'.

Previous history
His mum had had an uncomplicated pregnancy and he was delivered with the aid of forceps after the second stage had become a little prolonged. He suffered no particular childhood diseases and was not prone to colic or ENT conditions as a baby or young child. However, he was generally uncoordinated, with 'wobbly limbs and an ungainly run'. At school he was very slightly behind, his reading and writing being a little below average. He was, however, a happy child, who strove to be 'just like his dad' and be good at sports. Despite his general lack of coordination, he was reasonably successful at sports and enjoyed them a lot.

On examination
This boy stood unevenly. He had a slightly kyphotic posture, with the right shoulder being held higher than the left and with the right arm more inwardly rotated than the left. Both knees were slightly flexed, inwardly rotated, with both feet having a loss of their medial arches. The right ilium was strongly rotated anteriorly. The right knee was in genu valgum and the left in relative genu varum. Both tibial tuberosities were tender to the touch and the quadriceps muscles were tense. The patella did not track evenly on either femur. Both feet were quite tense, and the plantar fascia quite tender.

In the spine, the lumbosacral spine was extended and the sacrum was quite bound between the ilia. His lower thoracic spine appeared very compressed and his upper thoracic spine was slightly scoliotic and held in tension between the shoulder girdle pattern and the pelvic pattern of restriction. The O/A joints were both very tight and restriction, with some degree of condylar strain in the basiocciput. The cartilaginous portions of the cranial base were compressed in a rotatory pattern and there was some general tension and torsion within the vault, which was in a contrary direction to this basilar pattern.

Discussion
It appeared that, because of the compressive forces occurring during the prolonged second stage and his subsequent delivery by forceps, a degree of intraosseous strain had developed within the cranium and upper cervical spine. This had left him with a torsion pattern in the upper cervical articulations, giving him a spinal scoliotic pattern, which extended through to the pelvis. Some of the spinal restrictions were due to a few knocks and bumps he had sustained during sports – particularly when he had tried playing rugby (which was his dad's favourite, but one the son couldn't play any more due to his knee pain). Overall, the spinal patterns and torsion in the dural membranes were creating an uneven gait pattern, which was

leading to a poor alignment of the legs, poor patellar tracking and adverse tension at the level of the tibial tuberosities. He was also quite upset that he could not play sports like his dad, and whenever he talked about this his shoulder girdle tension pattern was exaggerated.

Interestingly, when one sat him down to draw a few pictures, while taking his case history with the aid of his parents, it was clear that he held his pens and generally oriented himself quite awkwardly at the desk and over his work. He was apparently always contorted into some posture or other, and had always written/drawn like that.

The tensions he sustained early in life had not only led to an adapted gait and the tibial apophysitis but might also be contributing to his general lack of coordination. As hand–eye coordination and cross-crawl coordination develop, neural reflexes become established between the various parts of the body. The pattern of activity established within this young lad seemed to have adapted itself around the upper cervical restrictions (in particular) and he could not easily hold his head to look at whatever he was drawing without tilting or twisting his head to one side. Also, whenever he crawled, walked or ran, he could not do so without being constrained by some degree of soft tissue tension and therefore his interlimb coordination became somewhat adapted as a result. None of these factors would have helped his progress at school.

Treatment

Over a couple of months, a lot of treatment was given to the cranial base and bones of the upper cervical spine. This was coupled with functional work to the structures of the vault and the dural membranes throughout the spinal column to the pelvis. Articulation and soft tissue work was given to the upper and lower thoracic spines and functional work was applied to the clavicles. Exercises and massage were prescribed for his legs and quadriceps in particular, and the whole family discussed how much sport he was doing and whether they thought this was in fact too much, or just enough!

Gradually his knee symptoms reduced and he also became more relaxed at school. His reading and writing improved and he seemed generally much more integrated into a range of school activities than before. He ran in a more neat and coordinated way and, provided he did not do too much running, his knees soon remained symptom-free.